TAFT STRATEGIC ATLAS

U.S. HEALTH CARE REFORM

Also by Frederick Taft

Stan Mahoney: The Adventures of a Working Man

Welcome to the Friday Forum

TAFT STRATEGIC ATLAS

U.S. HEALTH CARE REFORM

FREDERICK I. TAFT

First Edition - April 1993

Published by
Public Strategy Company
2000 Huntington Building
Cleveland, Ohio 44115-1496

Additional copies of the Chart of the Debate are available from the publisher for a small charge.

This book was bound by Steffen Bookbinders, Macedonia, Ohio using the Otabind™ process. This process uses a flexible glue which permits the book to open nearly flat.

Printed in the United States of America

ISBN: 0-9635808-0-9

For Susan Hoefflinger Taft

CONTENTS

Preface xiii

Acknowledgments xvii

1. A Guide to the Atlas 1

2. Glossary 7

3. Chart of the Debate 63

Key Concepts Presented in the Chart . . 69

Fold-out Chart 75

4. Refining the Key Concepts 77

General Principles

Cautionary Principles 83

The Individual Perspective 91

Specific Proposals

Expand Employer-Sponsored Insurance . 102

Make Limited Medicaid Coverage More Widely Available 106

Help Underserved Areas 109

Restructure the Handling of Malpractice Claims 111

Reshape the Private Insurance Market . 113

Modify Antitrust Rules 119

Use Tax Credits to Cover More People . 120

Follow Managed Competition Principles. . 126

Control Costs with Global Budgets . . 142

Broaden Medicare to Achieve Universal Coverage 149

Achieve Equity and Efficiency with a Single Payer System 150

5. Health Care Reform Plans: Summaries and Key Concepts . . 155

Hawaii Plan 159

Oregon Plan 165

President Bush's Plan 169

Heritage Plan 175

Pauly Plan 181

Reinhardt Plan 187

American Nurses Association Plan . . 193

Health Insurance Association of America Plan 199

American Hospital Association Plan . . 205

Jackson Hole Group Plan 213

Conservative Democratic Forum Plan . 221

American Association of Retired Persons Plan 229

President Clinton's Plan 237

Stark Plan 243

Shortell Plan 249

American College of Physicians Plan . . 255

Aaron Plan 263

Catholic Health Association Plan . . 269

Hagan Plan 277

McDermott/Wellstone Plan . . . 283

6. Health Care Reform Plans: Original Text

6. Health Care Reform Plans: Original Text 291

Hawaii Plan 295

Oregon Plan 305

President Bush's Plan 339

Heritage Plan 373

Pauly Plan 389

Reinhardt Plan 411

American Nurses Association Plan . . 421

Health Insurance Association of America Plan 437

American Hospital Association Plan . . 451

Jackson Hole Group Plan 461

Conservative Democratic Forum Plan . 491

American Association of Retired Persons Plan 505

President Clinton's Plan 515

Stark Plan 539

Shortell Plan 559

American College of Physicians Plan . . 581

Aaron Plan 593

Catholic Health Association Plan . . 609

Hagan Plan 619

McDermott/Wellstone Plan 637

7. Bibliography 653
Access 657
Cost Containment 658
Effect on Small Businesses . . . 660
Ethics and Values 660
Health Care Reform: Overview . . . 661
Health Care Reform: Focused Discussion . 664
History 668
Insurance 669
International Health Care Systems . . 669
Managed Competition. 670
Political Action Committees (PACs) . . 672
Public Opinion 672
Statewide Reforms 673
Statistics 674

8. Index 677

PREFACE

Democracy lodges ultimate power in a general populace mostly made up of people too busy to pay more than passing attention to the exercise of this ultimate power. It follows that any mechanism which makes it easier for busy people to understand political issues and participate in their resolution will strengthen a democracy.

This Atlas aspires to be such a mechanism. Indeed, though the book deals specifically with the hottest potato in our political oven - health care reform - it aspires to do so in a way that creates a new mode of political inquiry.

The defining characteristic of this new mode is that it respects complexity but is committed to achieving simplicity. It seeks to ride this paradox by observing such rules as these:

- Choose a consequential issue of manageable scope.

- Begin with thorough and reasonably objective inquiry into what knowledgeable people are proposing be done to reckon with the issue.

- Look for the main ideas that underlie each proposal.

- Give these ideas a name (I call them Key Concepts) and phrase them in single sentences of limited complexity so they are whole, bounded thoughts.

- Organize and distill the ideas to show succinctly the full range of concepts being debated.

- Show graphically, or in some other clear way, which proponents support which ideas, but do not drown the reader in data.

- Respect theory, for it explains how the ideas of a proposal fit together and is the fountain of new ideas.

- Define terms, use plain English and reach out to the non-expert, but organize ideas in a way that will be valuable to lay person and expert alike.

- Search for the simplicity which reveals the forces shaping life's complexity.

A mode of inquiry devoted to achieving simplicity should itself have a simple name. I propose FACT, an acronym for Find A Clear Track. The full name evokes the task of weighing alternatives and therefore dealing in theory, while the acronym reminds one of the dispositive power of facts.

I hope to apply this FACTual approach to a range of complex issues in our political life and to see others, too, use all or part of the paradigm.

The hallmarks of success for any work in this new mode of inquiry will be adding clarity and order to public debate and bringing more people into the political process.

Cleveland, Ohio — Frederick I. Taft
1993

ACKNOWLEDGMENTS

The enterprise which today takes the form of this book has been trying to crack its way out of its eggshell for more than two decades. My wife, Susan, to whom this book is dedicated, could not help but wonder if the only thing to come out of so many years in an incubator would be an incubus.

I hope her patience during the incubator era is about to be rewarded with a politically interesting and economically viable product. Her contributions to this work are legion. As a health care practitioner and academic, she stimulated my own interest in the field. As a mother, she provided extra parenting for our children when I was immersed in this book. As an editor, she critiqued the drafts. As a co-breadwinner, she provided financial backing. I proclaim her support and counsel as the sine qua non of this venture.

My employee and compatriot in this endeavor has been Michael Salatka. His law degree, graduate work in epidemiology and administrative work and study in the nursing field enable him to see health care issues through several prisms. As Editor, he does everything from basic research and drafting to final paste-up. His unfailing enthusiasm, breadth of interest and ear for what is not yet right have been a great boon to me.

Mike's predecessor as my helper was Michele Lew. It was my receipt of her resume that peeled the scales from my eyes. Here was a talented young woman, fresh out of Yale College, who wanted a summer job in the public policy realm before going on to further study at the Kennedy School of Government. I realized that with an able employee I could create a book that would never come into being if I tried to create it by myself out of tag ends of time from around the edges of my legal practice.

As you might imagine, my training program for Michele when she arrived for work involved throwing her overboard into a sea of data. She not only didn't sink, she played like a dolphin in a bow wave.

Five good friends brought their health care expertise to bear as this book took shape:

> Case Western Reserve University Professor J.B. Silvers, a member of the Prospective Payment Assessment Commission for Medicare, gave me the benefit of his wide knowledge of health care reform theories and their advocates.

Roy Call, Vice President of External and Governmental Relations at SUMMA Health System in Akron, gave generously of his practical wisdom; in particular, he provided an insightful critique of every draft of the Glossary.

Gail Bromley, Vice President/Clinical Services at Lakewood Hospital, also reviewed the Glossary with a keen eye for proper nuance and provided the first enthusiastic review of this book in her Chair's column in the Midwest Alliance In Nursing newsletter.

Dr. Fred Robbins, Nobel Laureate and former Dean of the CWRU Medical School, made important suggestions about terminology and general approach.

Phyllis Yale, a health care consultant with Bain & Co., is the mother of the Chart of the Debate presented in Section 3. "Graph the Key Concepts against the plans," she said, and we gladly did.

The help by a friend which has gone furthest beyond the call of duty is that of Tom Rask, our advisor on graphic design and the computer wizard who stayed up with me one night past 4:00 a.m. completing the Chart for a presentation a few hours later.

The proponents of the various plans we analyze in the Atlas were also generous in making time available to review the Summaries and Key Concepts we prepared to describe their plans. In particular, Dr. Paul Ellwood, founder of the Jackson Hole Group, helped us capture accurately in our summary the spirit of the Group's managed competition proposal.

My law firm, Spieth, Bell, McCurdy & Newell Co., L.P.A., is structured in a way that has allowed me to devote substantial time to this book. The firm also let me use the empty office next to mine to house the venture.

For the help I received from all those I have mentioned above and many others I have not been able to mention, I offer this book as tangible evidence of our collaborative success and of my gratitude.

F.I.T.

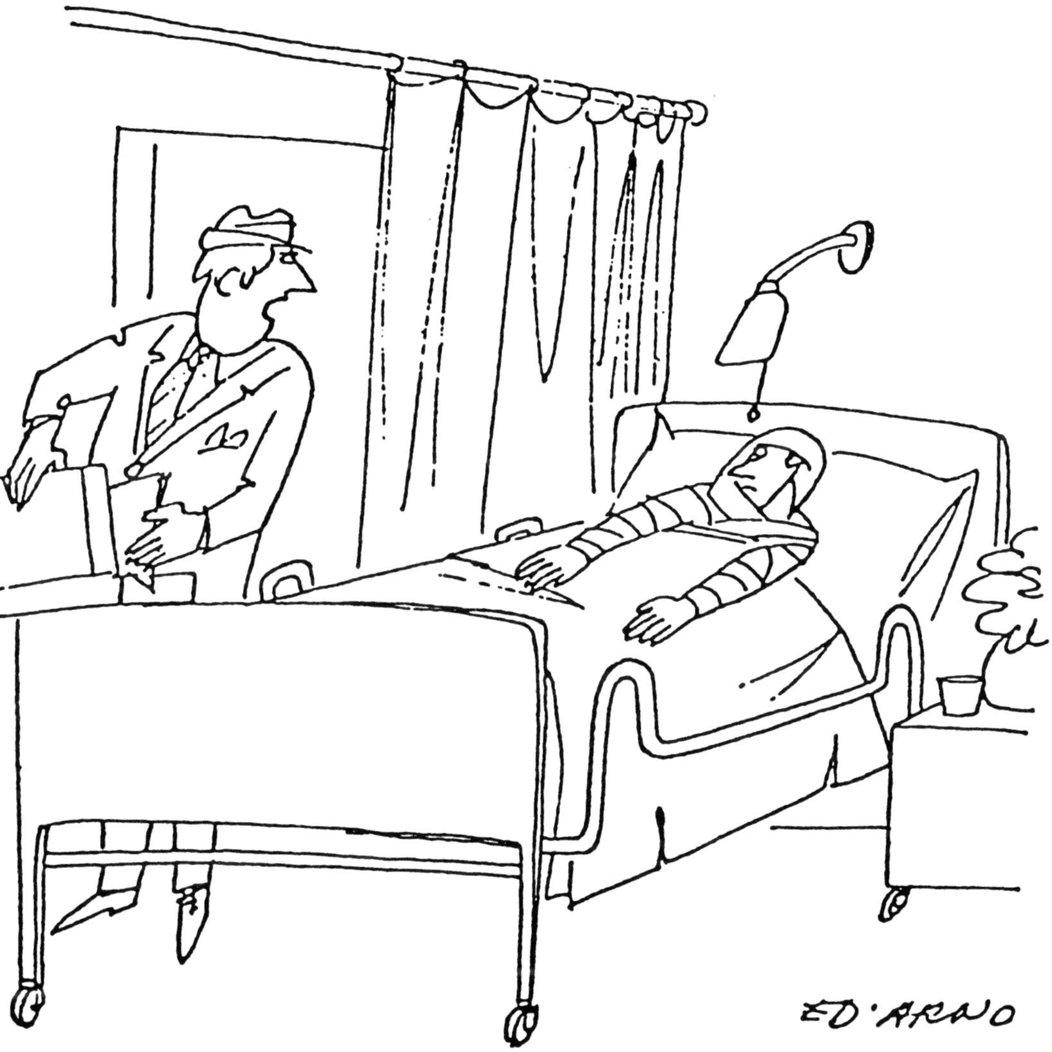

LOOK 9-8-70

"I'm sorry, but under the terms of your group policy, you don't collect unless the entire group is sick."

SECTION 1

A GUIDE TO THE ATLAS

A GUIDE TO THE ATLAS

The mission of this Atlas is to bring a new dimension of clarity and order to the health care reform debate in the United States and thereby to help both professionals and everyday citizens make this high-stakes exercise in democracy successful.

In carrying out this mission, we have sought to respect complexity, but achieve simplicity.

Our respect for the complexity of the U.S. health care reform debate was reflected in our search from one end of the political spectrum to the other for coherent reform plans. We finally selected twenty such plans. It is also out of respect for the complexity of the issue that we reprint in the Atlas previously published material describing each of those plans in the proponent's own words. These excerpts are presented in **Section 6 - Original Text**.

Achievement of simplicity was the greater challenge.

We devised a three-part format for describing each of the twenty plans:

- First we present a box of short phrases that sketch the plan's main points, then a summary of each plan no more than three pages long. The ideas are packed into these summaries fairly tightly, but the style is readable.

- Next we cite our principal sources and tell you a little about the plan's proponents.

- Finally we extract from each plan its essential ideas in easy-to-understand, single-sentence form. We call these essential ideas **Key Concepts**.

This treatment - summary, background data, and Key Concepts - is presented for each of the twenty plans in **Section 5 - Summaries and Key Concepts**.

By preparing these summaries and Key Concepts we had achieved some simplification within each plan, but the picture of the overall debate remained jumbled.

So we printed out all the Key Concepts from the twenty plans, and chopped them apart with a paper cutter. This gave us 173 slips of paper, one Concept to a slip. Then we looked for identical or closely related ideas and pulled them together into a group. Eventually 36 piles emerged, each composed of a single Key Concept or several Concepts that varied in wording and particulars but shared a common idea. For each such pile we crafted a sentence that expressed the single Concept or captured the common idea of the group.

In this way we brought the original sprawl of 173 Concepts down to a non-duplicative family of 36. **We believe these 36 Concepts together define the theoretical landscape of the U. S. health care reform debate.** The distillation process that yielded this set of ideas is presented in **Section 4 - Refining the Key Concepts**.

The extraction of Key Concepts from the plans in Section 5 and the refining of those Concepts in Section 4 form the intellectual heart of the Atlas. In those sections we abstract and distill ideas to the point of simplicity while seeking to preserve their vital spark - their capacity to ignite further thought.

Since we had drawn 36 Concepts from twenty plans, what could be more natural than to graph the Concepts against the plans? Now an Atlas full of words had a chart to provide a global picture of the health care reform debate. In **Section 3 - Chart of the Debate**, the contents of the Chart are described and the Chart itself folds out from page 75.

The Chart is the pinnacle of a pyramid of information presented in this Atlas. You can stay near the top of the pyramid and use the Chart to scan the whole environment of health care reform - to look at the panoply of ideas and their supporters. Or you can use it to help you penetrate the pyramid and explore in depth any of the 36 Concepts presented in the Chart.

To make this in-depth exploration, pick out on the Chart a Key Concept of interest to you, then look across the columns to trace the origins of the Concept to the plans which support it. You can then read in Section 5 the summary of each supportive plan and, if you wish, the plan's original text in Section 6.

At the beginning of the Atlas is **Section 2 - Glossary**, a source of user-friendly, non-technical definitions of terms commonly used in the health care debate.

At the end of the book are **Section 7 - Bibliography** (organized by topic) and **Section 8 - Index**.

Frederick I. Taft, Author
Michael A. Salatka, Editor

SECTION 2

GLOSSARY

GLOSSARY

This section provides easily understood definitions of terms commonly used in the health care reform debate. The terms are drawn from many fields, including law, medicine, and insurance, but in this Glossary they are given the meaning they have in the health care context.

Accountable Health Plan:

A managed care organization (that is, a health plan which carries out both the insurance and health care delivery functions) that complies with the various managed competition rules which the Jackson Hole Group advocates.

This term was coined by the Conservative Democratic Forum, a group of conservative and moderate Democrats in the U.S. House of Representatives.

[The Conservative Democratic Forum plan for health care reform and the Jackson Hole Group plan are described in the Summaries and Key Concepts section of this Atlas.]

Acute Care:

[See also "Chronic Care."]

Health care for illnesses or injuries that have a rapid onset and relatively severe symptoms.

Examples:

- Care for food poisoning, heart attacks, accidents, etc.

Adverse Selection:

The natural tendency of high-risk individuals (i.e., individuals who anticipate using the health care system as a whole, or a particular part of it, more than the average individual) to take such opportunities as they may have to buy insurance coverage at premiums that are low in relation to their risk of filing health insurance claims against the insurance company.

Effect:

- Over time, the high-risk individuals will file higher-than-average claims against the insurance company. If such individuals are relatively numerous in the covered group, the insurer will encounter higher costs and lower profits.

The insurer will then either raise the premiums or change its underwriting policies. If the insurance company raises premiums, low-risk individuals (who have already been paying high premiums in relation to their risk) will tend to drop out of the plan, which drives up premium costs even further. Alternatively, the insurer may seek to cut claims by broadening its preexisting medical condition exclusion or making other changes in its underwriting practices.

Antitrust:

A type of federal or state law that prohibits activities, such as monopolies, price-fixing, or anticompetitive mergers, that place unacceptable constraints on competition in a market.

This is a major area of concern for hospitals wishing to discuss a possible merger or collaborative arrangement, such as shared ownership of high-cost equipment or joint creation of a managed care plan.

In general, a rule of reason is applied to the facts of a particular situation to determine if anticompetitive effects of a course of conduct will be

[CONTINUED]

severe enough to create an antitrust law violation. Antitrust authorities have, in applying this rule to the recent wave of hospital mergers, decided to challenge only a small number of the mergers.

Balance Billing:

The practice by physicians, hospitals, and other providers of billing patients for the balance (or remainder) of their health care bills after the insurance company has paid its portion. This practice occurs when physicians or hospitals charge and seek to collect more for health care services than the established payment rates under Medicaid, Medicare, or private insurance coverage.

Bundling:

The combining by an insurer of a set of services (for which a health care provider may seek to submit a set of separate bills) into one "bundled" service for which the insurer makes a single payment.

Rationale:

- Insurance companies may group (bundle) related health care services into a single treatment category for reimbursement purposes to avoid excessive billing by health care providers for component parts of the overall treatment.

Buy Into:

To spend one's own money to purchase, perhaps at a subsidized rate, the right to participate in a publicly-sponsored insurance program (such as Medicaid).

Capitation:

A method of payment for health care services in which a health care plan receives a fixed monthly fee for each enrolled individual regardless of the extent of service actually provided to that person. This contrasts with a fee-for-service payment system in which providers are paid separately for each service provided to the patient. Under a capitation system, hospitals and physicians join together and are paid as one entity, then allocate the fees among themselves.

[CONTINUED]

Goal:

- A capitation system for reimbursement creates financial incentives for a health care plan to keep its enrollees healthy and provide only necessary services. It has this effect because the monthly fee is fixed and does not increase when more services are provided.

Catastrophic Care:

Extremely costly treatment of life-threatening conditions.

Example:

- Heart transplant.

Certificate of Need (CON):

The Health Planning and Resource Development Act of 1974 required that all states receiving federal health resources enact certificate-of-need laws to provide for state review and approval of capital investments by health care institutions. This was designed to avoid costly overbuilding and to assure that only needed health care services were provided to patients. In 1986, federal CON requirements for state funding were dropped because their impact on cost containment was generally viewed as minimal. Some states, however, continue to use CON requirements as part of a strategy to contain costs and to avoid unnecessary duplication of expensive, high technology services.

CHAMPUS:

CHAMPUS (Civilian Health and Medical Program of the Uniform Services) is a federal government health insurance program which covers medical care provided by civilian health care providers to dependents of active duty, retired, or deceased military service personnel.

Chronic Care:

[See also "Acute Care."]

Health care for illnesses of long duration.

Example:

- Nursing home care.

Claim:

A request to an insurer by a patient (or by a provider on behalf of a patient) for payment of benefits under an insurance contract.

Closed Panel:

[See also "Open Panel."]

A type of managed care plan in which the enrollees can, in general, only use the physicians employed by the managed care plan.

Coinsurance:

[See also "Copayment."]

A provision in an insurance policy that limits the percentage of a health care expense that an insurer will pay. The portion not covered by insurance must be paid by the individual out of his or her own pocket.

Example:

- If the insurance company limits the amount of health care coverage to 80 percent, then the individual must pay the remaining 20 percent of the bill.

Community Rating:

[See also "Experience Rating."]

A method by which commercial insurers calculate premiums for individuals and families that reflect the health status and claims experience of the entire community, not the health status of some more narrowly-defined group.

Setting premiums based on the health care history of a more narrowly-defined group is called experience rating.

Continuous Quality Improvement (CQI):

A systems approach to achieving continuous improvement in the quality of an organization's performance. The approach calls for careful inquiry into and management of an organization's internal structure, processes and patient outcomes. CQI relies on a set of tools - flow charts, graphs, statistical monitoring, etc. - to organize data and aid in scientific analysis of an organization's processes. Many hospitals have adopted CQI approaches in recent years.

[CONTINUED]

Example:

- To meet CQI goals, a hospital may require regular review of a patient's care as it is being provided in order to properly sequence the components of care, coordinate their delivery and see if the intended outcome of each caregiver's service is achieved.

Coordinated Care:

[See also "Managed Care."]

One of several health care delivery models, such as a health maintenance organization (HMO) and preferred provider organization (PPO), in which providers collaborate to deliver care to an enrolled population for a monthly fee per enrollee rather than on a fee-for-service basis.

Goals:

- To enable a group of physicians and other providers to coordinate their clinical decisions concerning patient care.
- To closely integrate the financing and delivery of health care.

Copayment:

[See also "Coinsurance" and "Cost Sharing."]

The portion of a medical expense that an insurance policy holder must pay out of his or her own pocket because the insurance policy does not cover it. Copayments are often a fixed amount, such as $5.00 or $10.00 for an office visit in an HMO.

Purpose:

- To foster reasonable restraint in the use of health care services by those who are eligible to receive them.

Cost Containment:

Control of health care costs, especially by the reduction of inefficiencies in consumption, allocation, or production of health care services.

Cost Sharing:

Requiring patients to pay part of the cost of the health care that they receive.

Cost Shifting:

This occurs when one patient group pays to a hospital or other provider less than the group's real share of the provider's costs while another group pays the provider more than its real share.

Cost shifting enables providers to draw money from groups with private insurance to make up for financial losses from uncompensated or undercompensated care.

Example:

- Hospitals that treat Medicare patients are often not fully reimbursed by the government for the actual cost of the services provided. In order to compensate for the loss, the hospitals bill at higher rates and receive increased payments from the insurance carriers for non-Medicare patients.

Deductible:

The amount of health care expense that an insured person must pay out of his or her pocket during each year or other coverage period before any amount will be paid by the insurer.

Diagnosis-Related Grouping System (DRG System):

A system adopted by Medicare in 1983 which categorizes all possible medical diagnoses into 478 groupings. Each diagnostic category has a fixed rate of reimbursement per hospital stay. The intent of the DRG System is to categorize patients into groups that are homogeneous with respect to resource use and statistically similar in their length of stay.

Categorization Method:

- Based on the principal diagnosis, the need for surgery and type of procedure, risk of complications, and other relevant criteria.

Benefits:

- Hospitals that contain costs below the DRG prospective payment rates may keep the diffcrence. If hospital costs exceed the DRG rates, the hospital bears the added expense.

[CONTINUED]

Problems:

- Government in recent years has set reimbursement rates based on budget goals and not necessarily on the real cost of care.

- Hospitals have an incentive to maneuver patients into more highly compensated DRG categories (this is called "DRG creep") and to avoid treating the most severely ill cases within a DRG category.

Disability:

A physical or mental condition which results from a congenital problem, sickness or injury, and which limits a person's ability to perform tasks. A disability may be partial or total. A partial disability prevents an individual from performing one or more job functions. A total disability prevents an individual from performing substantially all his or her work duties.

Disability income insurance provides periodic payments to replace income when a person is unable to work as a result of a disability.

ERISA:

The Employee Retirement Income Security Act of 1974. This federal law governs employee pension and welfare plans.

A pension plan provides retirement income or deferred income to employees. A welfare plan provides health care coverage and other benefits in the event of sickness, accident, disability, death or unemployment.

ERISA sets standards for disclosure, trustee conduct, vesting of rights, etc. The law also precludes certain kinds of state experimentation with employee benefits law. A state "play or pay" law, for instance, would not be allowed without an ERISA exemption.

Exclusion:

[See also "Preexisting Condition."]

A provision in an insurance policy which states there is no coverage for a particular illness or condition (such as a condition which existed before the individual was covered by the policy) or for a particular kind of care (such as routine physicals).

Exclusive Provider Organization (EPO):

An entity which contracts to provide health care services only through a selected group of participating providers.

Non-emergency services which a patient elects to receive from a health care provider outside of the EPO are not covered.

Experience Rating:

A method by which commercial insurers calculate premiums for covered individuals that reflect the health status of the insured group. The premiums charged in one year are affected by the costs incurred for the relevant group in previous years. In other words, the new rates reflect past experience.

Effects:

- Tends to lower rates for groups with a disproportionate number of healthy young workers and men.
- Tends to increase rates for groups with a disproportionate number of older workers, women (due principally to their potential for pregnancy) and people with serious medical conditions.

- Means an insurer may drastically raise the premiums or cancel the policy for a group with a small number of members if a member of the group develops a serious illness.

- Means an insurer may deny coverage at any price to certain groups with a history of high claims.

Federal Poverty Level:

The level of annual income below which the federal government considers an individual to be "poor." The federal poverty level is used to assess eligibility for Medicaid and other entitlement programs.

Example:

- In 1991, the federal poverty level was $6,620 for an individual and $13,400 for a family of four.[1]

---

[1] Fisher GM. Poverty Guidelines for 1992. *Social Security Bulletin.* 55(1); Spring 1992:43-46.

Fee-for-service:

A method of delivering and paying for services in which a health care provider receives a separate fee for each service provided to the patient. Services can be small (follow-up visit or laboratory test) or substantial (surgical procedure).

Problem:

- Since the provider's income depends on the volume and price of the services rendered, there is no economic incentive to limit the services provided.

Gatekeeper:

[See also "Primary Care Physician."]

A primary care physician, in some cases, who also serves as a patient's point-of-entry for other health services covered by the patient's health care plan. The gatekeeper seeks to respond appropriately to the patient's needs and preferences with referrals, where medically indicated, to specialists and other available health services. If the patient obtains services without going through the gatekeeper, insurance coverage for those services will be reduced or eliminated.

Goals:

- Cost control.

- To protect patients from unnecessary treatment.

Examples:

- Family practitioner.
- General internist.
- General pediatrician.
- Obstetrician-gynecologist.

Global Budget:

A budget established for an entire health care system or health care facility which is intended to limit overall spending.

Gross Domestic Product (GDP):

A broad measure of all the goods and services produced within the borders of a nation. Using GDP rather than GNP is appropriate when there is no need to measure production by a nation outside its borders.

Gross National Product (GNP):

The total value of goods and services a nation produces, domestically and abroad, in a given year.

Health Care Financing Administration (HCFA):

The division of the federal government's Department of Health and Human Services which is responsible for overseeing and monitoring the Medicare and Medicaid programs.

Health Care Provider:

An individual or organization that provides health care services.

Examples:

- Physician.
- Hospital.
- Nursing home.
- Nurse practitioner.
- Chiropractor.
- Dentist.
- Psychotherapist.

Health Insurance:

A form of protection for individuals which provides payment for costs incurred to treat sickness or injury. Sometimes used broadly to include disability and accidental death or dismemberment insurance.

Health Maintenance Organization (HMO):

A prepaid, fixed fee, comprehensive health plan which is regulated by state and federal laws.

How it works:

- Instead of paying for each visit to the doctor or other health care provider, the individual pays a monthly fee to the HMO. In general, only medical care from the HMO personnel and hospitals is covered by the fee. However, HMO doctors sometimes refer patients outside the system for certain specialty care at no additional cost to the patient.

Benefits:

- Treatment costs are held down because the physicians' economic incentives are aligned with those of the HMO that employs them.

[CONTINUED]

- Although choice of doctors is limited, patients can still choose a particular primary care provider from the HMO panel.

Growth of HMO's:

- In 1980, 235 HMOs covered 9 million Americans.
- In 1990, 650 HMOs covered 36 million Americans.[2]

Health Insurance Purchasing Cooperative (HIPC) or Health Plan Purchasing Cooperative (HPPC):

An organization designed to collectively bargain for and purchase health insurance plans on behalf of individuals and small businesses.

Structure:

- Nonprofit.
- Voluntary membership.
- Board elected by members of the cooperative.

This concept is integral to managed competition proposals for health care reform.

---

[2] Coddington DC, Keen DJ, Moore KD, Clarke RL. *The Crisis in Health Care: Costs, Choices, and Strategies.* San Francisco: Jossey-Bass Publishers, 1990: 6.

Hospice:

A public agency or private organization that provides on an inpatient or at home basis pain relief, symptom management, and social support to terminally ill patients and their families. The hospice emphasis on providing a dignified and comfortable death for the terminally ill means that many disorders are left untreated.

Independent Practice Association (IPA):

An association of individual, independent physicians (or small groups of physicians) that has been formed for the purpose of contracting with one or more health care organizations to deliver medical services to that organization's enrolled population. IPAs serve several important functions for HMOs and other managed care organizations:

- IPAs provide a mechanism for translating capitation payments made to an HMO into another form of physician payment.

[CONTINUED]

- IPAs help managed care organizations attract broad panels of participating physicians.

- IPAs provide a vehicle for implementing peer review, quality assurance, and utilization management programs on behalf of managed health care organizations.

Insurable Risk:

A hazard against which an insurance company is willing to provide insurance coverage. Several conditions must be present in order to make a risk insurable, such as:

- the risk must produce a definite loss not under the control of the individual to be insured.

- the loss must be calculable and the cost of insuring against it must be economically feasible.

- the loss must be of the sort that will not affect all insured individuals simultaneously.

- there must be a large number of individuals who are exposed to the same risk.

International Classification of Diseases, Ninth Revision, Clinical Modification (ICD-9-CM):

A diagnosis and classification system designed to facilitate collection of uniform and comparable health information. The ICD-9-CM is the ninth version; the first in the series was issued in 1979. This classification system is the basis for grouping patients into the diagnosis-related groupings (DRGs).

Job Lock or Lock-in:

The feeling that one cannot quit a job or change employers for fear of losing one's health insurance or exposing oneself to preexisting condition exclusions under a new employer's insurance plan.

Joint Commission on Accreditation of Healthcare Organizations (JCAHO):

A private, not-for-profit organization that evaluates and accredits more than 5,000 hospitals as well as 3,600 other health care organizations which provide home care, mental health services, long-term care, etc. To participate in the Medicare program, hospitals must be accredited by JCAHO or the Health Care Financing Administration.

Accreditation is voluntary and JCAHO does not levy sanctions or fines, but some states require JCAHO accreditation for state licensure and operation.

A JCAHO team surveys each accredited hospital at least every three years and will conduct interim surveys at the request of hospitals found to be out of compliance with some standards.

Long-term Care:

A variety of ongoing health and social services provided for individuals who need assistance on a regular, continuing basis because of physical or mental disability.

A broad range of long-term care services are commonly provided to the elderly, the chronically ill, or disabled individuals. Health care services may be provided on an inpatient basis (nursing home, rehabilitation facility, or mental hospital), outpatient basis, or home health care arrangement.

Managed Care:

[See also "Coordinated Care."]

A system of delivering health care in which the provider and insurer work in concert with the goal of providing cost effective treatment that meets the patient's overall health care needs.

Goals:

- To control health care costs.
- To organize the health care plan around keeping the patient healthy.

Applicability:

- The term "managed care" applies to several types of health care organizations and management practices. For example, managed care is used in reference to:

[CONTINUED]

- managed care systems
  -- Health Maintenance Organization
  -- Preferred Provider Organization
  -- Exclusive Provider Organization

- management practices
  -- utilization review
  -- case management
  -- outcomes management
  -- quality assurance
  -- continuous quality improvement

- capitation

- discount arrangements
  -- point of service plans

A managed care organization may be a hybrid of the different systems listed above and may use its own blend of managed care management practices.

Managed Competition:

A strategy developed by the Jackson Hole Group which seeks to structure the health care market so that cost- and quality-conscious consumers can choose among competing managed care plans, all of which must meet federal standards.

Goals:

- To control health care costs and render quality care through limited government intervention which shapes and invigorates a highly competitive private market.

[The Jackson Hole Group Plan is described in the Summaries and Key Concepts section of this Atlas.]

Medicaid:

A health insurance program financed and run jointly by the federal and state governments for eligible low-income people of all ages who do not have the money or insurance to pay for health care services.

Goal:
- To provide medical and other health care services to all eligible individuals so they are not burdened with excessive health care costs and can maintain as much self-sufficiency as possible.

Administration:
- Federal level - Health Care Financing Administration (HCFA).
- State level - Departments of human services.
- Payments are made directly by states to the health care provider.

Eligibility:
- Determined by federal and state rules
- Varies from state to state, but generally includes:
    - Families on Aid to Dependent Children (ADC).
    - Some low-income pregnant women and their children not on ADC.

- Some low-income elderly.
- Low-income blind or disabled persons.
- Low-income persons in nursing homes.

What is covered:

- In general, health care services based on medical necessity, such as most hospital services, care in nursing homes or hospices, and certain prescription drugs.

Medicare:

A federally funded and administered program that provides health insurance to over 35 million elderly and disabled Americans.

Managed by:

- Health Care Financing Administration

Eligibility:

- Most persons over age 65, persons with disability status, or persons with irreversible kidney failure.

What is covered:

Part A:

- Inpatient hospital services, home health care, and limited skilled nursing facility care.

Part B:

- Outpatient hospital services, a portion of physician services, outpatient dialysis, and medical supplies and durable equipment.

Medigap:

A type of private supplemental insurance that covers certain costs excluded from Medicare coverage.

Multiple Payer System:

[See also "Single Payer System."]

A health care system in which many different insurers pay physicians and hospitals under many different kinds of health insurance.

This contrasts with a single payer system, which has only one insurance payer (generally the national government) in the health care system.

Open Panel:

[See also "Closed Panel."]

A system in which a managed care plan allows its subscribers to use independent physicians affiliated with the plan as well as any physicians employed by the plan. All the physicians to whom a subscriber has access together constitute the open panel.

A physician may affiliate with an open panel plan by agreeing to treat its subscribers and be paid according to an agreed fee schedule.

Effects:

- A physician may be affiliated with and see patients through several managed care plans.
- From the patient's perspective, a large open panel yields a broad choice of physician.

Outcomes Management:

An approach to managing patient care in which the desired outcome for the patient is determined first, then the necessary health care resources are allocated to achieve the desired outcome.

Example:

- For a patient who is about to have coronary artery bypass surgery, the hospital's desired outcome may be discharge of the patient in appropriately better health 7 days after surgery. In order to achieve this desired outcome, the hospital must schedule and manage the necessary caregiver services and other resources for each day of the intended course of care.

Payer:

[See "Third Party Payer."]

The person or organization responsible for paying for health care. This term usually refers to an insurance company (a "third party payer"), but it can be applied to an employer or a patient who pays the health care provider directly.

Peer Review Organization (PRO):

A statewide, federally mandated organization that is responsible for reviewing the quality and appropriateness of care rendered to Medicare patients.

Goals:

- To determine whether Medicare should make payments to doctors and to health care facilities.
- To monitor quality of care and contain costs.

Administration:

- PROs have contracts with the Health Care Financing Administration.

Penalties:

- If a case fails peer review, Medicare may deny payment for that case and penalize the physician involved.

Future:

- PROs have been criticized for an undue focus on individual instances of unnecessary treatment, excessive length of stay, etc. Some PROs have begun to look instead for inappropriate patterns of care and to shift more attention to overall quality enhancement.

Play or Pay:

A health care reform approach that guarantees employer-sponsored health insurance to all workers and their non-working dependents.

How it works:

- Employers either buy private insurance for their workers ("play") or contribute to a public plan that covers the workers ("pay").
- The price for public plan coverage is a percentage of the employer's payroll. To promote private coverage, the percentage needs to be set high enough to give employers a financial incentive to provide their own health insurance benefit package, rather than using the public plan for their employees.

Point of Service Plans:

This type of health insurance plan furnishes different levels of coverage depending on whether the member uses the health care providers designated by the plan or goes outside the plan for health care services.

Example:

- A Preferred Provider Organization (PPO) may be a point of service plan. Plan members receive a greater level of coverage if they use the PPOs designated (or "preferred") providers than if they use providers not affiliated with the PPO.

Political Action Committee (PAC):

An organization permitted by the state and federal election laws to gather political contributions from many individuals with similar interests and donate the money to the campaign funds of political candidates. State and federal laws set various limits on the amounts which can be contributed to PACs and by them to candidates.

The health care industry has organized over 200 political action committees, which have contributed more than $60 million to congressional campaigns over the past decade.[3]

Portability:

The ability to move between jobs or in and out of employment while continually keeping one's health insurance.

3 Common Cause News, Washington, D.C.: October 16, 1991

Preexisting Condition:

[See also "Exclusion."]

A medical condition that an individual has prior to obtaining insurance coverage. The insurer may take a preexisting condition into account when determining premiums or the extent of coverage for that individual.

Effects:

- Many insurers have preexisting condition provisions that involve one or more of the following:
  - Waiting periods before coverage for the condition begins.
  - Exclusion of coverage for prior medical conditions.
  - A look-back period during which insurers may investigate for preexisting illness (ranging from three months to an indefinite time period).
  - Higher rates for individuals with preexisting conditions.

[CONTINUED]

- Preexisting condition clauses can make it extremely difficult for uninsured patients with conditions which may require costly care (e.g., cancer, pregnancy, Grave's disease) to secure the coverage they need; even if they receive health insurance benefits from, say, a new job, the insurance policy may well exclude coverage for their condition.

Preferred Provider Organization (PPO):

A health insurance plan in which an insurer contracts with a group of health care providers who agree to furnish services at lower than usual fees in return for prompt payment of claims and a certain guaranteed volume of patients. Plan members may go to a provider with whom the PPO does not have a contract, but the coverage for that service is at a lower level. This type of managed health care plan is similar to an HMO but offers more flexibility for the patient to choose, at some additional cost, a private practice physician or a hospital outside of the PPO.

Goals:

- To negotiate discounts from hospitals and doctors. Those who agree to give the discount become "preferred providers."

	• The discount is sometimes coupled with controls on the utilization of health care services. For example, pre-authorization may be required before certain services are provided.
Key characteristics:	• Fee-for-service. • Discounted fee schedule negotiated by the PPO with preferred providers. • Designated panel of preferred providers. • Incentives to use preferred providers. • Utilization review.
Number of PPOs:	• In 1990, approximately 700 PPOs covered 50 million Americans.[4]

Primary Care Physician or Primary Caregiver:

[See also "Gatekeeper."]

A physician or other caregiver, such as a nurse practitioner, who provides general rather than specialized care and who can help determine what specialized care a patient may need.

[CONTINUED]

---

[4] Coddington, DC, Keen DJ, Moore KD, Clarke RL. *The Crisis in Health Care: Costs, Choices, and Strategies.* San Francisco: Jossey-Bass Publishers, 1990:7.

Some health care plans require a patient to secure approval by such a primary care provider prior to hospital admission or care by a specialist.

Examples:

- Family practitioner
- Nurse practitioner
- General internist
- General pediatrician
- Obstetrician-gynecologist

Prospective Payment System (PPS):

A method of paying for health care services in which the provider receives a fixed payment for treating a given medical condition or occurrence. The reimbursement rates are established in advance, and providers are paid these amounts regardless of the costs they actually incur. Medicare reimburses hospitals on a PPS basis, paying a set amount per hospital discharge based on the Diagnosis-Related Grouping (DRG) which is involved.

Goals:

- To provide a financial incentive for efficient use of hospital services.
- To promote cost containment.

Origin:

- Medicare enacted the PPS system in 1983, coupling it with a DRG system (see Diagnosis-Related Grouping System).

Quality Assurance (QA):

[See also "Continuous Quality Improvement" and "Total Quality Management."]

A management process used by health care providers to monitor and improve the quality of patient care. QA is associated with monitoring performance of individuals on tasks of recognized consequence, locating and correcting problems, and upgrading of skills through education, improved techniques, etc.

By comparison with QA, Continuous Quality Improvement is more focused on fundamental analysis and redesign of the way services are rendered and Total Quality Management is more focused on strategic reshaping of the organization as a whole.

Rationing:

Limiting the type of health care service that will be covered by an insurer or the number of treatments of a certain type that will be allowed in a system.

Examples:

- Care can be rationed by limiting the availability of special services, such as by limiting the number of open heart surgery units or

[CONTINUED]

Magnetic Resonance Imaging (MRI) scanners in a community.

- In Great Britain, the national health insurance program does not pay for certain kinds of surgery beyond established age thresholds.

Reinsurance:

[See also "Stop Loss."]

Insurance provided by one or more secondary insurers (the reinsurers) to a primary insurer which provides primary insurance coverage against a risk. Reinsurance allows the primary insurer to cut down its own exposure by spreading the risk of loss onto other insurance companies.

Resource-Based Relative Value System (RBRVS):

A physician reimbursement system instituted on January 1, 1992 by the federal government for the Medicare program. The relative values established for different physician services are intended to give fair weight to both cognitive and procedural skills.

Examples:

- Primary care physicians are paid more under RBRVS than they were previously for their cognitive skills (such as those used in diagnosis).
- Surgeons, radiologists, and anesthesiologist are paid less than they were previously for their procedural skills.

Risk Pool:

A group of individuals who have the same health insurance coverage from the same insurer. The insurer is able to use the premium income from all the members of the pool to offset the cost of claims paid to particular insured individuals.

Self-insurance:

A form of group health insurance in which the benefits are financed entirely through the internal resources of the entity, such as a large employer, which makes the insurance available. Only large entities can safely self-insure rather than purchase coverage from commercial insurance carriers.

Single Payer System:

[See also "Multiple Payer System."]

A health insurance system in which one entity, usually the national government, serves as the source of health care insurance for everyone and hence the sole payer to health care providers.

Sometimes a market for supplemental health insurance coverage is also allowed, in which case the "single" payer is the dominant, but not the only, payer in the system.

Skilled Nursing Facility:

An institution that provides inpatient nursing care and rehabilitative services to patients with acute care needs. These are often patients in transition from a hospital to their home or a nursing home.

Medicare will reimburse a skilled nursing facility for many acute care expenses, but generally will not cover long-term care in a nursing home.

Stop Loss:

[See also "Reinsurance."]

A form of reinsurance purchased by a health care plan to provide protection, generally on a year-to-year basis, against medical expenses above a certain limit. Such reinsurance may apply to expenses incurred by an entire health plan over a stated period of time or by any single component of its operations.

Example:

- A health plan may have stop-loss reinsurance for cases whose cost exceeds $100,000. After costs in a case reach $100,000, the plan receives from the reinsurance company for the rest of the year all or a stated percentage of its expenses in that case in excess of $100,000.

Supplemental Insurance:

Insurance which is in addition to a primary insurance policy.

Example:

- For Medicare beneficiaries, a private health insurance plan, such as a Medigap or post-retirement health benefit policy, which supplements Medicare coverage.

Tax Credit:

An amount which is credited against a tax owed (such as an income tax). Each dollar of the credit reduces the tax by one dollar.

Tax Deduction:

An amount which reduces the income against which a tax percentage applies. Each dollar of the deduction reduces the tax only by an amount equal to the tax percentage times one dollar.

Examples :

- Businesses which buy health insurance for their employees are allowed a federal tax deduction against their corporate income for the entire insurance premium.
- For a limited period which ended July 1, 1992, self-employed individuals were allowed to take a federal tax deduction for 25% of the cost of their health insurance.

Tax Exclusion:

In the health care context, the exclusion from an employee's taxable compensation of the value of any employer-provided health insurance.

Many reform proposals would require that a portion or all of the employer-paid health insurance premium be considered as taxable income of the employee.

Tax Exemption:

In the health care context, this term may be used interchangeably with tax exclusion to refer to the exclusion of the value of employer-sponsored health benefits from the taxable compensation of an employee.

In a more general context, this term may refer to the right accorded certain organizations, such as universities or churches, to pay no tax on their net income or on the real estate they own.

Third Party Payer:

An insurer who pays a provider for health care rendered to a patient. The patient and provider are the first two parties to a health care "transaction," and the insurer is considered the third party.

Total Quality Management (TQM):

[See "Continuous Quality Improvement " and "Quality Assurance."]

A management philosophy and a set of practices derived from it that call for a commitment to strategic planning, excellent customer service and quality-enhancing innovation. Senior management is expected to take the lead, but the ultimate goal of TQM is to make the pursuit of excellence a part of the organization's culture at every level.

UCR (Usual, Customary, and Reasonable):

Identifies a method for determining what a health insurer will pay for a particular covered service, such as an office visit or anesthesia during an appendectomy. The UCR rate is intended to be the locally prevailing rate for that service.

This payment method was used more widely in the 1960s and 1970s than it is today.

Uncompensated Care:

Health care provided without full payment from either the patient, a private insurer or a government program.

Examples:

- Charity care, which is provided without the expectation of payment.
- Care yielding a bad debt, that is, care for which the provider has made an unsuccessful effort to collect from the patient or other source deemed able to pay.

[CONTINUED]

- Care for which the provider receives from a government program or other insurer less than the cost of the services provided; sometimes this is called "undercompensated care."

Underwriting:

The process by which a health insurer decides whether or not to accept an insurance application and, if the application is acceptable, the premium to be charged as well as any conditions to be placed on the coverage. Health insurance underwriting involves an assessment of an individual's health status and applicable risk factors.

Uninsurable Risk:

A risk posed by a condition or a person where the likelihood of a substantial claim is so great that it is not practical for an insurance company to offer insurance against the risk.

Universal Access:

A kind of health care system in which everyone is insured, often under a government program, and therefore has ready access to health care.

Utilization Review (UR):

The process of reviewing the health services provided to (utilized by) patients. The review considers issues such as medical necessity, appropriateness of the delivery setting, and conformity with proper standards of patient care. The review may be conducted prior to delivery of services (prospective UR), concurrently with the provision of services, or after their delivery (retrospectively).

Goals:

- Cost effectiveness and quality control.

What it includes:

- Utilization review involves examination of such factors as the following:
  - Pre-admission testing and certification.
  - Case management for high-cost treatment.
  - Required second opinions before elective surgery.
  - Monitoring of patient's treatment and length of stay in the hospital.
  - Follow-up after discharge.

Value-added Tax:

Sometimes called a national sales tax, this is a type of consumption tax which is common in Europe. It is like a retail sales tax in its cumulative effect, but it is collected from each party that handles an item on its journey from raw material to finished good sold to the end-user. Each party along the way must pay a tax (which in Europe commonly amounts to over 10 percent), but the tax is payable only on the increment of value added to the item by that party.

SECTION 3

CHART OF THE DEBATE

CHART OF THE DEBATE

A Guide to this Section

The contents of the Chart of the Debate are described in this section and the Chart itself folds out from page 75.

The vertical dimension of the Chart is formed by a list of 36 Key Concepts that together define the theoretical landscape of the U.S. health care reform debate. Because of its importance, this family of Concepts is also presented in the first part of this section.

Across the horizontal dimension of the Chart are listed the twenty reform plans examined by this Atlas.

CONTINUED

CONTINUED FROM PREVIOUS PAGE

They are ordered left to right from those which call for the least structural change in the health care system to those which call for the most.

The Chart graphs health care reform ideas against the plans from which the ideas are derived. It shows which plans support (or oppose) which ideas.

- If a plan **supports** a Key Concept presented in the Chart, a dot (•) appears where the column for that plan meets the row for that Concept.

- If a plan **opposes** a Key Concept, an X appears at the appropriate intersection of column and row.

- If no dot or X appears, it means that the plan was not found, through the process described below, to support or oppose the Key Concept.

Support or opposition for purposes of the Chart is determined by reference to Section 4 - Refining the Key Concepts.

That section takes a large group of Key Concepts (let us call them the "Unrefined Concepts") drawn from the health care reform plans themselves and refines them into the 36 Key Concepts which are presented in the Chart (the "Refined Concepts").

CONTINUED

CONTINUED FROM PREVIOUS PAGE

The results of this refining process are graphically displayed on the Chart in the following way:

- If a plan contributes in Section 4 an Unrefined Concept that supports a particular Refined Concept, a dot appears in the appropriate box on the Chart.

- If a plan contributes an Unrefined Concept that opposes a particular Refined Concept, an X appears in the appropriate box on the Chart.

Browsing through Section 4 will help you see this pattern of support or opposition emerging as the Unrefined Concepts are refined.

Key Concepts Presented in the Chart . . 69

Fold-out Chart 75

KEY CONCEPTS PRESENTED IN THE CHART

CAUTIONARY PRINCIPLES

1. **Health care reforms should preserve successful aspects of our present system.**

2. **Comprehensive health care reform may need to be achieved in stages.**

3. **Reform of the health care system should not raise the federal deficit.**

4. **Federal leadership in shaping the health care system is appropriate, but the system must be allowed to adapt to state and local realities.**

5. **Avoid detailed regulation of the provider-patient relationship.**

THE INDIVIDUAL PERSPECTIVE

6. **Consumers should be made conscious of health care costs and given incentives to make cost-effective choices about their care.**

7. **Americans value highly the opportunity to make choices about the kind of health care they will receive.**

8. **Primary care should be available in accessible, friendly settings to lower barriers to timely care.**

9. **More attention and resources need to be devoted to wellness promotion and preventive care.**

10. **Everyone should have basic health insurance coverage.**

EXPAND EMPLOYER-SPONSORED INSURANCE

11. Require all employers to provide basic health insurance as a job benefit or pay an equivalent tax to enroll employees in a public plan ("Play or Pay").

12. Require all employers to provide basic health insurance as a job benefit ("Play").

MAKE LIMITED MEDICAID COVERAGE MORE WIDELY AVAILABLE

13. Ration limited Medicaid funding to cover only those health services that achieve a publicly-determined threshold of cost-effectiveness.

14. Expand Medicaid to cover those just above the poverty level.

HELP UNDERSERVED AREAS

15. Rural, inner city and other areas underserved by the health care system need expanded government subsidies for facilities and personnel.

RESTRUCTURE THE HANDLING OF MALPRACTICE CLAIMS

16. Medical practice guidelines, alternative dispute resolution and other measures are needed to lessen defensive medicine and control the cost of handling malpractice claims.

RESHAPE THE PRIVATE INSURANCE MARKET

17. **Standardize and streamline health insurance claims procedures.**

18. **Assure individuals access to health insurance without regard to preexisting conditions, and prohibit or narrowly limit the use of experience rating to vary premiums.**

19. **Eliminate underpayments by public health care programs that shift cost burdens onto privately insured patients.**

CLARIFY ANTITRUST RULES

20. **Clarify antitrust rules that govern how competing health care providers may share expensive equipment, create managed care organizations, or collaborate in other appropriate ways.**

USE TAX CREDITS TO COVER MORE PEOPLE

21. **To bring the poor and the less affluent into the health insurance market, create a federal tax credit usable for health insurance only which yields a refund for the poor but gradually diminishes as income rises.**

22. **Those who do not secure private insurance should be assigned to a public health insurance plan and, if they are above the poverty level, required to pay a premium scaled to income.**

23. **Treat all employee health benefits as taxable compensation.**

FOLLOW MANAGED COMPETITION PRINCIPLES

24. Preserve the private market core of our health care system and devise procompetitive measures to correct its societal inequities and other market failures.

25. Form an independent national commission to establish a uniform set of health benefits and to monitor and improve the health care system.

26. The federally-determined minimum benefits package must include a lifetime continuum of primary, acute and long-term care.

27. Involve experts and the general public in determining an acceptable minimum health benefits package.

28. Encourage the formation of integrated health care delivery and financing networks that provide managed care for a set fee per individual, then structure the market so these networks must compete against each other.

29. Promote health insurance purchasing cooperatives to pool individual and small business buying power.

30. Require health care providers to disclose cost and performance data.

31. Limit the income tax exclusion for health benefits to the cost of buying the federally-determined minimum benefits package from a local managed care provider.

32. Allow payments to health plans to qualify for favorable tax treatment only if the plans comply with the managed competition rules.

CONTROL COSTS WITH GLOBAL BUDGETS OR EXPENDITURE TARGETS

33. Use global budgets or expenditure targets at the national and state levels to control the growth of health care costs.

34. Establish health promotion and accountability regions to set budgets, assess needs, and manage the health care system in a way that is responsive to local realities.

BROADEN MEDICARE TO ACHIEVE UNIVERSAL COVERAGE

35. Achieve universal health care coverage by expanding Medicare and abolishing Medicaid.

ACHIEVE EQUITY AND EFFICIENCY WITH A SINGLE PAYER SYSTEM

36. Use a single national payer for the health care system to control costs, limit unnecessary treatment, and bargain for good access to care for the underserved.

SECTION 4

REFINING THE KEY CONCEPTS

REFINING THE KEY CONCEPTS

A Guide to this Section

In Section 5 of this Atlas, twenty health care reform plans are described. For each plan, a series of Key Concepts are presented which capture the essential ideas in the plan.

In this section all the Key Concepts from all the plans - a total of 173 Key Concepts - are brought together, sorted and refined.

The Concepts are sorted by content into 36 categories. Each category is composed of a single Key Concept or several Concepts that vary in wording and particulars but share a common idea.

Within each of the categories the single idea or related group of ideas is refined to yield a new Key Concept which succinctly reexpresses the single idea or captures the common idea of the group.

This section thus shows how a sprawling domain of 173 Key Concepts drawn from twenty plans yields a non-duplicative family of 36 refined Key Concepts.

CONTINUED

CONTINUED FROM PREVIOUS PAGE

These 36 refined Concepts together define the theoretical landscape of the U.S. health care reform debate. They are presented here in the following sequence:

- The whole family of ideas is divided into two categories. Concepts fitting the category of General Principles are presented first, since they have broad application, then come the ideas that embody Specific Proposals.

- Within both General Principles and Specific Proposals, the Concepts are grouped under topic headings. The headings are listed below as part of the table of contents for this section.

- Within Specific Proposals, the ideas are ordered from those which call for the least structural change in the health care system to those which call for the most.

To see this family of 36 refined Concepts presented alone, look at the first part of Section 3 - Chart of the Debate or at the Chart itself, which folds out from page 75.

GENERAL PRINCIPLES

Cautionary Principles 83

The Individual Perspective . . . 91

SPECIFIC PROPOSALS

Expand Employer-Sponsored Insurance . 102

Make Limited Medicaid Coverage More Widely Available 106

Help Underserved Areas 109

Restructure the Handling of Malpractice Claims 111

Reshape the Private Insurance Market . 113

Clarify Antitrust Rules 119

Use Tax Credits to Cover More People . 120

Follow Managed Competition Principles . 126

Control Costs with Global Budgets or Expenditure Targets 142

Broaden Medicare to Achieve Universal Coverage 149

Achieve Equity and Efficiency with a Single Payer System 150

CAUTIONARY PRINCIPLES

1. HEALTH CARE REFORMS SHOULD PRESERVE SUCCESSFUL ASPECTS OF OUR PRESENT SYSTEM.

President Bush's Plan

Government regulation of private business should be kept to a minimum in order to allow market forces to work effectively.

Heritage Plan

Government health programs such as Medicare and Medicaid should remain largely intact because they function adequately to cover the cost of health care for the elderly and poor.

Heritage Plan

Health care reforms should preserve successful aspects of our present system.

Pauly Plan

Political feasibility and use of existing systems in health care and government are important factors to consider in reforming the health care delivery system.

CONTINUED

CAUTIONARY PRINCIPLES - CONTINUED

CONTINUED FROM PREVIOUS PAGE

Pauly Plan

While the obligation to obtain coverage is on individual citizens, many will choose to satisfy this obligation by continuing with or initiating the purchase of insurance through employment-related groups.

CAUTIONARY PRINCIPLES - CONTINUED

2. COMPREHENSIVE HEALTH CARE REFORM MAY NEED TO BE ACHIEVED IN STAGES.

American College of Physicians Plan

Comprehensive changes may need to be made gradually, particularly those changes that have significant financial impact.

CAUTIONARY PRINCIPLES - CONTINUED

3. REFORM OF THE HEALTH CARE SYSTEM SHOULD NOT RAISE THE FEDERAL DEFICIT.

Heritage Plan

Health care reform should be budget neutral and not raise the federal deficit.

Aaron Plan

Reform of the health care finance system cannot wait until the federal budget deficit is brought under control, so health care financing reform must raise enough revenue so it causes no increase in the deficit.

CAUTIONARY PRINCIPLES - CONTINUED

4. FEDERAL LEADERSHIP IN SHAPING THE HEALTH CARE SYSTEM IS APPROPRIATE, BUT THE SYSTEM MUST BE ALLOWED TO ADAPT TO STATE AND LOCAL REALITIES.

Hawaii Plan

Federal leadership in health promotion, cost containment and expanding access to health care is needed, but the states should be given room to experiment and find locally appropriate solutions.

Oregon Plan

The health care system must be allowed to adapt to varying local and regional circumstances.

American Nurses Association Plan

Shape the delivery system to respond to local needs and realities.

Catholic Health Association Plan

No task should be absorbed by a higher, more centralized level of the health care system if that task can be performed adequately at a lower level.

CONTINUED

CAUTIONARY PRINCIPLES - CONTINUED

CONTINUED FROM PREVIOUS PAGE

Catholic Health Association Plan

While the states should define local health care needs, set priorities, and manage competition, the federal government, through an independent public agency, should coordinate and finance the national health care system and guarantee universal access.

CAUTIONARY PRINCIPLES - CONTINUED

5. AVOID DETAILED REGULATION OF THE PROVIDER-PATIENT RELATIONSHIP.

American Hospital Association Plan

Health care providers must be given greater freedom to make decisions without micro-management by government payers and insurers in order to focus more energy on patient care and less on administrative details.

American College of Physicians Plan

Physicians will accept cost constraints in a reformed health care system if there is an end to the overwhelming regulatory intrusion that currently dominates medical practice.

American College of Physicians Plan

There is an appropriate role for regulation at the macro-level, such as governing the supply of health resources, but micro-level regulation of the physician-patient relationship has failed.

CONTINUED

CAUTIONARY PRINCIPLES - CONTINUED

CONTINUED FROM PREVIOUS PAGE

Catholic Health Association Plan

Improve and coordinate health care for individual families and communities by realigning the financial incentives which providers face rather than through a burdensome regulatory structure.

THE INDIVIDUAL PERSPECTIVE

6. CONSUMERS SHOULD BE MADE CONSCIOUS OF HEALTH CARE COSTS AND GIVEN INCENTIVES TO MAKE COST-EFFECTIVE CHOICES ABOUT THEIR CARE.

Pauly Plan

Consumers who are conscious of health care costs will use preventive services more and emergency services less.

American Nurses Association Plan

Give consumers incentives and the means to be cost-conscious about health care and actively involved in their own health care decisions.

American Hospital Association Plan

Because most consumers have insurance and do not pay directly for the cost of health care, they have little incentive to conserve their use of health care resources, compare potential benefits to cost, or shop for the most cost-effective providers.

CONTINUED

THE INDIVIDUAL PERSPECTIVE - CONTINUED

CONTINUED FROM PREVIOUS PAGE

Conservative Democratic Forum Plan

Basic health insurance policies should require copayments to make consumers cost-conscious.

THE INDIVIDUAL PERSPECTIVE - CONTINUED

7. AMERICANS VALUE HIGHLY THE OPPORTUNITY TO MAKE CHOICES ABOUT THE KIND OF HEALTH CARE THEY WILL RECEIVE.

Heritage Plan

Changes in the health care system should maximize the opportunity for individuals to make choices about the kind of health care they will receive.

Heritage Plan

The success of the "consumer choice" health benefits program which covers over nine million federal government workers indicates that American consumers will be capable of making sound choices on health insurance plans if they are provided with adequate information.

Reinhardt Plan

Some tiering of the quality of health care services by income class is inherent in such ideas as consumer choice and managed competition.

CONTINUED

THE INDIVIDUAL PERSPECTIVE - CONTINUED

CONTINUED FROM PREVIOUS PAGE

Reinhardt Plan

Assure low income individuals a basic comprehensive health care benefit package, but allow higher-income groups to enroll in more comprehensive plans.

American Hospital Association Plan

The freedom of individuals to choose a primary caregiver supports a traditional American value and ensures a convenient point of entry into the health care system.

Jackson Hole Group Plan

The freedom to choose health care providers and bargain for health insurance is important to consumers and ingrained in the American health care delivery system.

American Association of Retired Persons Plan

Cost containment efforts should not unreasonably limit a patient's choice of health care provider, because the freedom to make choices regarding one's health care provider is a valued element of our present system.

CONTINUED

THE INDIVIDUAL PERSPECTIVE - CONTINUED

CONTINUED FROM PREVIOUS PAGE

Catholic Health Association Plan

Health care consumers and individual providers must have meaningful opportunities to participate in the shaping and governance of the health care system.

McDermott/Wellstone Plan

Each individual should be free to choose among independent practitioners or to enroll in a managed care plan.

THE INDIVIDUAL PERSPECTIVE - CONTINUED

8. PRIMARY CARE SHOULD BE AVAILABLE IN ACCESSIBLE, FRIENDLY SETTINGS TO LOWER BARRIERS TO TIMELY CARE.

American Nurses Association Plan

Deliver primary health care in community-based settings, such as schools, work sites and community health centers.

American Hospital Association Plan

Health care is a local concern because people generally seek medical care and develop relationships with primary care providers in their own community.

American Hospital Association Plan

Individuals must be encouraged to obtain care when they need it and in an appropriate health care setting.

[CONTINUED]

THE INDIVIDUAL PERSPECTIVE - CONTINUED

[CONTINUED FROM PREVIOUS PAGE]

American Association of Retired Persons Plan

Easy access to health care will encourage individuals to use needed services, especially primary and preventive services such as maternal and child health care, immunizations, and screening programs.

THE INDIVIDUAL PERSPECTIVE - CONTINUED

9. MORE ATTENTION AND RESOURCES NEED TO BE DEVOTED TO WELLNESS PROMOTION AND PREVENTIVE CARE.

American Nurses Association Plan

Focus the health care system on wellness promotion, especially for women and children.

American Hospital Association Plan

The basic health benefits package should emphasize preventive services, such as health education and screening for early detection of disease.

THE INDIVIDUAL PERSPECTIVE - CONTINUED

10. EVERYONE SHOULD HAVE BASIC HEALTH INSURANCE COVERAGE.

President Bush's Plan

The health care insurance market must be restructured to achieve portability, wide access, and renewable coverage for all citizens.

Pauly Plan

Health care is a service which the nonpoor in the community are concerned about providing to the poor.

Reinhardt Plan

U.S. health care reform should achieve universal coverage, portable health insurance, simplicity and administrative cost control.

Reinhardt Plan

All taxpayers should pay a small tax to help finance health insurance for the poor.

CONTINUED

THE INDIVIDUAL PERSPECTIVE - CONTINUED

CONTINUED FROM PREVIOUS PAGE

Clinton Plan

Provide all Americans affordable access to high quality health care.

Shortell Plan

In addition to cost containment, health care reform must address unmet health care needs and quality of service rendered.

American College of Physicians Plan

All persons living in the United States would through private or public insurance have access to the same benefits - all medically effective and appropriate care.

Aaron Plan

The federal government can use its regulatory powers to achieve near universal coverage of working people and their families through private, employer-sponsored insurance and its taxing powers to assure coverage for those with too slender a connection with the workforce.

Catholic Health Association Plan

Basic health care should be viewed not as a commodity but as a fundamental right.

CONTINUED

THE INDIVIDUAL PERSPECTIVE - CONTINUED

CONTINUED FROM PREVIOUS PAGE

Catholic Health Association Plan

Every human life has intrinsic worth and should not be ranked as more or less important than any other.

Catholic Health Association Plan

To assure decent health care for the poor and uninsured, create a health care system in which their fate is linked to that of the average American.

McDermott/Wellstone Plan

Achieve universal coverage through a single payer system.

EXPAND EMPLOYER-SPONSORED INSURANCE

11. REQUIRE ALL EMPLOYERS TO PROVIDE BASIC HEALTH INSURANCE AS A JOB BENEFIT OR PAY AN EQUIVALENT TAX TO ENROLL EMPLOYEES IN A PUBLIC PLAN ("PLAY OR PAY").

American Nurses Association Plan

Achieve universal coverage for a federally-defined minimum benefits package by requiring employment-based health insurance (or an equivalent tax payment by the employer) and covering the rest of the population with a public health insurance program.

American Association of Retired Persons Plan

Employers should pay a health care payroll tax unless they opt out by providing a federally-defined comprehensive health benefits package of private insurance to their employees.

CONTINUED

EXPAND EMPLOYER-SPONSORED - CONTINUED

CONTINUED FROM PREVIOUS PAGE

American College of Physicians Plan

Employers must "play or pay," but the private insurance must be designed so it will generally be cheaper for an employer to play (provide private insurance) than to pay the tax to enroll employees in the public plan.

Aaron Plan

The federal government should mandate that employers either sponsor coverage for all workers employed at least twenty-five hours a week, or pay a tax equal to roughly 9 percent of total payroll.

OPPOSING CONCEPT

President Bush's Plan

The "play or pay" approach would hurt small businesses, increase costs for government, force employers to reduce wages or cut employees, and eventually cascade into a form of national health insurance.

EXPAND EMPLOYER-SPONSORED - CONTINUED

12. REQUIRE ALL EMPLOYERS TO PROVIDE BASIC HEALTH INSURANCE AS A JOB BENEFIT ("PLAY ").

Hawaii Plan

Mandated employer-sponsored health insurance covering a basic benefits package is the practical foundation for universal health insurance, because it leaves a manageable gap to be filled between Medicaid and private insurance.

Health Insurance Association of America Plan

To achieve universal health insurance coverage, have all employers sponsor health insurance for their employees, publicly fund care for the poor, and require all others to purchase their own coverage.

CONTINUED

EXPAND EMPLOYER-SPONSORED - CONTINUED

CONTINUED FROM PREVIOUS PAGE

American Hospital Association Plan

Universal coverage should be gradually achieved by requiring employment-based health insurance and consolidating and enlarging the Medicaid and Medicare programs.

OPPOSING CONCEPTS

Reinhardt Plan

Employers should not be required to provide health insurance for employees, because the cost of such a mandate is simply shifted to customers (in the form of higher prices), to employees (in the form of lower wages or reductions in other fringe benefits) or, least likely, to owners (in the form of lower profits).

Reinhardt Plan

All health care dollars are ultimately drawn from the budgets of individual households.

MAKE LIMITED MEDICAID COVERAGE MORE WIDELY AVAILABLE

13. RATION LIMITED MEDICAID FUNDING TO COVER ONLY THOSE HEALTH SERVICES THAT ACHIEVE A PUBLICLY-DETERMINED THRESHOLD OF COST-EFFECTIVENESS.

Oregon Plan

Practical limits on health care resources mean that not every beneficial service can be included in a basic health care package to be assured to everyone.

Oregon Plan

Explicit ranking of all health care services to determine which services will be funded and which lower priority services will be denied is an honest and effective way to allocate limited funds for health care of the poor.

CONTINUED

MEDICAID COVERAGE - CONTINUED

CONTINUED FROM PREVIOUS PAGE

Aaron Plan

Since society has never placed an infinite value on human life, the right to health care services necessarily has limits.

MEDICAID COVERAGE - CONTINUED

14. EXPAND MEDICAID TO COVER THOSE JUST ABOVE THE POVERTY LEVEL.

Conservative Democratic Forum Plan

Medicaid should be transformed into a new federal program that will pay health plan premiums for those in poverty and provide a premium subsidy on a sliding scale for those with incomes between 100 and 200 percent of the poverty level.

Stark Plan

Medicaid should be gradually expanded to provide assistance to individuals with incomes up to 200 percent of the federal poverty level.

HELP UNDERSERVED AREAS

15. RURAL, INNER CITY AND OTHER AREAS UNDERSERVED BY THE HEALTH CARE SYSTEM NEED EXPANDED GOVERNMENT SUBSIDIES FOR FACILITIES AND PERSONNEL.

President Bush's Plan

In order to increase the number of doctors and clinics in inner city and rural areas and increase preventive care, funding should be expanded for community health centers, Migrant Health Centers and the National Health Service Corps.

Conservative Democratic Forum Plan

Funding to assist rural and other underserved areas should be substantially increased.

CONTINUED

UNDERSERVED AREAS - CONTINUED

CONTINUED FROM PREVIOUS PAGE

American College of Physicians Plan

To control costs and provide universal access to medically effective care, enhanced investment is needed in training generalist physicians, in medical research and in management of medical information.

McDermott/Wellstone Plan

Greater emphasis should be placed on the delivery of primary and preventive care, especially in underserved areas.

RESTRUCTURE THE HANDLING OF MALPRACTICE CLAIMS

16. MEDICAL PRACTICE GUIDELINES, ALTERNATIVE DISPUTE RESOLUTION AND OTHER MEASURES ARE NEEDED TO LESSEN DEFENSIVE MEDICINE AND CONTROL THE COST OF HANDLING MALPRACTICE CLAIMS.

Hawaii Plan

Tort reform will help control the cost of defensive medicine.

President Bush's Plan

Incentives that encourage malpractice litigation and defensive medicine can be changed by eliminating joint and several liability, excluding double recovery, promoting alternative dispute resolution, and requiring structured payments for malpractice awards.

CONTINUED

MALPRACTICE REFORM - CONTINUED

CONTINUED FROM PREVIOUS PAGE

Health Insurance Association of America Plan

Limit defensive medicine through clinical practice guidelines and malpractice litigation reforms.

Conservative Democratic Forum Plan

Reform of the system for handling malpractice claims is needed to reduce the costs of expensive litigation and defensive medicine.

President Clinton's Plan

Medical practice guidelines and other measures are needed to control the cost of dealing with malpractice.

RESHAPE THE PRIVATE INSURANCE MARKET

17. STANDARDIZE AND STREAMLINE HEALTH INSURANCE CLAIMS PROCEDURES.

President Bush's Plan

Administrative costs in health care can be reduced through regulatory reforms that streamline the paperwork and by market reforms that allow small businesses to share administrative costs through group purchasing.

Health Insurance Association of America Plan

Handle claims with a user-friendly, paperless system.

Jackson Hole Group Plan

Standardizing health care insurance practices will improve cost-effectiveness by encouraging competition and creating administrative simplicity.

CONTINUED

RESHAPE THE PRIVATE INSURANCE MARKET - CONTINUED

CONTINUED FROM PREVIOUS PAGE

Conservative Democratic Forum Plan

Federal standards should be developed for health claim forms and electronic transmission of health claims data.

President Clinton's Plan

Administrative burdens must be reduced by streamlining procedures.

Stark Plan

Uniform claims-handling procedures and electronic networks among providers and payers should be established by the federal government to control the cost of administering the health care system.

RESHAPE THE PRIVATE INSURANCE MARKET - CONTINUED

18. ASSURE INDIVIDUALS ACCESS TO HEALTH INSURANCE WITHOUT REGARD TO PREEXISTING CONDITIONS, AND PROHIBIT OR NARROWLY LIMIT THE USE OF EXPERIENCE RATING TO VARY PREMIUMS.

Hawaii Plan

Insurers must insure all employees, regardless of risk, and community rating must be required unless it naturally prevails.

Oregon Plan

Require participation by insurance companies in state-run high-risk pools to increase access to coverage for individuals whose preexisting medical conditions would otherwise leave them "uninsurable."

Heritage Plan

Assure that individuals can renew health insurance with limited premium increases regardless of health problems.

CONTINUED

RESHAPE THE PRIVATE INSURANCE MARKET - CONTINUED

CONTINUED FROM PREVIOUS PAGE

American Nurses Association Plan

Reform private insurance practices to require community rating and eliminate preexisting condition exclusions.

Health Insurance Association of America Plan

Insurers must issue and renew health care coverage for all, regardless of health, financial or employment status.

Health Insurance Association of America Plan

Allow limited experience rating of health insurance premiums to preserve cost control incentives, but do not allow drastic premium disparities for demographically similar groups.

Conservative Democratic Forum Plan

Health plans should not be allowed to exclude coverage of preexisting conditions or use experience rating.

CONTINUED

RESHAPE THE PRIVATE INSURANCE MARKET - CONTINUED

CONTINUED FROM PREVIOUS PAGE

President Clinton's Plan

To widen access to health insurance, new rules must require community rating, open enrollment without regard to preexisting conditions, and availability of a basic benefits package.

Stark Plan

To protect wide access to health insurance, new rules for health insurers should eliminate most preexisting condition exclusions and require community rating.

American College of Physicians Plan

Insurance plans should be required to offer the same benefits, pay providers according to the same fee schedule, and accept all enrollees, so they would be forced to compete on price charged and on value delivered.

RESHAPE THE PRIVATE INSURANCE MARKET - CONTINUED

19. ELIMINATE UNDERPAYMENTS BY PUBLIC HEALTH CARE PROGRAMS THAT SHIFT COST BURDENS ONTO PRIVATELY INSURED PATIENTS.

Health Insurance Association of America Plan

Eliminate underpayments by public health care programs that shift cost burdens onto privately insured patients.

CLARIFY ANTITRUST RULES

20. CLARIFY ANTITRUST RULES THAT GOVERN HOW COMPETING HEALTH CARE PROVIDERS MAY SHARE EQUIPMENT, CREATE MANAGED CARE ORGANIZATIONS, OR COLLABORATE IN OTHER WAYS.

President Bush's Plan

Antitrust rules should provide clearer guidelines for health care providers on sharing of medical technology and services, peer review activities, and pooling arrangements.

USE TAX CREDITS TO COVER MORE PEOPLE

21. TO BRING THE POOR AND THE LESS AFFLUENT INTO THE HEALTH INSURANCE MARKET, CREATE A FEDERAL TAX CREDIT USABLE FOR HEALTH INSURANCE ONLY WHICH YIELDS A REFUND FOR THE POOR BUT GRADUALLY DIMINISHES AS INCOME RISES.

President Bush's Plan

The use of tax credits and deductions to assist in the purchase of insurance plans will protect consumer choice and increase awareness of health care costs.

Heritage Plan

Require everyone not covered by a public program to buy basic health insurance and use a tax credit that diminishes as income rises to fund purchases by those with low incomes.

CONTINUED

TAX CREDITS - CONTINUED

CONTINUED FROM PREVIOUS PAGE

Pauly Plan

A health care tax credit that diminishes with rising income and that yields a refund for the poor should be substituted for the current tax exclusion of health care benefits.

TAX CREDITS - CONTINUED

22. THOSE WHO DO NOT SECURE PRIVATE INSURANCE SHOULD BE ASSIGNED TO A PUBLIC HEALTH INSURANCE PLAN AND, IF THEY ARE ABOVE THE POVERTY LEVEL, REQUIRED TO PAY A PREMIUM SCALED TO INCOME.

Pauly Plan

To increase awareness of health care costs and to invigorate the market for health insurance, individuals should be required to bargain for and purchase a minimum package of health insurance.

Pauly Plan

Since there are limits to an individual's willingness or capacity to obtain health care insurance, the government must provide a mechanism for ensuring basic health insurance coverage for individuals who do not arrange coverage on their own.

CONTINUED

TAX CREDITS - CONTINUED

CONTINUED FROM PREVIOUS PAGE

Pauly Plan

People may not recognize or accurately evaluate their own need for health care or health insurance coverage, so the government must establish a minimum required level of coverage.

Reinhardt Plan

Those individuals who do not have private insurance should pay a progressive tax to fund insurance to be provided to them by the government, which will bargain for such insurance as a powerful buyer.

TAX CREDITS - CONTINUED

23. TREAT ALL EMPLOYEE HEALTH BENEFITS AS TAXABLE COMPENSATION.

Heritage Plan

In order for individuals to become more aware of the costs of health care insurance and to raise money to cover the cost of a tax credit program, employer-paid health insurance benefits should be included in the employee's taxable wages.

Pauly Plan

Individuals will shop more aggressively for value in spending their health care insurance dollars, if they see and feel the insurance being purchased with pre-tax dollars.

Pauly Plan

Exclusion of health care benefits from income tax distorts employee bargaining behavior in favor of compensation through untaxed health care insurance and gives an inequitable tax break to employees who work for firms with health care benefits as opposed to those who work for firms without such benefits.

CONTINUED

TAX CREDITS - CONTINUED

CONTINUED FROM PREVIOUS PAGE

Reinhardt Plan

Keeping the present system in which most people secure health insurance through their work is fine, but employees should be taxed on the value of the insurance.

FOLLOW MANAGED COMPETITION PRINCIPLES

24. PRESERVE THE PRIVATE MARKET CORE OF OUR HEALTH CARE SYSTEM AND DEVISE PROCOMPETITIVE MEASURES TO CORRECT ITS SOCIETAL INEQUITIES AND OTHER MARKET FAILURES.

Health Insurance Association of America Plan

Use procompetitive public regulations to foster a flexible, pluralistic system of delivering and financing health care.

Jackson Hole Group Plan

Preserve the private market core of the American health care system and pair it with appropriate regulation by government to encourage competition among provider organizations and correct market failures.

CONTINUED

MANAGED COMPETITION - CONTINUED

CONTINUED FROM PREVIOUS PAGE

President Clinton's Plan

The government must intervene in the health care system to adjust societal inequities which market forces cannot adequately correct because the free enterprise system does not serve the poor as well as it serves the wealthy.

MANAGED COMPETITION - CONTINUED

25. FORM AN INDEPENDENT NATIONAL COMMISSION TO ESTABLISH A UNIFORM SET OF HEALTH BENEFITS AND TO MONITOR AND IMPROVE THE HEALTH CARE SYSTEM.

Health Insurance Association of America Plan

A national commission should establish a basic benefits package and rules of conduct for the health care marketplace.

American Hospital Association Plan

An independent federal commission should establish the basic health benefits package and capitation fee guidelines.

Jackson Hole Group Plan

To enhance the nation's capacity to get data on and evaluate services provided to patients, a national health board and several private sector boards should be established that would work together to monitor and improve the health care system.

CONTINUED

MANAGED COMPETITION - CONTINUED

CONTINUED FROM PREVIOUS PAGE

Conservative Democratic Forum Plan

Form an independent national board to establish a uniform set of effective health benefits and monitor system performance.

American Association of Retired Persons Plan

The federal government should establish a comprehensive health care benefits package to which all individuals are entitled.

American College of Physicians Plan

A national health care commission with representation from patients, providers, employers, insurers, government and other key sectors of society should determine a minimum package of health care benefits.

MANAGED COMPETITION - CONTINUED

26. THE FEDERALLY-DETERMINED MINIMUM BENEFITS PACKAGE MUST INCLUDE A LIFETIME CONTINUUM OF PRIMARY, ACUTE, AND LONG-TERM CARE.

American Association of Retired Persons Plan

Health promotion, disease prevention, and acute and long-term care should be coordinated to ensure a continuum of care throughout the lifetime of an individual.

American Association of Retired Persons Plan

An important element of a long-term care program is assisting families and friends who act as informal caregivers but who themselves need supportive services such as respite care and adult day care.

CONTINUED

MANAGED COMPETITION - CONTINUED

CONTINUED FROM PREVIOUS PAGE

American Association of Retired Persons Plan

By setting reasonable levels of cost-sharing by patients and spreading the rest of the cost of long-term care across the entire population through an expanded Medicare program, all individuals can receive long-term care when they need it.

Catholic Health Association Plan

The federally-determined minimum benefits package must include a lifetime continuum of primary, acute, and long-term care.

McDermott/Wellstone Plan

A comprehensive basic health benefits package should extend to such services as substance abuse treatment, mental health programs and long-term care.

MANAGED COMPETITION - CONTINUED

27. INVOLVE EXPERTS AND THE GENERAL PUBLIC IN DETERMINING AN ACCEPTABLE MINIMUM HEALTH BENEFITS PACKAGE.

Oregon Plan

Broad public participation in the development of a basic health care package allows the shared values of the community to shape the outcome and should give those individuals who will be most affected a chance to express their views.

Jackson Hole Group Plan

Since health care resources are limited, the government should, in setting a minimum acceptable stardard of health benefits coverage, draw on both expert data and general public commentary.

MANAGED COMPETITION - CONTINUED

28. ENCOURAGE THE FORMATION OF INTEGRATED HEALTH CARE DELIVERY AND FINANCING NETWORKS THAT PROVIDE MANAGED CARE FOR A SET FEE PER INDIVIDUAL, THEN STRUCTURE THE MARKET SO THESE NETWORKS MUST COMPETE AGAINST EACH OTHER.

Reinhardt Plan

On the supply side, the government should encourage the development of managed care options, though a role will remain for more expensive fee-for-service arrangements.

Health Insurance Association of America Plan

Successful cost containment depends on fostering competition among managed care plans that are accountable to patients and the community.

CONTINUED

MANAGED COMPETITION - CONTINUED

CONTINUED FROM PREVIOUS PAGE

American Hospital Association Plan

Health care networks that offer the needed continuum of health care services should be organized at the community level because communities differ in terms of health care needs, medical practice patterns, regulation of health care providers, and available resources.

American Hospital Association Plan

Collaboration of providers within health care networks and competition among networks is a good formula for cost containment.

Jackson Hole Group Plan

To provide more cost-effective benefits to society, the government should foster the development of integrated health care delivery and financing systems and structure the market so these systems must compete with each other.

CONTINUED

MANAGED COMPETITION - CONTINUED

CONTINUED FROM PREVIOUS PAGE

Conservative Democratic Forum Plan

By using strong tax incentives to encourage insurers and providers to form integrated health care plans, the health care market can be managed more effectively and competition can be fostered.

American Association of Retired Persons Plan

The growth of managed care plans should be encouraged.

Shortell Plan

Health care providers should be clinically accountable for the health care services they deliver and should be financially rewarded for enhancing the health status of the population they serve.

Catholic Health Association Plan

State Health Organizations should oversee the shaping of health care resources into competing integrated delivery networks.

MANAGED COMPETITION - CONTINUED

29. PROMOTE HEALTH INSURANCE PURCHASING COOPERATIVES TO POOL INDIVIDUAL AND SMALL BUSINESS BUYING POWER.

Oregon Plan

Promote health insurance purchasing networks to pool individual and small business buying power.

President Bush's Plan

The use of health insurance networks to pool buying power recognizes that individual consumers and small businesses are limited in terms of bargaining power and resources.

Reinhardt Plan

The federal government should reconfigure the health care system to organize and strengthen the collective bargaining power of consumers on the "demand side" of the health care equation.

CONTINUED

MANAGED COMPETITION - CONTINUED

CONTINUED FROM PREVIOUS PAGE

Jackson Hole Group Plan

Since small businesses and individuals, especially the uninsured, have limited expertise and ability to bargain for health insurance coverage, they should have the opportunity to join purchasing cooperatives that will collectively bargain on their behalf for such coverage.

Conservative Democratic Forum Plan

Create large regional health insurance purchasing cooperatives to give individuals and small businesses the benefits of greater buying power.

President Clinton's Plan

Health insurance purchasing cooperatives must be fostered to pool small business and individual buying power.

Stark Plan

Promote health insurance purchasing cooperatives to bargain for managed care plans and increase buying power for individuals and small businesses.

MANAGED COMPETITION - CONTINUED

30. REQUIRE HEALTH CARE PROVIDERS TO DISCLOSE COST AND PERFORMANCE DATA.

Hawaii Plan

Providers must be required to publish cost and performance data so those who purchase health care can bargain intelligently.

American Hospital Association Plan

Networks should be accountable to their communities for cost-effectiveness and for maintaining and improving the health status of the community they serve.

Jackson Hole Group Plan

The government should require health care providers to make available standardized health outcomes and cost data.

Hagan Plan

Providers must be required to disclose cost and performance data to the state-run health care plan.

MANAGED COMPETITION - CONTINUED

31. LIMIT THE INCOME TAX EXCLUSION FOR HEALTH BENEFITS TO THE COST OF BUYING THE FEDERALLY-DETERMINED MINIMUM BENEFITS PACKAGE FROM A LOCAL MANAGED CARE PROVIDER.

Hawaii Plan

To make all parties cost-conscious, specific limits should be set on the value of health insurance benefits which can be excluded from an employee's taxable income.

Health Insurance Association of America Plan

To promote tax equity and to help fund health care coverage for the poor, any employee health benefits in excess of the basic benefits package should be treated as taxable income to the employee.

CONTINUED

MANAGED COMPETITION - CONTINUED

CONTINUED FROM PREVIOUS PAGE

Jackson Hole Group Plan

To achieve greater equity and promote effective bargaining for health insurance, the income tax exemption for individuals' health insurance premiums paid by employers or by the self-employed should be limited to the cost of the minimum benefits package.

Conservative Democratic Forum Plan

Employers should be allowed to deduct basic health plan costs, but not the excess costs of policies which cover more than the basic benefits package.

Conservative Democratic Forum Plan

All individuals, including the self-employed, should be allowed to exclude from taxable income 100 percent of the cost of a basic health benefits package.

MANAGED COMPETITION - CONTINUED

32. ALLOW PAYMENTS TO HEALTH PLANS TO QUALIFY FOR FAVORABLE TAX TREATMENT ONLY IF THE PLANS COMPLY WITH THE MANAGED COMPETITION RULES.

Conservative Democratic Forum Plan

To keep tax-favored status, health plans must offer the standard benefits package, comply with insurance reforms and disclose information on medical outcomes, cost-effectiveness and consumer satisfaction.

CONTROL COSTS WITH GLOBAL BUDGETS OR EXPENDITURE TARGETS

33. USE GLOBAL BUDGETS OR EXPENDITURE TARGETS AT THE NATIONAL AND STATE LEVELS TO CONTROL THE GROWTH OF HEALTH CARE COSTS.

American Hospital Association Plan

When health care providers are held publicly accountable for health outcomes and financially responsible for maintaining a predetermined budget, there are proper incentives to maintain patient health and keep costs to a minimum.

American Association of Retired Persons Plan

Cost containment can be achieved by setting expenditure targets at the national and state level and by establishing uniform reimbursement rates for both the new Medicare system and private insurers.

CONTINUED

GLOBAL BUDGETS - CONTINUED

CONTINUED FROM PREVIOUS PAGE

President Clinton's Plan

Use of global budgets at the national and state levels set by a national health care board is necessary to control growth of health care costs.

Stark Plan

A global health care budget for the nation operating in conjunction with a federal rate-setting system for all health care services is necessary to control health care costs.

Stark Plan

An independent agency established by the federal government should set prices for all health care services.

Shortell Plan

Areawide health care budgets and a controlled price for a basic benefits package are necessary measures for cost-effective management of the health care system.

CONTINUED

GLOBAL BUDGETS - CONTINUED

CONTINUED FROM PREVIOUS PAGE

American College of Physicians Plan

Global budgeting will promote cooperation and compel providers and payers to explicitly negotiate how to meet each community's needs with limited dollars - a function largely missing in an open-ended, fee-for-service system that rewards excessive care.

American College of Physicians Plan

Exceeding budgets will sometimes be justified, since global budgeting is a device to introduce fiscal discipline and to evaluate whether expenditures reflect expected costs, not a mechanism to cut off necessary health care.

Aaron Plan

Efficient allocation of health care resources is better attained through a global budget than through controls on price per unit of service, because price limits provide no incentive to deny low-benefit care.

Catholic Health Association Plan

To control health care costs, use national expenditure caps and risk-adjusted capitated payments to competing integrated health plans.

CONTINUED

GLOBAL BUDGETS - CONTINUED

CONTINUED FROM PREVIOUS PAGE

Hagan Plan

Requiring institutional providers to negotiate a single annual budget will create appropriate incentives to control cost.

McDermott/Wellstone Plan

Contain health care costs through national, state and institutional budgets, negotiated provider fee schedules, and limitations on prescription drug prices.

McDermott/Wellstone Plan

A state's share of the national health budget should be based on population, cost of living, proportion of rural or medically underserved areas, and any special conditions affecting health status.

OPPOSING CONCEPTS

Hawaii Plan

A national health care budget and federal price controls are unwieldy, unnecessary and politically unappealing.

[CONTINUED]

GLOBAL BUDGETS - CONTINUED

[CONTINUED FROM PREVIOUS PAGE]

Heritage Plan

Health care costs are better controlled through consumer choice than through price controls.

Jackson Hole Group Plan

Top down price controls in the form of global budgets are impractical and would undermine an effort to achieve cost control through managed competition.

GLOBAL BUDGETS - CONTINUED

34. ESTABLISH HEALTH PROMOTION AND ACCOUNTABILITY REGIONS TO SET BUDGETS, ASSESS NEEDS, AND MANAGE THE HEALTH CARE SYSTEM IN A WAY THAT IS RESPONSIVE TO LOCAL REALITIES.

Shortell Plan

To manage the health care system in a way that is responsive to local realities, states should charter Health Promotion and Accountability Regions (HPARs), that is, regional partnerships among health care system participants.

Shortell Plan

An epidemiological assessment of an HPAR's population will be an important step in determining the health care needs, basic benefits package, and overall health care budget of the region.

CONTINUED

GLOBAL BUDGETS - CONTINUED

CONTINUED FROM PREVIOUS PAGE

Shortell Plan

HPARs may themselves need backup insurance to cover underestimates of health care use caused by natural disasters or other unexpected events.

Catholic Health Association Plan

Each State Health Organization should serve an appropriate region, which could be all or part of a state, or a metropolitan region in more than one state.

BROADEN MEDICARE TO ACHIEVE UNIVERSAL COVERAGE

35. ACHIEVE UNIVERSAL HEALTH CARE COVERAGE BY EXPANDING MEDICARE AND ABOLISHING MEDICAID.

American Association of Retired Persons Plan

The Medicaid program should be abolished and the Medicare program should be expanded and strengthened to ensure universal health care access for all individuals, regardless of age, income or employment status.

ACHIEVE EQUITY AND EFFICIENCY WITH A SINGLE PAYER SYSTEM

36. USE A SINGLE NATIONAL PAYER FOR THE HEALTH CARE SYSTEM TO CONTROL COSTS, LIMIT UNNECESSARY TREATMENT, AND BARGAIN FOR GOOD ACCESS TO CARE FOR THE UNDERSERVED.

Aaron Plan

Since market competition does not function well in small communities or inner city urban areas with a limited number of health care providers, a single payer system supervised by regional agents is needed to monitor patterns of care and bargain for good health care access even in underserved areas.

CONTINUED

SINGLE PAYER SYSTEM - CONTINUED

CONTINUED FROM PREVIOUS PAGE

Aaron Plan

A wholly public plan is not obtainable because Congress would be unwilling to shift current private health care expenditures and disbursements to public budgets and to displace current health care arrangements for most Americans.

Aaron Plan

Although federal action is necessary to set a floor under the provision of insurance coverage and set global budgets, states should act as financial agents to shape health care spending and health care benefits to meet local needs.

Aaron Plan

Global budgeting requires that control over health care spending be concentrated in one or a few hands.

Catholic Health Association Plan

Fragmentation in the sources of health care funding fosters a similar fragmentation of the delivery system.

CONTINUED

SINGLE PAYER SYSTEM - CONTINUED

CONTINUED FROM PREVIOUS PAGE

Hagan Plan

Instead of using a patchwork system of premiums, deductibles, copayments, and out-of-pocket expenditures to finance health care, a financing structure which uses payroll and excise taxes will distribute costs more efficiently.

Hagan Plan

The most direct route to universal coverage and acceptable cost control is through a state-run, single-payer health care insurance system.

Hagan Plan

A single payer mechanism will control health care cost inflation and unnecessary medical treatment more effectively than a multiple payer system, because a single payer can conduct systemic analysis and limit payments to providers.

McDermott/Wellstone Plan

A single payer system should be administered by the states under the direction of a national health board.

CONTINUED

SINGLE PAYER SYSTEM - CONTINUED

CONTINUED FROM PREVIOUS PAGE

McDermott/Wellstone Plan

A single payer national health system which replaces most private health insurance, Medicare and Medicaid will be more efficient than the current multiple payer system.

McDermott/Wellstone Plan

A state-based single payer program will simplify and streamline the health care system and lower administrative waste.

OPPOSING CONCEPTS

President Bush's Plan

Because health care services would have to be rationed and prices controlled, a government-run single payer system would destroy diversity and flexibility in the financing, organization, and delivery of care.

Pauly Plan

Individuals with varying preferences about health care and insurance will be dissatisfied with a single payer, government-run system, because their range of choice of health care services and insurance coverage will be sharply reduced.

SECTION 5

SUMMARIES AND KEY CONCEPTS

HEALTH CARE REFORM PLANS: SUMMARIES AND KEY CONCEPTS

A Guide to this Section

This section describes twenty plans for reform of the U.S. health care system. The plans were selected for their coherence, political visibility and variety. They are presented in order of proposed structural change - that is, from the plan which proposes the least structural change to the plan which proposes the most. The description of each plan has three parts:

- A short summary preceded by a box sketching the plan's main points.
- A list of principal sources used and a brief description of the plan's proponents.
- A series of Key Concepts, each no more than one sentence long, which together capture in simple language the essential ideas of the plan.

Hawaii Plan 159

Oregon Plan 165

President Bush's Plan 169

Heritage Plan 175

Pauly Plan 181

Reinhardt Plan 187

American Nurses Association Plan . . . 193

Health Insurance Association of America Plan . 199

American Hospital Association Plan . . . 205

Jackson Hole Group Plan 213

Conservative Democratic Forum Plan . . 221

American Association of Retired Persons Plan . 229

President Clinton's Plan 237

Stark Plan 243

Shortell Plan 249

American College of Physicians Plan . . . 255

Aaron Plan 263

Catholic Health Association Plan . . . 269

Hagan Plan 277

McDermott/Wellstone Plan 283

HAWAII PLAN

- HAWAII PREPAID HEALTH INSURANCE ACT
- STATE HEALTH INSURANCE PROGRAM
- FEDERAL AND STATE MEDICAID PROGRAM

This strategy provides nearly universal access to health care through three separate mechanisms.

First, under Hawaii's Prepaid Health Care Act of 1974, employers are required to provide health insurance coverage for all employees working more than 19 hours per week. (Insisting that all employers provide health insurance required a congressional exemption from ERISA; Congress has been unwilling to grant such an exemption to any other state.) Employees may be required to pay up to 1.5 percent of their monthly wages toward the premium, but not over half the cost. Employers are required to pay the balance. Dependent coverage is optional; it is commonly provided with employer and employee sharing the cost. To assist businesses that demonstrate hardship in complying, the law created a premium supplementation fund, but it has been used only five times in eighteen years. Insurers must accept all employees, regardless of preexisting conditions; in part due to this requirement, community rating has emerged as the dominant way to determine premiums.

The second way Hawaii has expanded health insurance coverage is through the State Health Insurance Plan (SHIP). The program was created to subsidize health care premiums for those individuals in the gap between Medicaid and employer-sponsored insurance. Individuals with incomes up to 300 percent of the federal poverty level are eligible, but must pay monthly premiums which increase as income rises. An average monthly premium for an adult is $20.00. Under this plan, primary and preventive care is well-covered, but inpatient care is limited. SHIP health benefits are not as comprehensive as those required under the Prepaid Health Care Act. Hawaii contracts for SHIP insurance with the state's two largest insurers which together cover over 70 percent of the population. One insurer, The Hawaii Medical Services Association, currently provides a fee-for-service SHIP plan but may develop a managed care system in the near future. The other insurer, Kaiser Permanente, is a health maintenance organization which subsidizes a portion of the costs of coverage for SHIP enrollees.

The third mechanism for providing health care coverage is the federally-supported Medicaid program. Hawaii's Medicaid program is generous. It covers people with incomes up to 62.5 percent of the federal poverty level (45 percent is the average for other states). Special programs extend coverage to elderly and disabled persons with incomes up to 100 percent of the poverty level, children under age six with income up to 133 percent of the poverty level, and pregnant women and infants up to 185 percent of the poverty level.

The Prepaid Health Care Act, SHIP, and Medicaid together provide health coverage to 98 percent of the population.

SOURCES: State of Hawaii. Prepaid Health Care Act. 393 HRS §§1-48.

State of Hawaii Department of Health. Report to the Legislature: State Health Insurance Program. January 1992.

Lewin JC. Reflections on National Health Care Reform Based on Hawai`i's Experience. Honolulu: Hawaii Department of Health; March 1992. [Reprinted in Section 6.]

Lewin JC. The Implementation of National Health Care Reform: Lessons from Hawai`i. Presented at the Conference on the Implementation of National Health Care Reforms; Washington, D.C.: June 12, 1992.

For more information, contact: John C. Lewin, M.D., Director, Hawaii State Department of Health, 1250 Punchbowl Street, Honolulu, Hawaii 96813 (808) 548-6505.

PROPONENT:

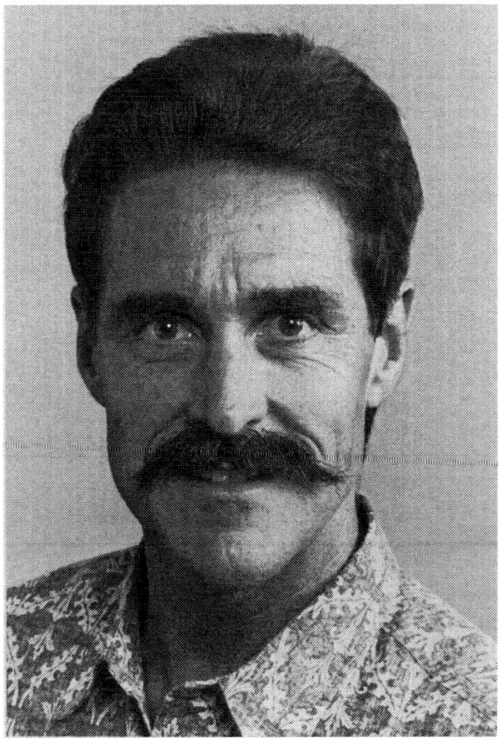

JOHN C. LEWIN is the Director of Hawaii's Department of Health. He serves as the chief health and environmental official for the state. He is past president of the Association of State and Territorial Health Officials, ASTHO, the national organization of state commissioners and directors of health. He is also a clinical professor of International Health at the University of Hawaii, School of Public Health. Prior to his current position, he was in private practice on Maui and was the medical director of Kula Hospital as well as the chief of family practice at Maui Memorial Hospital.

HAWAII PLAN
KEY CONCEPTS

Mandated employer-sponsored health insurance covering a basic benefits package is the practical foundation for universal health insurance, because it leaves a manageable gap to be filled between Medicaid and private insurance.

Hawaii Plan

Insurers must insure all employees, regardless of risk, and community rating must be required unless it naturally prevails.

Hawaii Plan

A national health care budget and federal price controls are unwieldy, unnecessary and politically unappealing.

Hawaii Plan

Federal leadership in health promotion, cost containment and expanding access to health care is needed, but the states should be given room to experiment and find locally appropriate solutions.

Hawaii Plan

Providers must be required to publish cost and performance data so those who purchase health care can bargain intelligently.

Hawaii Plan

To make all parties cost-conscious, specific limits should be set on the value of health insurance benefits which can be excluded from an employee's taxable income.

Hawaii Plan

Tort reform will help control the cost of defensive medicine.

Hawaii Plan

OREGON PLAN

- EMPLOYER-PROVIDED HEALTH INSURANCE
- RATIONING HEALTH CARE SERVICES
- PUBLIC DEBATE ON BASIC HEALTH CARE BENEFITS PACKAGE
- HIGH-RISK INSURANCE POOLS

This strategy, which primarily stems from the Oregon Basic Health Services Act of 1989, establishes three mechanisms for increasing access to health insurance.

One measure establishes high-risk insurance pools with state-subsidized premiums for those individuals who do not qualify for private insurance because of preexisting health conditions.

Another part of the law encourages and eventually requires employers to provide health insurance to their employees or make mandatory contributions to a state fund for purchasing insurance. Businesses receive tax credits for providing insurance.

The most ambitious portion of the law undertakes to reshape and expand Oregon's Medicaid program. The goal of the law is to expand the state's Medicaid program to include a minimum level of coverage for all residents with incomes up to 100 percent of the federal poverty level. A premise of the plan is that to cover more poor individuals with roughly the same funding, some services previously covered will need to be cut. A Health Services Commission was charged with the task of consulting with professionals and the general public to develop a priority list for all health care services. A list of 709 condition-treatment pairs was generated, and federal permission was sought for a Medicaid project that would have covered only the top 587 services.

In August of 1992 Secretary of Health and Human Services Louis Sullivan denied the requested permission on the ground that the ranking process discriminated against the disabled in a way forbidden by the Americans with Disabilities Act. In March 1993, the Clinton administration indicated that a revised proposal would be accepted.

SOURCES: Garland MJ. (1991). Setting Health Care Priorities in Oregon. *Health Matrix.* 1(2):139-156. [Reprinted in Section 6.]

Mason T. (1992). Sullivan Made the Right Choice in Rejecting the Oregon Plan. *Health Matrix.* 2(1) 85-88. [Reprinted in Section 6.]

Congress of the United States. *Evaluation of the Oregon Medicaid Proposal.* Washington, D.C.: Office of Technology Assessment. 1992. [Excerpts reprinted in Section 6.]

For more information, contact: The Honorable John Kitzhaber, M.D., State Capitol, S-203, Salem, Oregon 97310 (503) 378-8173.

OREGON PLAN
KEY CONCEPTS

Practical limits on health care resources mean that not every beneficial service can be included in a basic health care package to be assured to everyone.

Oregon Plan

The health care system must be allowed to adapt to varying local and regional circumstances.

Oregon Plan

Broad public participation in the development of a basic health care package allows the shared values of the community to shape the outcome and should give those individuals who will be most affected a chance to express their views.

Oregon Plan

Promote health insurance purchasing networks to pool individual and small business buying power.

Oregon Plan

Explicit ranking of all health care services to determine which services will be funded and which lower priority services will be denied is an honest and effective way to allocate limited funds for health care of the poor.

Oregon Plan

PRESIDENT BUSH'S PLAN

- TAX CREDITS AND DEDUCTIONS
- HEALTH INSURANCE NETWORKS (HINs)
- INSURANCE REFORM
- MALPRACTICE AND ANTITRUST REFORM

This strategy focuses on market reform and would coordinate health care while maintaining the viability and competitive environment of the private sector in the current health care delivery system.

The plan would make health insurance more affordable for individuals and small businesses by using health insurance networks to pool consumer resources for greater purchasing power. Employees would be guaranteed access to insurance coverage and the right to renew it without prohibitive premium increases. Preexisting medical condition limits on the coverage of individuals would be eliminated.

A health insurance tax credit or deduction would be available for moderate and low income citizens to purchase a basic health benefits package. Specifically, a tax credit of up to $3,750 would be available to low income families, a tax deduction of up to $3,750 would be available to middle income families, and an increase to 100 percent in the tax deduction for health insurance premiums would be available to self-employed individuals. The tax credit would diminish to zero as the family's income increased. Each state would be required to develop a basic health insurance package that could be purchased with the tax credit. Consumers, however, would be free to purchase other insurance if they preferred.

Other aspects of the plan include antitrust and medical malpractice reform as well as encouragement of health promotion and disease prevention.

SOURCE: The President's Comprehensive Health Reform Program. Washington, D.C.; February 6, 1992. [Excerpts reprinted in Section 6.]

Author's Note:

Proponents of health care reform plans that focus on tax credits and related changes in the income tax system generally have in common a preference for market forces over government decision-making as a way of allocating the resources of our society. A forceful statement of this preference and thorough presentation of a health care reform plan based upon it is made in *Patient Power: Solving America's Health Care Crisis* by John C. Goodman and Gerald Musgrave (Washington, D.C.: Cato Institute, 1992). The book advocates, for example, privatizing much of Medicare through such devices as Medical IRA's (tax-favored accounts through which individuals could save for their retirement health care costs and retain control of the way the money is ultimately spent).

PRESIDENT BUSH'S PLAN
KEY CONCEPTS

Because health care services would have to be rationed and prices controlled, a government-run single payer system would destroy diversity and flexibility in the financing, organization, and delivery of care.

President Bush's Plan

The "play or pay" approach would hurt small businesses, increase costs for government, force employers to reduce wages or cut employees, and eventually cascade into a form of national health insurance.

President Bush's Plan

Government regulation of private business should be kept to a minimum in order to allow market forces to work effectively.

President Bush's Plan

The health care insurance market must be restructured to achieve portability, wide access, and renewable coverage for all citizens.

President Bush's Plan

The use of tax credits and deductions to assist in the purchase of insurance plans will protect consumer choice and increase awareness of health care costs.

President Bush's Plan

The use of health insurance networks to pool buying power recognizes that individual consumers and small businesses are limited in terms of bargaining power and resources.

President Bush's Plan

Administrative costs in health care can be reduced through regulatory reforms that streamline the paperwork and by market reforms that allow small businesses to share administrative costs through group purchasing.

President Bush's Plan

Antitrust rules should provide clearer guidelines for health care providers on sharing of medical technology and services, peer review activities, and pooling arrangements.

President Bush's Plan

Incentives that encourage malpractice litigation and defensive medicine can be changed by eliminating joint and several liability, excluding double recovery, promoting alternative dispute resolution, and requiring structured payments for malpractice awards.

President Bush's Plan

In order to increase the number of doctors and clinics in inner city and rural areas and increase preventive care, funding should be expanded for community health centers, Migrant Health Centers and the National Health Service Corps.

President Bush's Plan

HERITAGE PLAN

- TAX CREDITS
- CONSUMERS PURCHASE INSURANCE COVERAGE
- BASIC HEALTH BENEFITS PACKAGE
- INSURANCE REFORM

This strategy allows consumers to choose their own health care plan and relies on competition among insurance and health care providers to efficiently allocate resources and control costs.

The plan would require every individual to purchase a basic health benefits package, unless the person were covered by Medicaid, Medicare, or other government health programs. Congress would specify the minimum benefits package required by law.

Employers who continue to provide insurance coverage for their employees would include the health benefits contribution as taxable income to the employee. The current tax exclusion for employer-sponsored health insurance coverage would be replaced with a tax credit for individuals to cover health insurance and out-of-pocket medical expenses. The tax credit would diminish as income rises.

If an employee chooses a plan different from his or her employer's, the employer is required to pay the employee in wages what the employer would have contributed to the employee's health insurance coverage.

Insurers would be required to guarantee annual renewals while limiting annual premium increases to the average increase which the insurer charges all individuals covered under the insurer's plan. Increases in premium due to changes in health status would be prohibited. "Uninsurable" individuals would be randomly assigned to insurers in order to spread the cost of insuring high-risk individuals.

SOURCE: Butler SM. A Policy Maker's Guide To The Health Care Crisis - Part II: The Heritage Consumer Choice Health Plan. In: Heritage Talking Points. Washington, D.C.: The Heritage Foundation: March 5, 1992. [Excerpt reprinted in Section 6.]

Although this health care reform plan is entitled "The Heritage Plan," it was written by Stuart M. Butler and does not necessarily reflect the views of The Heritage Foundation.

For more information, contact: Stuart M. Butler, The Heritage Foundation, 214 Massachusetts Avenue, N.E., Washington, D.C. 20002-4999 (202) 546-4400.

Author's Note:

For a thorough presentation of a health care reform plan based on tax credits and related changes in the income tax system, see *Patient Power: Solving America's Health Care Crisis* by John C. Goodman and Gerald Musgrave (Washington, D.C.: Cato Institute, 1992), which is briefly discussed on page 170 in this section.

PROPONENT:

STUART M. BUTLER is the Director of Domestic Policy Studies and the Roe Institute for Economic Policy Studies at the Heritage Foundation.

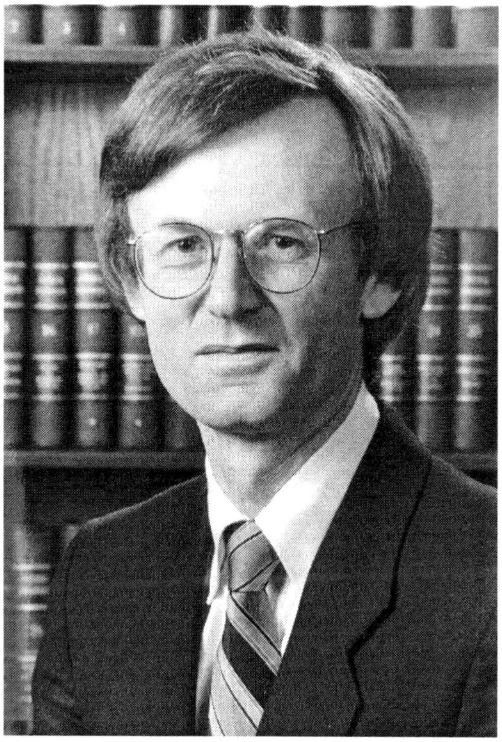

HERITAGE PLAN
KEY CONCEPTS

Require everyone not covered by a public program to buy basic health insurance and use a tax credit that diminishes as income rises to fund purchases by those with low incomes.

Heritage Plan

Assure that individuals can renew health insurance with limited premium increases regardless of health problems.

Heritage Plan

Changes in the health care system should maximize the opportunity for individuals to make choices about the kind of health care they will receive.

Heritage Plan

In order for individuals to become more aware of the costs of health care insurance and to raise money to cover the cost of a tax credit program, employer-paid health insurance benefits should be included in the employee's taxable wages.

Heritage Plan

Health care reforms should preserve successful aspects of our present system.

Heritage Plan

Government health programs such as Medicare and Medicaid should remain largely intact because they function adequately to cover the cost of health care for the elderly and poor.

Heritage Plan

The success of the "consumer choice" health benefits program which covers over nine million federal government workers indicates that American consumers are capable of making sound choices on health insurance plans if they are provided with adequate information.

Heritage Plan

> Health care costs are better controlled through consumer choice than through price controls.
>
> Heritage Plan

> Health care reform should be budget neutral and not raise the federal deficit.
>
> Heritage Plan

PAULY PLAN

- TAX CREDITS
- FOCUS ON MARKET FORCES
- CONSUMERS PURCHASE INSURANCE COVERAGE
- USE OF EXISTING GOVERNMENT PROGRAMS

This strategy would enhance the private market sector of our health care system and build on existing government programs to achieve universal health insurance coverage. Every person would be required to obtain his or her own basic coverage through an individual or family insurance plan. The required minimum policy would include catastrophic coverage, acute care services and preventive services that are beneficial to the consumer and cost-effective for the health care delivery system as a whole.

If people in any income level fail to obtain basic coverage in a timely fashion, the government arranges "fallback coverage" with insurers in each geographic market.

Low income individuals would be entitled to a tax credit or voucher to cover the cost of a basic insurance policy. The tax credit diminishes to zero as the individual's income rises. Any employer health insurance premium payments would be treated as taxable income of the employee.

SOURCE: Pauly MV, Danzon P, Feldstein PJ & Hoff J. *Responsible National Health Insurance.* Washington, D.C.: AEI Press, 1992:3-21. [Excerpt reprinted in Section 6.]

For more information, contact: Dr. Mark V. Pauly, 203 Colonial Penn Center Building, 3641 Locust Walk, University of Pennsylvania, Philadelphia, Pennsylvania 19104-6218 (215) 898-2838.

Author's Note:

For a thorough presentation of a health care reform plan based on tax credits and related changes in the income tax system, see *Patient Power: Solving America's Health Care Crisis* by John C. Goodman and Gerald Musgrave (Washington, D.C.: Cato Institute, 1992), which is briefly discussed on page 170 in this section.

PROPONENT:

MARK V. PAULY holds the Bendheim Professorship and is professor of health care systems, insurance, public management, and economics at the Wharton School, University of Pennsylvania. He is the director of research for the Leonard Davis Institute of Health Economics, University of Pennsylvania. He received his Ph.D. in economics from the University of Virginia.

PAULY PLAN
KEY CONCEPTS

To increase awareness of health care costs and to invigorate the market for health insurance, individuals should be required to obtain a minimum package of health insurance.

Pauly Plan

Individuals will shop more aggressively for value in spending their health care insurance dollars, if they see and feel the insurance being purchased with pre-tax dollars.

Pauly Plan

While the obligation to obtain coverage is on individual citizens, many will choose to satisfy this obligation by continuing with or initiating the purchase of insurance through employment-related groups.

Pauly Plan

Individuals with varying preferences about health care and insurance will be dissatisfied with a single payer, government-run system, because their range of choice of health care services and insurance coverage will be sharply reduced.

Pauly Plan

Consumers who are conscious of health care costs will use effective preventive services more and emergency services less.

Pauly Plan

Since there are limits to an individual's willingness or capacity to obtain health care insurance, the government must provide a mechanism for ensuring basic health insurance coverage for individuals who do not arrange coverage on their own.

Pauly Plan

People may not recognize or accurately evaluate their own need for health care or health insurance coverage, so the government must establish a minimum required level of coverage.

Pauly Plan

Health care is a service which the nonpoor in the community are concerned about providing to the poor.

Pauly Plan

Exclusion of health care benefits from income and payroll taxation distorts employee bargaining behavior in favor of compensation through untaxed health care insurance and gives an inequitable tax break to employees who work for firms with health care benefits as opposed to those who work for firms without such benefits.

Pauly Plan

A health care tax credit that diminishes with rising income and that yields a refund for the poor should be substituted for the current tax exclusion of health care benefits.

Pauly Plan

Political feasibility and use of existing systems in health care and government are important factors to consider in reforming the health care delivery system.

Pauly Plan

REINHARDT PLAN

- PREMIUMS PAID THROUGH THE INCOME TAX SYSTEM
- TAX FOR INDIGENT CARE
- WAYS FOR THE GOVERNMENT TO BUY INSURANCE

Under this strategy, the government would insist that every individual carry basic, comprehensive health insurance coverage. Employers would be free to decide whether or not to provide health insurance as part of their total compensation package for employees.

Collection of money from individuals for an insurance fund would be accomplished through the tax system. Taxpayers would pay a progressive income-based premium for basic health insurance coverage that would automatically be provided to the taxpayer by the government. However, if an individual attached evidence of a private policy at least as comprehensive as the basic health insurance package provided by the government, the taxpayer would be excused from paying the premium tax.

All taxpayers, even if privately insured, might be required to pay a small, progressive tax earmarked for indigent care.

These funds would supplement the premiums collected from low income families.

There are at least three cost-effective ways the government could procure the health insurance it is to provide to the public. First, the federal government could use the insurance funds to enroll all people who are not privately insured in an expanded Medicare program. This approach shares some features with the single payer strategy.

Second, the federal government could distribute the insurance funds to the states in the form of capitation payments that would be adjusted for age, sex, and regional cost variations. Each state could then disburse these capitation amounts to health care providers in a manner that suits local preferences. A state might instead opt to enroll individuals without private insurance in a state-run program similar to Medicaid.

Third, some states might prefer to process the capitation payments through the private insurance sector by letting uninsured families choose from a selection of privately managed health care plans. This would resemble the managed competition approach proposed by the Jackson Hole Group.

Rules governing the private health care insurance industry would be designed to prevent the enrollment of a disproportionate number of high-risk people in the public insurance pool.

SOURCE: Reinhardt UE. An "All American"™ Health Reform Proposal. Princeton, NJ: Princeton University; August 1992. [Reprinted in Section 6.]

For more information, contact: Uwe E. Reinhardt, Ph.D., Woodrow Wilson School of Public and International Affairs, Princeton University, Robertson Hall, Princeton, NJ 08544-1013 (609) 258-4830.

PROPONENT:

UWE E. REINHARDT has taught at Princeton University since September, 1968. His research and writing has focused on health economics. He has also published articles on accounting and corporate finance issues. He received his Ph.D. in Economics from Yale in 1970. He was born in Osnabrueck, West Germany and has lived in the United States since 1964.

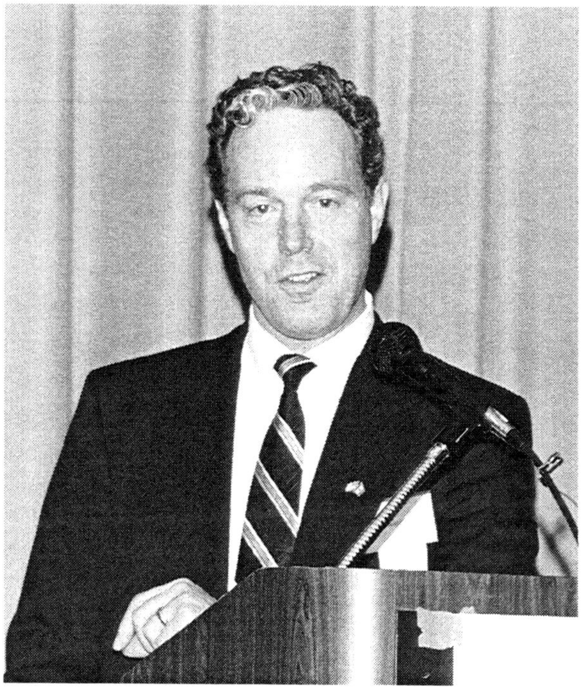

REINHARDT PLAN
KEY CONCEPTS

U.S. health care reform should achieve universal coverage, portable health insurance, simplicity and administrative cost control.

Reinhardt Plan

The federal government should reconfigure the health care system to organize and strengthen the collective bargaining power of consumers on the "demand side" of the health care equation.

Reinhardt Plan

On the supply side, the government should encourage the development of managed care options, though a role will remain for more expensive fee-for-service arrangements.

Reinhardt Plan

Keeping the present system in which most people secure health insurance through their work is fine, but employees should be taxed on the value of the insurance.

Reinhardt Plan

Employers should not be required to provide health insurance for employees, because the cost of such a mandate is simply shifted to customers (in the form of higher prices), to employees (in the form of lower wages or reductions in other fringe benefits) or, least likely, to owners (in the form of lower profits).

Reinhardt Plan

All health care dollars are ultimately drawn from the budgets of individual households.

Reinhardt Plan

Those individuals who do not have private insurance should pay a progressive tax to fund insurance to be provided to them by the government, which will bargain for such insurance as a powerful buyer.

Reinhardt Plan

All taxpayers should pay a small tax to help finance health insurance for the poor.

Reinhardt Plan

Some tiering of the quality of health care services by income class is inherent in such ideas as consumer choice and managed competition.

Reinhardt Plan

Assure low income individuals a basic comprehensive health care benefit package, but allow higher-income groups to enroll in more comprehensive plans.

Reinhardt Plan

AMERICAN NURSES ASSOCIATION PLAN

- PLAY OR PAY
- FEDERALLY-DEFINED BASIC HEALTH BENEFITS PACKAGE
- PUBLIC AND PRIVATE HEALTH CARE PLANS
- EMPHASIS ON CONSUMER RESPONSIBILITY

Universal access to a federally defined basic health care benefits package is a goal of this strategy. It would be achieved in stages by expanding a public health insurance plan so it eventually covers everyone who does not have private coverage.

The public plan would be administered by the states and provide coverage for the poor and high-risk populations. Employers and individuals would have the option of purchasing this plan as their source of coverage. Private plans would be required to offer at least the federally mandated basic benefits. Both public and private plans would make use of deductibles and copayments to provide financial incentives for the economical use of health services. Managed care options would be encouraged.

Employers would be required to provide basic coverage for employees or pay into the public plan.

Delivery of primary health care services would occur in local community settings to promote a more consumer-friendly system. Although a package of essential health services would be mandated at the federal level, health services delivery would be decentralized to foster greater consumer orientation. In addition, health outcomes information would be disseminated to providers and consumers to assist them in making effective choices about care and treatment. Adequate access to preventive care, especially for children and pregnant women, and patient education on caring for oneself are high priorities.

Insurers would be required to use community rating and discontinue preexisting condition exclusions. Protection for individuals against catastrophic health care expenses, including those due to long-term care needs, would be available. A variety of taxing mechanisms could be used to raise needed funds.

SOURCE: American Nurses Association. Nursing's Agenda for Health Care Reform. Washington, D.C.: ANA; 1991. [Reprinted in Section 6.]

For more information, contact: American Nurses Association, 600 Maryland Avenue, SW, Suite 100 West, Washington D.C. 20024-2571 (202) 554-4444.

The American Nurses Association was formally incorporated in 1901 as the Nurses Associated Alumnae of the United States and changed its name to the American Nurses Association (ANA) in 1911. With more than 200,000 members, the ANA is a full-service professional association for the nation's 2 million registered nurses. ANA establishes and implements nursing's political and legislative programs, fosters a professional and equitable work environment, and develops standards that ensure high quality patient care in institutions and the community. Nursing's Agenda for Health Care Reform is currently endorsed by 67 national nursing and health-related organizations, which represent approximately 1 million registered nurses.

AMERICAN NURSES ASSOCIATION PLAN KEY CONCEPTS

Give consumers incentives and the means to be cost-conscious about health care and actively involved in their own health care decisions.

American Nurses Association Plan

Achieve universal coverage for a federally-defined minimum benefits package by requiring employment-based health insurance (or an equivalent tax payment by the employer) and covering the rest of the population with a public health insurance program.

American Nurses Association Plan

Focus the health care system on wellness promotion, especially for women and children.

American Nurses Association Plan

> Deliver primary health care in community-based settings, such as schools, work sites and community health centers.
>
> American Nurses Association Plan

> Shape the delivery system to respond to local needs and realities.
>
> American Nurses Association Plan

> Reform private insurance practices to require community rating and eliminate preexisting condition exclusions.
>
> American Nurses Association Plan

HEALTH INSURANCE ASSOCIATION OF AMERICA PLAN

- MANDATORY EMPLOYER-SPONSORED HEALTH INSURANCE
- GOVERNMENT FUNDS COVERAGE OF THE POOR
- INSURERS ISSUE AND RENEW COVERAGE FOR ALL
- USE MANAGED CARE FOR COST CONTROL
- MINIMUM HEALTH CARE BENEFITS PACKAGE

Under this strategy, the federal government would require all individuals to carry, and all employers to offer, a minimum health care benefits package. The government would fund health care coverage for the poor and would pay providers at fair rates that do not shift costs to the private sector.

A federally-chartered commission made up of health care system participants would establish procompetitive, flexible rules of conduct that support a pluralistic system. The commission would shape a basic benefits package providing good primary and preventive services as well as catastrophic coverage. Consumers would have the option to purchase supplemental coverage for additional benefits.

Cost containment would rely heavily on competition among a variety of managed care plans, though provider rate regulation and expenditure targets could be explored. New approaches would be designed to discourage excessive doctor visits and unnecessary use of technology, while encouraging healthy lifestyles and preventive care. To permit value comparison, managed care plans would be required to publish cost and performance data.

Enrollment of Medicare and Medicaid patients as regular-price participants in managed care plans would be a goal.

Legal restraints to systemic health care reform - such as state impediments to managed care and undue ERISA constraints - would be removed. A user-friendly, paperless system is envisioned. Clinical practice guidelines and reform of the malpractice litigation system would help limit defensive medicine.

Insurers would be required to issue and renew health care coverage for all, regardless of health, financial or employment status. With portable coverage, job lock would end. Insurers would retain limited rights to calibrate premiums to risk, since pure community rating hides costs so much that it works against cost containment. Reinsurance, risk-sharing, and other means of protecting insurer solvency would be important.

Two factors essential to keeping the health care system open to innovation are employer involvement in selecting health care coverage for employees and government rules that allow for reasonable variation in benefit plans. Business participation in insurance purchasing cooperatives would be voluntary.

To promote tax equity, premiums paid for a minimum benefits package would be excluded from the taxable income of an employee or a self-employed person, but premiums paid by an employer for health benefits in excess of the minimum package would be deemed taxable income to the employee. Funding to pay for coverage of people below the federal poverty level would come in part from such elimination of favorable tax treatment for benefits that go beyond the minimum benefits package and in part from new taxes.

SOURCE: Health Insurance Association of America. Health Care Reform Proposal, Washington, D.C.: HIAA; February 1993. [Reprinted in Section 6.]

For more information, contact: Health Insurance Association of America, 1025 Connecticut Avenue, N.W., Washington D.C. 20036-3998 (202) 223-7780 or FAX (202) 223-7896.

The Health Insurance Association of America (HIAA) is a trade association for commercial health insurers. It serves as a forum for the development of policy that reflects broad consensus and support within the industry. Conducting health insurance research and publishing technical literature and policy analyses on developments and trends in health insurance are among HIAA's most important functions.

HEALTH INSURANCE ASSOCIATION OF AMERICA PLAN

KEY CONCEPTS

To achieve universal health insurance coverage, have all employers sponsor health insurance for their employees, publicly fund care for the poor, and require all others to purchase their own coverage.

Health Insurance Association of America Plan

Successful cost containment depends on fostering competition among managed care plans that are accountable to patients and the community.

Health Insurance Association of America Plan

To promote tax equity and to help fund health care coverage for the poor, any employee health benefits in excess of the basic benefits package should be treated as taxable income to the employee.

Health Insurance Association of America Plan

Use procompetitive public regulations to foster a flexible, pluralistic system of delivering and financing health care.

Health Insurance Association of America Plan

A national commission should establish a basic benefits package and rules of conduct for the health care marketplace.

Health Insurance Association of America Plan

Insurers must issue and renew health care coverage for all, regardless of health, financial or employment status.

Health Insurance Association of America Plan

Allow limited experience rating of health insurance premiums to preserve cost control incentives, but do not allow drastic premium disparities for demographically similar groups.

Health Insurance Association of America Plan

Handle claims with a user-friendly, paperless system.

Health Insurance Association of America Plan

Limit defensive medicine through clinical practice guidelines and malpractice litigation reforms.

Health Insurance Association of America Plan

Eliminate underpayments by public health care programs that shift cost burdens onto privately insured patients.

Health Insurance Association of America Plan

AMERICAN HOSPITAL ASSOCIATION PLAN

- COMMUNITY CARE NETWORKS
- EMPLOYER-BASED COVERAGE
- BASIC HEALTH CARE BENEFITS PACKAGE
- CONSOLIDATING AND EXPANDING MEDICAID AND MEDICARE

This strategy is based on the premise that health care is a local concern and that lasting reform can be accomplished by restructuring consumer and provider incentives to coordinate patient care on a community level. Universal access to coverage for health care would be accomplished through a combination of private employer-based coverage and a single public program which would consolidate and expand Medicare and Medicaid.

The health care delivery system would be restructured by establishing community care networks under a set of national guidelines to meet local health care needs. The networks would consist of local health care providers, and possibly others, such as insurers and community agencies, working together to deliver health care in the local community. Providers in the network would administer health care services to an enrolled population. They would be paid a fixed annual fee for each person enrolled in the network.

Required employment-based coverage would be phased in and preceded by insurance reforms. Certain underwriting practices by insurers would change; for example, pre-existing condition clauses would be eliminated. Reinsurance mechanisms and insurance pools would be developed to spread the risk so that small businesses and medically uninsurable individuals could afford insurance coverage. Hardship funds would also be available for qualifying small businesses. Private employers providing coverage would be free to negotiate payment agreements with the network of their choice or with insurers offering more traditional products.

This strategy proposes combining Medicare and Medicaid into a new public program with an independent supervisory commission setting capitated rates to be paid to the networks. The independent commission would also define the basic health care benefits package that the public program would cover and that would serve as the floor for private coverage. Congress would set a national budget to cover the public portion of health care spending but would not be responsible for determining specific network payments. The specific capitated payment might be set by a state-level entity.

In the private sector, network payment rates would be negotiated between the networks and employers. Individual states would be left to decide whether to regulate the private sector.

Insurers could either play the traditional role of underwriting the risks of an enrolled population within a network or try such roles as marketing networks to individuals, providing reinsurance to networks, assisting networks in evaluating cost and quality performance data, contributing to regulatory compliance, and providing debt financing. These new roles would move insurers away from evaluating individual patient care decisions as part of claims processing and would focus more attention on the evaluation of the overall performance of the community care networks.

Training of an adequate number of general practice physicians, geographically appropriate distribution of health care providers, and increased development and dissemination of medical practice guidelines are also important goals of this plan.

SOURCES: American Hospital Association. National Health Care Reform: Refining and Advancing the Vision. Chicago:AHA; 1992. [Reprinted in Section 6.]

Davidson RJ. Community Care Networks: Cornerstone of Health Care Reform. *J Am Health Policy.* 1992; 14:12-15.

For more information, contact: American Hospital Association, 840 North Lakeshore Drive, Chicago, IL 60611 (312) 280-6000.

The American Hospital Association (AHA) has been in existence for over 90 years and has more than 5,000 institutional and associate members. The health care positions that AHA advocates in Washington are developed through a process involving consultation with all segments of AHA membership. The AHA staff in Washington presents these policy positions to Congress and federal agencies both formally - through written congressional testimony and comments on proposed federal regulations - and informally - in personal meetings with members of Congress, regulators, and their staffs.

AMERICAN HOSPITAL ASSOCIATION PLAN

KEY CONCEPTS

Universal coverage should be gradually achieved by requiring employment-based health insurance and consolidating and enlarging the Medicaid and Medicare programs.

American Hospital Association Plan

Health care is a local concern because people generally seek medical care and develop relationships with primary care providers in their own community.

American Hospital Association Plan

Health care networks that offer the needed continuum of health care services should be organized at the community level because communities differ in terms of health care needs, medical practice patterns, regulation of health care providers, and available resources.

American Hospital Association Plan

Networks should be accountable to their communities for cost-effectiveness and for maintaining and improving the health status of the community they serve.

American Hospital Association Plan

Collaboration of providers within health care networks and competition among networks is a good formula for cost containment.

American Hospital Association Plan

The freedom of individuals to choose a primary caregiver supports a traditional American value and ensures a convenient point of entry into the health care system.

American Hospital Association Plan

An independent federal commission should establish the basic health benefits package and capitation fee guidelines.

American Hospital Association Plan

The basic health benefits package should emphasize preventive services, such as health education and screening for early detection of disease.

American Hospital Association Plan

Individuals must be encouraged to obtain care when they need it and in an appropriate health care setting.

American Hospital Association Plan

Because most consumers have insurance and do not pay directly for the cost of health care, they have little incentive to conserve their use of health care resources, compare potential benefits to cost, or shop for the most cost-effective providers.

American Hospital Association Plan

When health care providers are held publicly accountable for health outcomes and financially responsible for maintaining a predetermined budget, there are proper incentives to maintain patient health and keep costs to a minimum.

American Hospital Association Plan

Health care providers must be given greater freedom to make decisions without micro-management by government payers and insurers in order to focus more energy on patient care and less on administrative details.

American Hospital Association Plan

JACKSON HOLE GROUP PLAN

- ACCOUNTABLE HEALTH PLANS
- MANAGED COMPETITION
- INFORMED PRICE-CONSCIOUS CONSUMERS
- HEALTH PLAN PURCHASING COOPERATIVES
- PROCOMPETITIVE REGULATORY FRAMEWORK

This strategy promotes managed competition, a blend of government regulation and competition among health care organizations. The government would establish rules for competition and provide support in the form of tax preferences and direct purchasing to those health care plans that conform with the rules.

The managed competition rules aim to reshape the delivery system to favor managed care organizations in which anyone can enroll. The rules give these organizations incentives to compete on the basis of risk management and health outcomes, not risk selection. Those that manage risk effectively and achieve better outcomes at a lower cost will be rewarded by the market with the most subscribers.

The Jackson Hole Group plan strives for consumers who are well-informed about health care cost and performance data, and who weigh these factors in their health care insurance choices. Comprehensive outcomes data would also be used by health care providers to help improve patient care.

Accountable Health Plans (AHPs) consisting of insurers and providers would provide managed care health benefit packages. AHPs would be required to disseminate information about the actual cost of patient care, medical outcomes achieved, and patient satisfaction.

Health Plan Purchasing Cooperatives (HPPCs) would function as collective purchasing agents on behalf of small employers and individuals. Federal law would be reformed to limit tax-free employer contributions to the amount which the local HPPC has bargained to pay an Accountable Health Plan for the minimum health benefits package. Employees who receive as a job benefit health insurance worth more than the HPPC-bargained amount in their area would pay income tax on the excess.

To help achieve this strategy, an independent federal agency and three standards-setting boards would be established. The federal agency would oversee the entire system and recommend a minimum health benefits package to Congress for approval. The minimum benefits package would take account of cost of services, value rendered to the consumer and society, and current medical technology.

The three standards-setting boards would assess medical technologies and treatments, underwriting practices, and methods of health services accounting. Appropriate standards would be set in each area.

Author's Note:

The above summary reflects two changes in terminology recently made by the Jackson Hole Group. The Group now prefers the term "Accountable Health Plan" over the term "Accountable Health Partnership" to refer to the managed care organizations which are intended to compete under the managed competition scheme. The Group also now prefers the term "Health Plan Purchasing Cooperative" over the term "Health Insurance Purchasing Cooperative" to refer to an association that collectively bargains for and purchases health insurance for small employers and individuals. The old terms have appeared in the Jackson Hole Group's published materials, including those reprinted in this Atlas. The new terms match those used in the managed competition legislation prepared by the Conservative Democratic Forum. The Conservative Democratic Forum plan is discussed next in this Atlas.

SOURCES: Ellwood PM, Enthoven AC, Etheredge L. (1992). The Jackson Hole Initiatives for a Twenty-First Century American Health Care System. *Health Economics.* 1:149-168. [Reprinted in Section 6.]

Enthoven A. (1992). Commentary: Measuring the Candidates on Health Care. *N Engl J Med.* 327:807-809. [Reprinted in Section 6.]

The plan for reform described above was developed by the Jackson Hole Group, an informal collection of health industry leaders, public officials, and health services researchers who have been meeting since the mid-1970s in Jackson Hole, Wyoming, where the founder of the group, Paul Ellwood, lives.
For more information, contact: The Jackson Hole Group, P.O. Box 350, Teton Village, Wyoming 83025 (307) 739-1176 FAX 307-739-1177.

PROPONENTS:

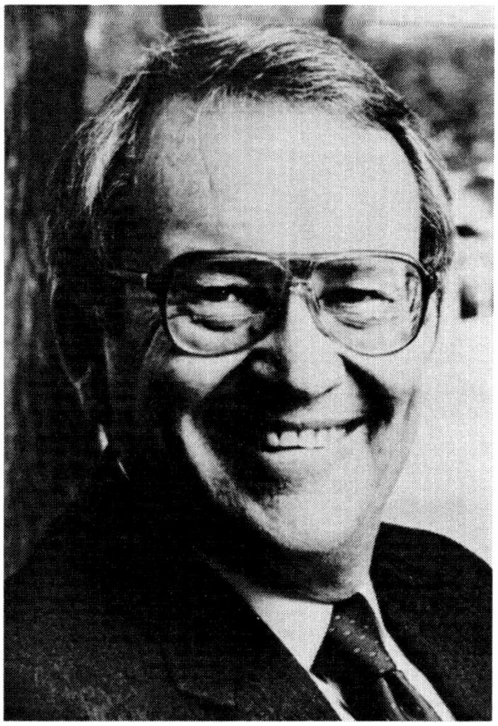

PAUL M. ELLWOOD is a graduate of Stanford Medical School and a Clinical Professor of Pediatrics, Neurology, and Physical Medicine and Rehabilitation at the University of Minnesota. He is also the CEO of InterStudy, a non-profit health policy research institute, and President of the Jackson Hole Group. He was in 1991 the first recipient of the U.S. Healthcare Quality Award. Dr. Ellwood practiced medicine for seventeen years and was co-editor of the *Handbook of Physical Medicine*.

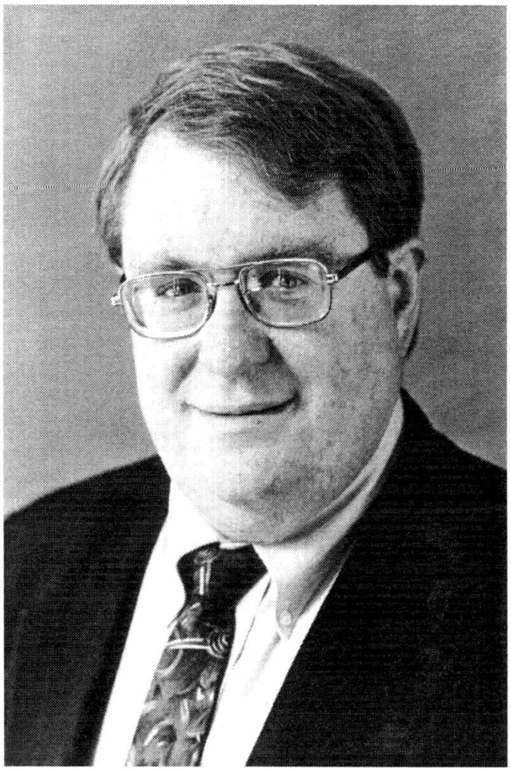

LYNN ETHEREDGE is an independent consultant who works with the public and private sectors on health care reform, income security, and government policy issues. He served in the federal Office of Management & Budget during four administrations, working on Medicare, Medicaid, and national health insurance. He was an associate director for health reform with the Clinton-Gore transition team and has been involved in state health policy reforms as a member of the National Governors Association health care task force. His recent articles include "Negotiating National Health Insurance" and "Managing a Pluralist Health System."

ALAIN C. ENTHOVEN is the Marriner S. Eccles Professor of Public and Private Management in the Graduate School of Business at Stanford University. He holds degrees in economics from Stanford, Oxford (where he was a Rhodes Scholar) and MIT. Among the positions he has held are Economist with the RAND Corporation, Assistant Secretary of Defense, and President of Litton Medical Products. In 1963, he received the President's Award for Distinguished Federal Civilian Service from John F. Kennedy. He is Chairman of the Health Benefits Advisory Council for CalPERS, the California Public Employees Retirement System, which sponsors health care plans. His latest book is *Theory and Practice of Managed Competition in Health Care Finance.*

JACKSON HOLE GROUP PLAN KEY CONCEPTS

Preserve the private market core of the American health care system while using appropriate government regulation to encourage competition among provider organizations and correct market failures.

Jackson Hole Group Plan

The freedom to choose health care providers and bargain for health insurance is important to consumers and ingrained in the American health care delivery system.

Jackson Hole Group Plan

To provide more cost-effective benefits to society, the government should foster the development of integrated health care delivery and financing systems and structure the market so these systems compete with each other.

Jackson Hole Group Plan

Top down price controls in the form of global budgets are impractical and would undermine an effort to achieve cost control through managed competition.

Jackson Hole Group Plan

To enhance the nation's capacity to collect data on and evaluate services provided to patients, a national health board and several private sector boards should be established that would work together to monitor and improve the health care system.

Jackson Hole Group Plan

The government should require health care providers to make available standardized health outcomes and cost data.

Jackson Hole Group Plan

Standardizing health care insurance practices will improve cost-effectiveness by encouraging competition and creating administrative simplicity.

Jackson Hole Group Plan

Since health care resources are limited, the government should, in setting a minimum acceptable standard of health benefits coverage, draw on both expert data and general public commentary.

Jackson Hole Group Plan

Since small businesses and individuals, especially the uninsured, have limited expertise and ability to bargain for health insurance coverage, they should have the opportunity to join purchasing cooperatives that will collectively bargain on their behalf for such coverage.

Jackson Hole Group Plan

To achieve greater equity and to promote effective bargaining for health insurance, the income tax exemption for individuals' health insurance premiums paid by employers or by the self-employed should be limited to the cost of the minimum benefits package.

Jackson Hole Group Plan

CONSERVATIVE DEMOCRATIC FORUM PLAN

- TAX INCENTIVES TO ENCOURAGE INSURER-PROVIDER PLANS
- BASIC HEALTH BENEFITS PACKAGE
- HEALTH PLAN PURCHASING COOPERATIVES
- DISCLOSURE OF HEALTH OUTCOMES INFORMATION

Using the managed competition approach, this strategy would establish insurer-provider partnerships called Accountable Health Plans (AHP) to offer health care and insurance coverage as a single product. The AHPs could offer a range of insurance programs, but would be required to offer at least a federally-defined basic health benefits package. AHPs would be also required to offer open enrollment and to disclose information about price and medical outcomes to consumers and employers so they could shop for the most cost-effective health care plan. Copayments would be required for all but preventive services.

To make coverage more available and spread the risk over a larger pool, individuals would be able to and small businesses would be required to join a state-chartered, not-for-profit organization called a Health Plan Purchasing Cooperative (HPPC). HPPCs would have their own exclusive geographic territory. Each state could charter one or more HPPCs within its borders. Individuals and small businesses would be able to choose from a variety of health plans offered by the HPPCs at lower costs than if the plans were purchased without the HPPCs help.

Employers would have the option of buying from an AHP insurance coverage more comprehensive than the basic package, but would only be allowed to deduct premiums paid up to the cost of the lowest priced AHP in the area that provided the basic package. Within this limit, tax deductibility of health insurance premiums paid by the self-employed would be increased from 25 to 100 percent.

However, if an individual or employer chose to purchase insurance coverage from a plan that did not qualify as an AHP, none of the premium would be tax deductible. For instance, if an insurer chose to engage in underwriting practices involving experience rating and preexisting medical conditions, employers could not deduct as a business expense the premiums paid for coverage from that insurer.

Medicaid would be replaced by a federal program which would purchase acute care coverage by an AHP for all individuals below the poverty line. In addition, a federal subsidy would be available to help individuals with incomes between 100 and 200 percent of the federal poverty level purchase insurance coverage from an AHP. The subsidy would diminish with rising income. The states would no longer have to finance Medicaid, but would gradually assume responsibility for funding long-term care for the poor.

Other aspects of the plan include malpractice reform, the promotion of preventive health care, the establishment of a national health board to oversee the health market, and increased funding to improve health care access for rural and inner city residents.

SOURCES: Conservative Democratic Forum Task Force on Health Care Reform. H.R. 5936: The Managed Competition Act of 1992 (Highlights). Washington, D.C.:CDF, September 1992. [Reprinted in Section 6.]

[This bill was introduced in the 102nd Congress. The Conservative Democratic Forum agreed to hold off introducing a managed competition bill in the 103rd Congress at the request of President Clinton's health transition team.]

American Hospital Association. (October 19, 1992). CDF Serves up Menu of Health-Plan Options for Consumers. *AHA News.* 28(42): 5. [Reprinted in Section 6.]

For more information, contact: Congressman Jim Cooper, 125 Cannon Building, Washington, D.C. 20515-4204 (202) 225-8831.

PROPONENT:

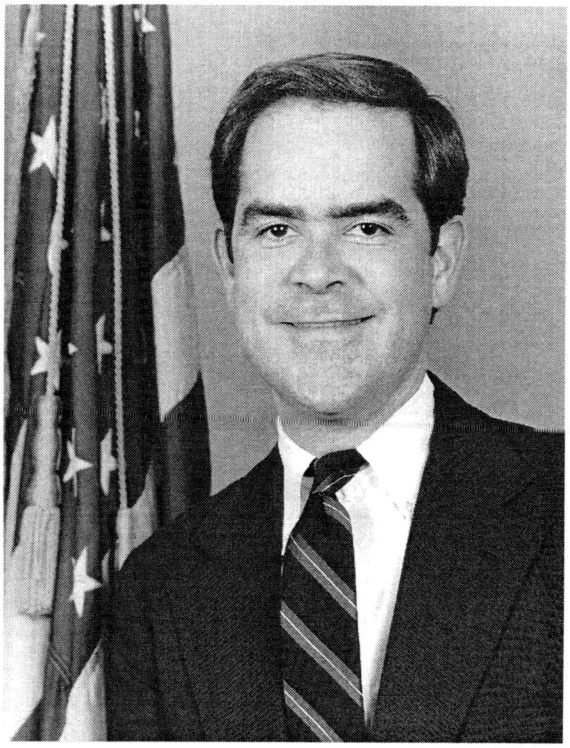

CONGRESSMAN JIM COOPER (D-Tenn.) is currently serving his fifth term in the House of Representatives. He serves on the House Budget Committee and the Energy and Commerce Committee. He graduated from the University of North Carolina, Oxford University in England, where he was a Rhodes Scholar, and Harvard Law School.

CONSERVATIVE DEMOCRATIC FORUM PLAN

KEY CONCEPTS

By using strong tax incentives to encourage insurers and providers to form integrated health care plans, the health care market can be managed more effectively and competition can be fostered.

Conservative Democratic Forum Plan

Create large regional health insurance purchasing cooperatives to give individuals and small businesses the benefits of greater buying power.

Conservative Democratic Forum Plan

Form an independent national board to establish a uniform set of effective health benefits and monitor system performance.

Conservative Democratic Forum Plan

To keep tax-favored status, health plans must offer the standard benefits package, comply with insurance reforms and disclose information on medical outcomes, cost-effectiveness and consumer satisfaction.

Conservative Democratic Forum Plan

Employers should be allowed to deduct basic health plan costs, but not the excess costs of policies which cover more than the basic benefits package.

Conservative Democratic Forum Plan

Basic health insurance policies should require copayments to make consumers cost-conscious.

Conservative Democratic Forum Plan

All individuals, including the self-employed, should be allowed to exclude from taxable income 100 percent of the cost of a basic health benefits package.

Conservative Democratic Forum Plan

Health plans should not be allowed to exclude coverage of preexisting conditions or use experience rating.

Conservative Democratic Forum Plan

Medicaid should be transformed into a new federal program that will pay health plan premiums for those in poverty and provide a premium subsidy on a sliding scale for those with incomes between 100 and 200 percent of the poverty level.

Conservative Democratic Forum Plan

Reform of the system for handling malpractice claims is needed to reduce the costs of expensive litigation and defensive medicine.

Conservative Democratic Forum Plan

Federal standards should be developed for health claim forms and electronic transmission of health claims data.

Conservative Democratic Forum Plan

Funding to assist rural and other underserved areas should be substantially increased.

Conservative Democratic Forum Plan

AMERICAN ASSOCIATION OF RETIRED PERSONS PLAN

- EXPAND MEDICARE AND ELIMINATE MEDICAID
- EXPENDITURE TARGETS
- MODIFIED PLAY OR PAY
- UNIVERSAL ACCESS TO COMPREHENSIVE BENEFITS

This strategy would expand Medicare to assure universal access to a comprehensive health care package, including long-term care, prescription drugs, and preventive care.

The AARP plan presents two alternative models. The first version proposes a modified "play or pay" approach. Employers would be required to pay an 8 percent payroll tax to enroll employees in the new Medicare program, but could opt out by providing private health insurance benefits to their employees that are the same or better than those offered in the new Medicare program. Preexisting condition exclusions would be prohibited in all private insurance plans.

The alternative model presented by AARP is a single-payer adaptation of the first. It would keep all the elements of the plan described below intact, but the federal government as single payer would assemble and pay out all health care funds. In this alternative model, the private insurance option is eliminated and all employers are required to pay a payroll tax to enroll their workers in the new Medicare program. Subsidies would be available to low-wage firms for a period of four years.

Cost containment would be achieved through a federal commission which would recommend for congressional approval national spending targets for acute and long-term health care. All payers for health services within each state, including the new Medicare program and any private, employer-sponsored insurance plans, would be required to reimburse providers according to the same rates and payment methods. Balance billing would be prohibited.

Individuals and families enrolled in the new Medicare program would be responsible for a monthly premium ($50 per adult, $125 maximum for a family) that would replace the existing Medicare premium. Copayments of 10 percent for most health care services would also be required up to an annual cap of $1,500 for individuals or $3,000 for families. Preventive care would be free. All persons with incomes at or below 200 percent of the federal poverty level would be eligible for subsidies covering all or a portion of their premiums and out-of-pocket health care costs.

The AARP plan calls for a comprehensive health care package that would integrate preventive care, acute care and long-term care into a wellness-promoting continuum. Managed care networks would be encouraged. The long-term care portion of the new Medicare program would be designed to help people stay at home as long as possible. Eligibility for long-term care benefits would be based solely on the need for care, not on the amount of a person's income or assets. Required copayments for long-term care would be limited.

Claims processing and billing would be handled by a uniform, national electronic system.

This strategy would be financed from five major sources: (1) existing federal revenues from Medicare, Medicaid, Veterans Administration, and other health care programs; (2) existing state health care spending; (3) an 8 percent payroll tax on all employers, except those opting for private insurance; (4) premiums and copayments paid by those enrolled in the new Medicare program; and (5) new taxes. It is estimated that the proposed health care system would require approximately $112 billion in new federal tax revenues, but this would be largely offset by reduced individual health care expenditures.

SOURCES: American Association of Retired Persons. Health Care America: The Draft Health Care Reform Proposal. Washington, D.C.:AARP; March 1992. [Excerpt reprinted in Section 6.]

For more information, contact: National Legislative Council, American Association of Retired Persons, 601 E Street, N.W., Washington, D.C. 20049 (202) 434-3770.

The American Association of Retired Persons (AARP) is a nonprofit organization whose purpose is to help older Americans achieve lives of independence, dignity and purpose. Founded in 1958, AARP is the nation's oldest and largest organization of older Americans, with a membership of more than 33 million. AARP develops legislative policy recommendations that are strictly nonpartisan with a focus on issues, not on candidates or their political affiliations. AARP serves a diverse population of workers and retirees; over one-third of the membership is in the work force.

AMERICAN ASSOCIATION OF RETIRED PERSONS PLAN

KEY CONCEPTS

The Medicaid program should be abolished and the Medicare program should be expanded and strengthened to ensure universal health care access for all individuals, regardless of age, income or employment status.

American Association of Retired Persons Plan

Easy access to health care will encourage individuals to use needed services, especially primary and preventive services such as maternal and child health care, immunizations, and screening programs.

American Association of Retired Persons Plan

Health promotion, disease prevention and acute and long-term care should be coordinated to ensure a continuum of care throughout the lifetime of an individual.

American Association of Retired Persons Plan

The federal government should establish a comprehensive health care benefits package to which all individuals are entitled.

American Association of Retired Persons Plan

The growth of managed care plans should be encouraged.

American Association of Retired Persons Plan

Cost containment can be achieved by setting expenditure targets at the national and state level and by establishing uniform reimbursement rates for both the new Medicare system and private insurers.

American Association of Retired Persons Plan

Cost containment efforts should not unreasonably limit a patient's choice of health care provider, because the freedom to make choices regarding one's health care provider is a valued element of our present system.

American Association of Retired Persons Plan

Employers should pay a health care payroll tax unless they opt out by providing a federally-defined comprehensive health benefits package of private insurance for their employees.

American Association of Retired Persons Plan

By setting reasonable levels of cost-sharing by patients and spreading the rest of the cost of long-term care across the entire population through an expanded Medicare program, all individuals can receive long-term care when they need it.

American Association of Retired Persons Plan

An important element of a long-term care program is assisting families and friends who act as informal caregivers but who themselves need supportive services such as respite care and adult day care.

American Association of Retired Persons Plan

PRESIDENT CLINTON'S PLAN

- GLOBAL BUDGETS
- MANAGED COMPETITION
- HEALTH INSURANCE PURCHASING COOPERATIVES
- COMPREHENSIVE BENEFITS PACKAGE
- INSURANCE REFORMS

Under this strategy, cost containment and universal coverage would be attained through managed competition with global budgets.

A National Health Board made up of consumers, providers, employers, labor, and government would be established to monitor system performance and set national and state health care budgets.

Insurers and providers would be encouraged to form competing managed care groups (collaborative care networks) to serve local or regional health care needs. In order to stay within its budget, each state would set an upper limit on the capitation fees that each network could charge. States would also set fee schedules for services provided by non-managed care providers.

A comprehensive health care benefits package would be established by the National Health Board and include ambulatory care, inpatient hospital care, prescription drugs, basic mental health care and preventive services. Insurers would be required to offer this benefits package as a minimum.

State-based insurance purchasing cooperatives would help small businesses and individuals bargain with competing private health care plans. Unemployed persons would be entitled to buy a plan on a publicly subsidized basis through the cooperatives.

To reform insurance practices, competition among insurers based on risk selection (favoring of low-risk groups) would be eliminated and insurers would be required to employ community rating instead of experience rating. Access to insurance would be guaranteed regardless of an individual's medical condition.

To cut administrative waste, insurers would be required to use a single claims form, standardized billing codes and electronic processing.

New medical practice guidelines and greater use of alternative dispute resolution methods would help diminish defensive medicine and cut the cost of handling malpractice claims.

Financing mechanisms for this plan have not yet been specified.

SOURCES: Clinton-Gore on Affordable, Quality Health Care. Little Rock: Clinton/Gore Campaign Headquarters; September 24, 1992. [Reprinted in Section 6.]

Magaziner I. Memorandum for the First Lady, *et al.* Preliminary Work Plan for the Interagency Health Care Taskforce. Washington, D.C.; January 26, 1993. [Excerpt reprinted in Section 6.]

For more information, contact: Health Care Task Force, Old Executive Office Building, Room 287, 1600 Pennsylvania Avenue, Washington, D.C. 20500 Attention: First Lady Hillary Rodham Clinton or Ira Magaziner, Senior Advisor for Policy Development (202) 456-1414.

PRESIDENT CLINTON'S PLAN
KEY CONCEPTS

The government must intervene in the health care system to adjust societal inequities which market forces cannot adequately correct because the free enterprise system does not serve the poor as well as it serves the wealthy.

President Clinton's Plan

Provide all Americans affordable access to high quality health care.

President Clinton's Plan

Use of global budgets at the national and state levels set by a national health care board is necessary to control growth of health care costs.

President Clinton's Plan

> To widen access to health insurance, new rules must require community rating, open enrollment without regard to preexisting conditions, and availability of a basic benefits package.
>
> President Clinton's Plan

> Health insurance purchasing cooperatives must be fostered to pool small business and individual buying power.
>
> President Clinton's Plan

> Administrative burdens must be reduced by streamlining procedures.
>
> President Clinton's Plan

> Medical practice guidelines and other measures are needed to control the cost of dealing with malpractice.
>
> President Clinton's Plan

STARK PLAN

- NATIONAL HEALTH EXPENDITURE BUDGET
- MANAGED COMPETITION
- HEALTH PLAN PURCHASING COOPERATIVES
- EXPANSIONS IN MEDICAID AND MEDICARE
- FEDERAL RATE-SETTING SYSTEM

This strategy would set a national health care expenditure budget that is estimated to stabilize at slightly more than 15 percent of the gross domestic product by 1999. Managed competition principles would guide a restructuring of the health care delivery system to assure that consumers have a choice of cost-effective health plans. In addition, there would be expansions in the Medicare program to cover more preventive health services and changes in the program to improve its operation. Savings achieved from cost containment under this strategy would be used when available to cxpand health insurance coverage and to improve Medicare benefits.

The national health care budget would be divided into categories dealing with different types of medical service. The

Secretary of Health and Human Services would set maximum payment rates for each type of health service. Current Medicare price-setting methods under the Diagnostic-Related Group (DRG) system would be used. The Resource-Based Relative Value Scale (RBRVS) would be used to determine the maximum payment rates for physician and other professional medical services. The federal government would also set maximum rates of payment for every prescription drug.

Health Plan Purchasing Cooperatives (HPPCs), one element of the managed competition scheme, would be established. Each HPPC would help small employers who chose to join it by bargaining collectively for them with health maintenance organizations and other qualified managed care plans. All health maintenance organizations and other care plans would have to offer a health benefits package meeting federally-defined standards.

Insurers would be required to offer health insurance on a year-round open enrollment basis and guarantee renewal coverage, regardless of medical status. Exclusion of coverage for preexisting conditions could only last for six months from the beginning of an individual's insurance coverage period. Any worker changing employment with less than a three-month break in insurance coverage could not have a new six-month exclusion period applied. Private insurers and HPPCs would be required to use community rating to set premiums.

Eligibility for some Medicaid assistance would be expanded in stages to include families with incomes up to 200 percent of the federal poverty level. Under this plan, 25 million of the 35 million uninsured Americans would be provided health insurance through the Medicaid program within the next decade.

Prevention benefits under Medicare would be expanded to include annual mammography screening, well-child care, immunizations, and many other preventive health procedures. National databases would be established in order to collect uniform information on health outcomes and patient satisfaction.

SOURCE: U.S. House of Representatives. H.R. 200 - Health Care Cost Containment and Reform Act of 1993. Washington, D.C.; Committee on Ways and Means; 1993:1-36. [Excerpt reprinted in Section 6.]

[This bill was introduced by Congressman Pete Stark in the 103d Congress on January 5, 1993.]

For more information, contact: Congressman Pete Stark, U.S. House of Representatives, Committee on Ways and Means, 1114 Longworth House Office Building, Washington, D.C. 20515 (202) 225-7785.

PROPONENT:

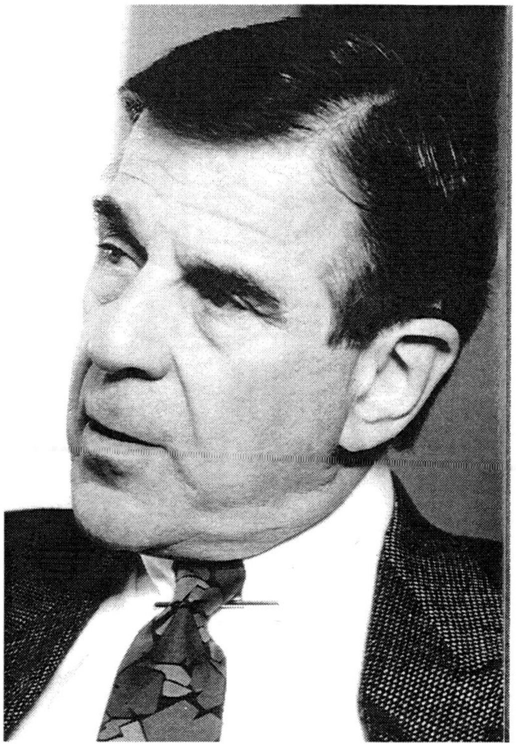

CONGRESSMAN PETE STARK (D-Cal.) was elected in 1990 to his 10th term in the U.S Congress. He represents the Ninth Congressional District of California. He is a senior member of the Ways and Means Committee and has chaired the Health Subcommittee since 1985. Prior to entering politics, he founded Security National Bank, which grew to have deposits of more than $100 million. He has been characterized as having a good understanding of the free enterprise system and a deep concern for social justice.

STARK PLAN
KEY CONCEPTS

A global health care budget for the nation operating in conjunction with a federal rate-setting system for all health care services is necessary to control health care costs.

Stark Plan

An independent agency established by the federal government should set prices for all health care services.

Stark Plan

Promote health insurance purchasing cooperatives to bargain for managed care plans and increase buying power for individuals and small businesses.

Stark Plan

To protect wide access to health insurance, new rules for health insurers should eliminate most preexisting condition exclusions and require community rating.

Stark Plan

Uniform claims-handling procedures and electronic networks among providers and payers should be established by the federal government to control the cost of administering the health care system.

Stark Plan

Medicaid should be gradually expanded to provide assistance to individuals with incomes up to 200 percent of the federal poverty level.

Stark Plan

SHORTELL PLAN

- PLAY OR PAY
- GLOBAL BUDGET
- INTEGRATED INSURER-PROVIDER HEALTH CARE PLANS
- HEALTH PROMOTION AND ACCOUNTABILITY REGIONS
- BASIC HEALTH BENEFITS PACKAGE

Under this strategy, state legislatures would create Health Promotion and Accountability Regions (HPARs). The more populous states would have several HPARs within them. HPARs would be governed by a board consisting of representatives from hospitals, physicians, insurers, employers, government, consumers and other groups. Each HPAR would have a technical staff trained in clinical epidemiology, statistics, planning and evaluation.

The HPAR would be responsible for shaping the health care market in its region. A basic health benefits package would be established by each HPAR.

Employers would be required to provide the basic health insurance coverage or contribute to a public plan. Tax incentives and coalitions would help small employers to participate in the play or pay approach.

Insurers doing business within the region would be required to offer the benefit package at or below the established premium and within recommended guidelines for income-related copayments and deductibles. Since all insurers would be offering the same benefits for essentially the same premiums, their financial success would depend on their ability to control costs.

Health care plans would be developed and offered by integrated insurer-provider entities. Each entity would be free to develop its own innovative approach to cost-effective care. The goal is competition among these entities for contracts based on the overall value of the plans they offer.

HPARs would also determine the overall budget required to meet the region's needs and enter into contracts with insurer-provider entities to deliver health care to those covered by the public plan. HPARs would monitor the performance of insurers and providers in the region and hold them accountable according to predetermined clinical and fiscal criteria.

SOURCE: Shortell SM. (1992). A Model For State Health Care Reform. *Health Affairs.* 11:108-127. [Reprinted in Section 6.]

For more information, contact: Dr. Stephen M. Shortell, Kellogg Graduate School of Management, 2001 Sheridan Road, Leverone Hall, Evanston, IL 60208-2001 (708) 491-5540.

PROPONENT:

STEPHEN M. SHORTELL is the A.C. Brehler Distinguished Professor of Health Services Management and professor of organization behavior in the Department of Organization Behavior at Northwestern University's J. L. Kellogg Graduate School of Management in Evanston, Illinois. He is also a member of the Center for Health Services and Policy Research. He holds a doctorate in the behavioral sciences from the University of Chicago and is an elected member of the Institute of Medicine of the National Academy of Sciences.

SHORTELL PLAN
KEY CONCEPTS

In addition to cost containment, health care reform must address unmet health care needs and quality of service rendered.

Shortell Plan

To manage the health care system in a way that is responsive to local realities, states should charter Health Promotion and Accountability Regions (HPARs), that is, regional partnerships among health care system participants.

Shortell Plan

Areawide health care budgets and a controlled price for a basic benefits package are necessary measures for cost-effective management of the health care system.

Shortell Plan

An epidemiological assessment of an HPAR's population will be an important step in determining the health care needs, basic benefits package, and overall health care budget of the region.

Shortell Plan

Health care providers should be clinically accountable for the health care services they deliver and should be financially rewarded for enhancing the health status of the population they serve.

Shortell Plan

HPARs may themselves need backup insurance to cover underestimates of health care use caused by natural disasters or other unexpected events.

Shortell Plan

AMERICAN COLLEGE OF PHYSICIANS PLAN

- NATIONAL HEALTH CARE BUDGET
- EMPLOYER AND PUBLICLY SPONSORED INSURANCE PLANS
- FEDERALLY-DEFINED BASIC HEALTH BENEFITS PACKAGE
- INSURANCE AND MALPRACTICE REFORM

This strategy calls for providing everyone a comprehensive health benefits package covering all medically effective services when they are appropriate for the patient. Public plans which now serve specific segments of the population would be consolidated and expanded to cover everyone not covered by employer-sponsored or other private insurance. To control costs, a national health care budget would be developed with a mixture of centralized and decentralized mechanisms to influence the price, volume, supply, and demand for health care services. A national health care commission would prepare the national budget and, in consultation with state authorities, an appropriate budget for each state.

Both the public and the private sector would sponsor and pay for health insurance plans. Employers would have the option to purchase insurance for employees up to 60 years of age or pay a tax which would permit those employees to enroll in a publicly-sponsored insurance plan. The employer's minimum contribution to the premium would be fifty percent, and the employee would be required to pay the rest. Anyone not covered by employer-sponsored insurance would enroll in a publicly sponsored plan. This group would include the unemployed, retirees, employees over 60 years of age, and employees whose employers chose not to offer plans.

Insurance reforms would include eliminating preexisting condition exclusions and using community rating instead of experience rating. Malpractice reforms would put a cap on awards for economic damages, eliminate joint and several liability, offset awards from collateral sources, modify statutes of limitations, and limit attorney contingency fees. Measures would also be instituted to enhance research, education, and medical information management.

SOURCE: Scott HD, Shapiro HB. (1992). Universal Insurance for American Health Care. *Ann Intern Med.* 117(6):511-519. [Reprinted in Section 6.]

For more information, contact: Department of Public Policy, American College of Physicians, 700 13th Street, N.W., Suite 250, Washington, D.C. 20005 (202) 393-1650.

The American College of Physicians, with 77,000 members practicing internal medicine, is the largest medical specialty society in the United States. Founded in 1915, the College's mission is to foster excellence in the practice of medicine through continuing education and the development and advocacy of public policies affecting public health and medical practice. The College publishes *Annals of Internal Medicine,* the most widely cited medical specialty journal in the world.

AMERICAN COLLEGE OF PHYSICIANS PLAN

KEY CONCEPTS

All persons living in the United States would through private or public insurance have access to the same benefits - all medically effective and appropriate care.

American College of Physicians Plan

A national health care commission with representation from patients, providers, employers, insurers, government and other key sectors of society should determine a minimum package of health care benefits.

American College of Physicians Plan

Employers must "play or pay," but the private insurance must be designed so it will generally be cheaper for an employer to play (provide private insurance) than to pay the tax to enroll employees in the public plan.

American College of Physicians Plan

Insurance plans should be required to offer the same benefits, pay providers according to the same fee schedule, and accept all enrollees, so they would be forced to compete on price charged and on value delivered.

American College of Physicians Plan

Global budgeting will promote cooperation and compel providers and payers to explicitly negotiate how to meet each community's needs with limited dollars - a function largely missing in an open-ended, fee-for-service system that rewards excessive care.

American College of Physicians Plan

Exceeding budgets will sometimes be justified, since global budgeting is a device to introduce fiscal discipline and to evaluate whether expenditures reflect expected costs, not a mechanism to cut off necessary health care.

American College of Physicians Plan

There is an appropriate role for regulation at the macro-level, such as governing the supply of health resources, but micro-level regulation of the physician-patient relationship has failed.

American College of Physicians Plan

Physicians will accept cost constraints in a reformed health care system if there is an end to the overwhelming regulatory intrusion that currently dominates medical practice.

American College of Physicians Plan

To control costs and provide universal access to medically effective care, enhanced investment is needed in training generalist physicians, in medical research and in management of medical information.

American College of Physicians Plan

Comprehensive changes may need to be made gradually, particularly those changes that have significant financial impact.

American College of Physicians Plan

AARON PLAN

- GLOBAL BUDGETING
- STATE OR REGIONAL AGENTS OPERATE AS SINGLE PAYERS
- EMPLOYER-SPONSORED HEALTH INSURANCE (PLAY OR PAY)
- PUBLIC HEALTH INSURANCE COVERAGE

This strategy would provide universal acute and long-term health care insurance coverage through a single payer health plan, but the role of the federal government as direct provider and manager of health insurance would be smaller under this plan than under the current system. Administration of health care plans would reside with state or regional agents rather than with federal agencies.

The federal government would establish general guidelines under which the states, acting alone or together, would create financial agents. Overall spending targets set by the federal government would limit total spending, but the financial agents in each region would determine how the region's allocation should be distributed among various health care providers. Financial agents would operate as the single payer in each region and be responsible for administering budgets, establishing payment schedules to health care providers, financing long-term care, and negotiating hospital reimbursements. In addition, the financial agents would be the channel for federal payments to provide health care coverage for those not covered by employer-sponsored plans.

All employers would be required to sponsor insurance coverage for workers and their dependents and pay roughly three-quarters of the premium cost or pay a tax equal to approximately nine percent of total payroll. The self-employed would also have to "play or pay." Workers with low incomes would be entitled to a refundable tax credit to prevent the cost of their share of the insurance premium from exceeding roughly five percent of their income.

Financial agents would have the responsibility for designing a gradual transition from experience rating to community rating by health insurers over a five-year period.

A federal trust fund would pay for insurance for all those not covered by employer-sponsored coverage. The fund would be financed by three main sources. The first source would be revenues currently collected to pay for Medicare and Medicaid. The second source would be payments by employers who elected to pay taxes rather than sponsor insurance. The third would consist of new tax revenues set aside for the financing of health care. Examples of possible new sources of tax revenue are a national value-added tax, higher tobacco taxes, and taxes raised by placing a limit on the exclusion of employee health care benefits from income tax.

SOURCE: Aaron HJ. *Serious and Unstable Condition: Financing America's Health Care..* Washington, D.C.:The Brookings Institution; 1991:140-152. [Excerpt reprinted in Section 6.]

For more information, contact: Henry J. Aaron, The Brookings Institution, 1775 Massachusetts Avenue, N.W., Washington, D.C., 20036 (202) 797-6000.

PROPONENT:

HENRY J. AARON is the Director of the Economic Studies program at The Brookings Institution in Washington D.C. He has served as Assistant Secretary for Planning and Evaluation at the Department of Health, Education, and Welfare. He holds a Ph.D. in economics from Harvard University. He is the author or editor of eleven books and co-author or co-editor of eleven others, including *Serious and Unstable Condition: Financing America's Health Care* and *Setting Domestic Priorities: What Can Government Do?*

AARON PLAN
KEY CONCEPTS

Efficient allocation of health care resources is better attained through a global budget than through controls on price per unit of service, because price limits provide no incentive to deny low-benefit care.

Aaron Plan

Global budgeting requires that control over health care spending be concentrated in one or a few hands.

Aaron Plan

Since market competition does not function well in small communities or inner city urban areas with a limited number of health care providers, a single payer system supervised by regional agents is needed to monitor patterns of care and bargain for good health care access even in underserved areas.

Aaron Plan

Reform of the health care finance system cannot wait until the federal budget deficit is brought under control, so health care financing reform must raise enough revenue so it causes no increase in the deficit.

Aaron Plan

Although federal action is necessary to set a floor under the provision of insurance coverage and set global budgets, states should act as financial agents to shape health care spending and health care benefits to meet local needs.

Aaron Plan

Since society has never placed an infinite value on human life, the right to health care services necessarily has limits.

Aaron Plan

The federal government can use its regulatory powers to achieve near universal coverage of working people and their families through private, employer-sponsored insurance and its taxing powers to assure coverage for those with too slender a connection with the workforce.

Aaron Plan

A wholly public plan is not obtainable because Congress would be unwilling to shift current private health care expenditures and disbursements to public budgets and to displace current health care arrangements for most Americans.

Aaron Plan

The federal government should mandate that employers either sponsor coverage for all workers employed at least twenty-five hours a week, or pay a tax equal to roughly 9 percent of total payroll.

Aaron Plan

CATHOLIC HEALTH ASSOCIATION PLAN

- UNIVERSAL HEALTH CARE COVERAGE
- NATIONAL TRUST FUND AS SINGLE SOURCE OF FINANCING
- GLOBAL BUDGETS
- BASIC HEALTH CARE BENEFITS PACKAGE
- CAPITATED PAYMENTS TO INTEGRATED DELIVERY NETWORKS

This plan is explicitly grounded in both Catholic moral precepts, such as the duty to care for the poor, and a market-oriented economic pragmatism.

To support universal coverage, centralized funding of the health care system through one national trust fund would be required. To maintain pluralism, the federally-assembled money would be distributed through independent State Health Organizations (SHOs) and the SHOs would encourage development of a wide variety of managed care plans. To achieve a more consumer-centered system and help control costs, all care would be rendered through competing managed care plans.

Managed care plans would be called Integrated Delivery

Networks (IDNs). Each IDN is to consist of a set of providers organized to deliver at a competitive price to any enrollee a basic health care benefits package. The minimum package would include a full continuum of health care services from preventive care through nursing home and hospice care. The goal is for every community to have several IDNs competing for subscribers by offering innovative client-oriented arrangements for efficient health care delivery.

Each IDN would receive risk-adjusted capitated payments - that is, per capita payments adjusted to reflect the health care needs of the enrolled population. The adjustment would be based on demographics of the enrolled group and perhaps even the presence of particular illnesses (e.g., AIDS) in the group. IDNs would compete for subscribers on the basis of quality and services, not price.

Individuals would select the IDN with the facilities and panel of practitioners they prefer and could change IDNs during an annual open season if dissatisfied. All providers would have to affiliate with one or more IDNs to participate in the health care system. Some physicians might join several IDNs constructed on the "open panel" model.

One or more State Health Organizations per state would be responsible for determining community needs, chartering IDNs within the state, and providing the IDNs with their capitated payments. The SHO would monitor performance of IDNs, but would leave them free to evolve a variety of internal structures and methods of operation.

A National Health Board (NHB), federally chartered but independent, would oversee the system. The NHB would develop a global budget and recommend expenditure levels to Congress, then allocate available funds to the SHOs based on the capitated payment amounts needed for each person in each state. The NHB would also determine a minimum health care benefits package. Individuals could supplement the package with private insurance, but the package itself would be sufficiently comprehensive to satisfy the health care needs of most Americans.

Existing public financing sources would be maintained but consolidated into a single health care trust fund. Revenues from Medicare, CHAMPUS, and the Veterans Administration, for example, would be transferred to a national trust fund. State money that now goes into Medicaid would also go into the trust fund.

Employers would pay a 6.9 percent payroll tax and employees would pay a 1.7 percent payroll tax. The remaining funds needed for the system would be collected through a combination of excise taxes and general revenues. Adoption of this plan would, after accounting for all cost savings, enlarge only slightly the overall cost of the health care system.

SOURCE: The Catholic Health Association. Setting Relationships Right: A Working Proposal for Systemic Healthcare Reform. Washington, D.C.: CHA; February 20, 1992. [Excerpt reprinted in Section 6.]

For more information, contact: Catholic Health Association, 1776 K Street, N.W., Suite 204, Washington, D.C., 20006 Attention: Jack Bresch (202) 296-3993.

The Catholic Health Association of the United States (CHA) is a 1,200 member organization of hospitals, long-term care facilities, dioceses, and individuals. CHA was founded in June 1915 in Milwaukee and moved to St. Louis in 1929. From its inception, CHA has worked to establish standards for Catholic hospitals, created educational programs for health care professionals, and conducted regular inspections to ensure that hospitals meet CHA's patient care standards.

CATHOLIC HEALTH ASSOCIATION PLAN KEY CONCEPTS

Basic health care should be viewed not as a commodity but as a fundamental right.

Catholic Health Association Plan

Every human life has intrinsic worth and should not be ranked as more or less important than any other.

Catholic Health Association Plan

To assure decent health care for the poor and uninsured, create a health care system in which their fate is linked to that of the average American.

Catholic Health Association Plan

No task should be absorbed by a higher, more centralized level of the health care system if that task can be performed adequately at a lower level.

Catholic Health Association Plan

Improve and coordinate health care for individual families and communities by realigning the financial incentives which providers face rather than through a burdensome regulatory structure.

Catholic Health Association Plan

Fragmentation in the sources of health care funding fosters a similar fragmentation of the delivery system.

Catholic Health Association Plan

State Health Organizations should oversee the shaping of health care resources into competing integrated delivery networks.

Catholic Health Association Plan

Each State Health Organization should serve an appropriate region, which could be all or part of a state, or a metropolitan region in more than one state.

Catholic Health Association Plan

While the states should define local health care needs, set priorities, and manage competition, the federal government, through an independent public agency, should coordinate and finance the national health care system and guarantee universal access.

Catholic Health Association Plan

To control health care costs, use national expenditure caps and risk-adjusted capitated payments to competing integrated health plans.

Catholic Health Association Plan

The federally-determined minimum benefits package must include coordinated delivery of primary, acute, and long-term care.

Catholic Health Association Plan

> Health care consumers and individual providers must have meaningful opportunities to participate in the shaping and governance of the health care system.
>
> Catholic Health Association Plan

HAGAN PLAN

- STATEWIDE HEALTH CARE BUDGET
- SINGLE PAYER SYSTEM
- PAYROLL AND EXCISE TAXES TO FINANCE TRUST FUND
- COMPREHENSIVE HEALTH CARE BENEFITS PACKAGE

[The strategy described below was embodied in the Universal Health Insurance for Ohio (UHIO) bill introduced in the Ohio House of Representatives in 1991 by Rep. Robert Hagan. This UHIO plan has served in a number of other states as a model for health care initiatives that call for a single payer system with universal access to health care.

Rep. Hagan has announced that he will introduce a substantially revised UHIO bill in the Ohio House in 1993.]

This strategy would create a single, publicly-financed statewide insurance program that would be administered by a Board of Governors representing consumers, labor, business, hospitals and physicians. Every Ohio resident would be eligible to receive comprehensive health care benefits covered under the statewide plan.

The plan would be financed by tax revenues from several sources. Each employer would pay 9 percent of payroll plus an additional tax of 0-4 percent of payroll depending on the number of its employees. Employees would pay 1 1/4 percent on wages. Taxes levied on tobacco products and alcoholic beverages would be increased. In accordance with rules to be established by a Board of Governors, the proceeds in the trust fund would be placed in several accounts. The Prevention Account would be used for establishing and maintaining primary community prevention programs. The Health Services Account would be used for paying providers participating in the plan. The Capital Account would be used to pay for construction, renovation and equipment for health care institutions. The Communication and Transportation Account would be used to cover the transportation of plan members from one institution to another for covered services and to facilitate communication and cooperation between providers. Finally, the Health Professional Education and Training Fund would be used to pay for educating and training health care professionals.

The plan would pay each institutional provider a single, comprehensive, annual budget negotiated between the provider and Board of Governors. Providers would be prohibited from charging rates higher than the negotiated reimbursement levels. Independent health care providers would be reimbursed on a fee-for-service basis with the fee levels to be negotiated on a profession-by-profession basis.

The health care benefits package is extensive and includes services such as inpatient and outpatient treatment, preventive services, mental health care services, substance abuse treatment, primary and acute dental services, and optical services for members 18 years of age or younger. Certain prescription drugs are covered, but long-term nursing home care is not included in the benefits package. Plan members can choose any participating provider.

Providers are required to disclose all information reasonably requested by the state for utilization review, cost containment, and similar purposes.

SOURCES: Ohio House of Representatives. Hagan Outlines New Health Care Reform Package. Columbus: House of Representatives; February 10, 1993. [news release] [Reprinted in Section 6.]

Hagan RF. The UHIO Health Security Act of 1993: Key Features. Columbus: House of Representatives; 1993. [Reprinted in Section 6.]

Hagan, Mallory, Sheerer, *et al.* HB 175: Universal Health Insurance for Ohio (UHIO). Columbus: House of Representatives; February 1991. [Reprinted in Section 6.]

For more information, contact: Representative Robert Hagan, Ohio House of Representatives, Riffe Center, 11th Floor, Columbus, Ohio 43266 (614) 466-9435.

PROPONENT:

ROBERT F. HAGAN, a Democrat, is the State Representative for the 53rd District in the Ohio House of Representatives. In 1990 he was named Legislator of the Year by the National Association of Social Workers. He serves on several House committees, including the Select Committee on Health Care Reform and the Committee on Health and Retirement.

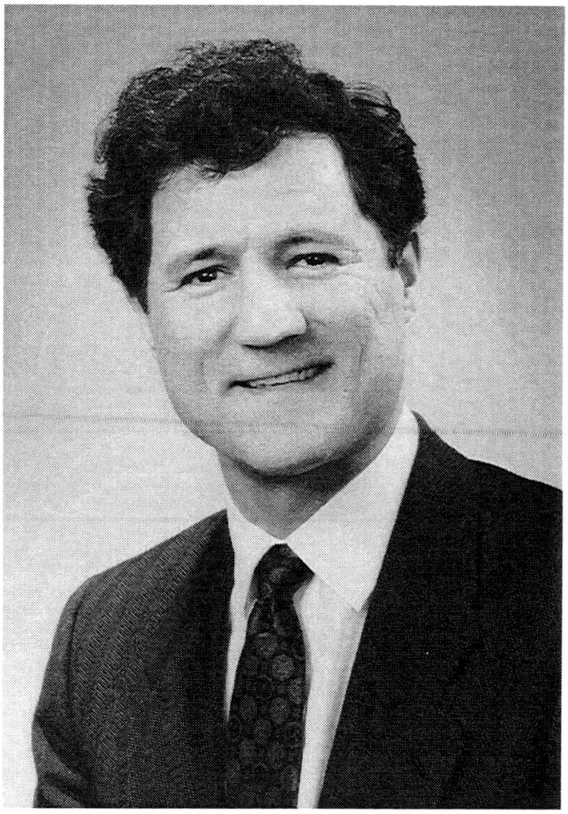

HAGAN PLAN
KEY CONCEPTS

The most direct route to universal coverage and acceptable cost control is through a state-run, single-payer health care insurance system.

Hagan Plan

A single payer mechanism will control health care cost inflation and unnecessary medical treatment more effectively than a multiple payer system, because a single payer can conduct systemic analysis and limit payments to providers.

Hagan Plan

Instead of using a patchwork system of premiums, deductibles, copayments, and out-of-pocket expenditures to finance health care, a financing structure which uses payroll and excise taxes will distribute costs more efficiently.

Hagan Plan

Requiring institutional providers to negotiate a single annual budget will create appropriate incentives to control cost.

Hagan Plan

Providers must be required to disclose cost and performance data to the state-run health care plan.

Hagan Plan

MCDERMOTT/WELLSTONE PLAN

- UNIVERSAL COVERAGE
- SINGLE PAYER
- NATIONAL, STATE AND INSTITUTIONAL BUDGETS
- FEE SCHEDULES
- COMPREHENSIVE HEALTH CARE BENEFITS

This proposal would provide universal access to comprehensive health care for all U.S. citizens and legal residents. This would be achieved through a single payer system (the American Health Security Program) administered by the states under standards set by a national health board. Most private health insurance, Medicare, and Medicaid would be replaced. Individuals would be covered regardless of employment status or place of residence.

Cost containment would be achieved through a national health care budget and corresponding state budgets. Each budget would serve as an expenditure target rather than a rigid cap; if, for instance, a state exceeded the target amount for a category, the state could lower the target for that category the following year.

The development of state health budgets from the national budget would be governed by the following factors: (1) state population; (2) differences among the states in prices of goods and services; (3) social, environmental or other conditions affecting the need for health care services; and (4) geographic distribution of population within the states, particularly the proportion of people who live in rural or medically underserved areas.

Payments to hospitals and nursing homes would be based on annual budgets established for each institution through negotiations with state agencies. Limits on new capital expenditures would reduce duplication of services and technology. Prescription drug prices would be set in negotiations with manufacturers. For health care professionals, negotiated fee schedules and volume performance standards would be established.

Consumers could choose their own health care providers from the same broad array available in the current system, including both accountable managed care plans and independent practitioners. Fees would be paid by the national fund, not the patient.

The comprehensive services assured to everyone would include primary and preventive services, inpatient and outpatient hospital care, nursing facility services for long-term care, hospice care, mental health and substance abuse treatment, and prescription medications. Strong emphasis would be placed on primary and preventive care services and the training of more primary care physicians. Community-based primary care clinics would be expanded to increase service to underserved rural and urban populations.

The single payer system would strive for progressive financing through a combination of increased payroll taxes, incomes taxes on higher income groups, income-adjusted premiums analogous to today's Medicare premiums, and revenue gained by closing loopholes in the tax code. Taxes would replace most private insurance premiums and out-of-pocket costs for patients. No copayments or deductibles would be necessary. All revenues collected for health care, including state funding at its present level, would be placed in an American Health Security Trust Fund and could only be used for health care expenses.

SOURCES: Wellstone P. The American Health Security Act of 1993: Bill Summary (S-491). Washington, D.C. 1993. [Reprinted in Section 6.]

[In March 1993, the American Health Security Act was introduced in the House of Representatives as H.R. 1200 by Congressman Jim McDermott and Congressman John Conyers and introduced in the Senate as S. 491 by Senator Paul Wellstone.]

For more information, contact: Congressman Jim McDermott, 1707 Longworth Building, Washington, D.C. 20516-4707 (202) 225-3106 or Senator Paul Wellstone, United States Senate, Washington, D.C. 20510-2303 (202) 224-5641.

OTHER SINGLE PAYER PLANS:

Himmelstein DU., Woolhandler S. *The National Health Program Chartbook.* Cambridge: The Center for National Health Program Studies, 1992.

Himmelstein DU., Woolhandler S. (1989). A National Health Program For The United States: A Physicians' Proposal. *N Engl J Med.* 320:102-108. [Reprinted in Section 6]

Citizen Action. Health Care Security For All: The Single-Payer Answer. Washington D.C.: Citizen Action, May 1992.

PROPONENTS:

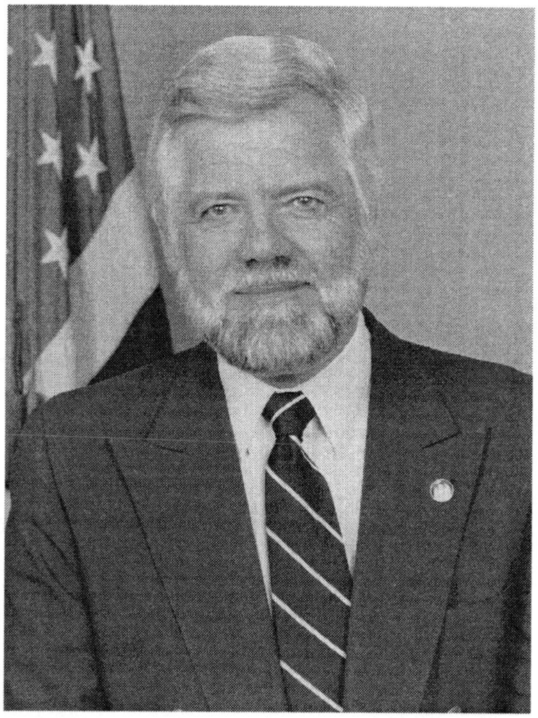

CONGRESSMAN JIM MCDERMOTT (D-Wash.), a graduate of University of Illinois Medical School, was appointed in 1992 to the Health Subcommittee of the Ways and Means Committee. He founded and co-chairs the Congressional Task Force on International HIV/AIDS and introduced the AIDS Housing Opportunities Act, a new program which authorizes $156 million for special housing assistance for people with AIDS. Rep. McDermott served in the U.S. Navy Medical Corps and worked as a Regional Medical Officer in

Kinshasa, Zaire for the U.S. Foreign Service.

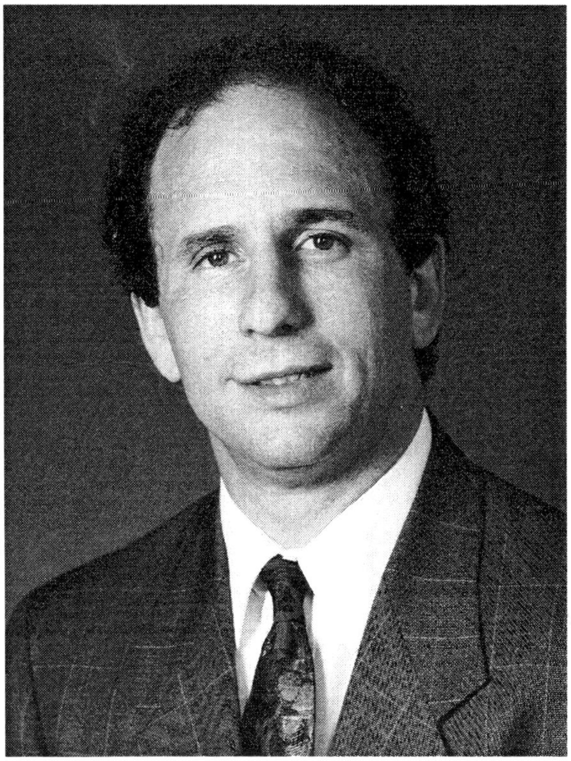

SENATOR PAUL WELLSTONE (D-Minn.) was elected to the U. S. Senate in 1990. He is a member of four committees (Labor and Human Resources, Energy and Natural Resources, Small Business, and Indian Affairs) and serves on eight subcommittees. Prior to being a senator, he was a professor of political science at Carleton College in Northfield, Minnesota, where he lived for over 20 years. He is a graduate of the University of North Carolina.

MCDERMOTT/WELLSTONE PLAN
KEY CONCEPTS

Achieve universal coverage through a single payer system.

McDermott/Wellstone Plan

A single payer system should be administered by the states under the direction of a national health board.

McDermott/Wellstone Plan

A single payer national health system which replaces most private health insurance, Medicare and Medicaid will be more efficient than the current multiple payer system.

McDermott/Wellstone Plan

Contain health care costs through national, state and institutional budgets, negotiated provider fee schedules, and limitations on prescription drug prices.

McDermott/Wellstone Plan

A state's share of the national health budget should be based on population, cost of living, proportion of rural or medically underserved areas, and any special conditions affecting health status.

McDermott/Wellstone Plan

A state-based single payer program will simplify and streamline the health care system and lower administrative waste.

McDermott/Wellstone Plan

Each individual should be free to choose among independent practitioners or to enroll in a managed care plan.

McDermott/Wellstone Plan

Greater emphasis should be placed on the delivery of primary and preventive care, especially in underserved areas.

McDermott/Wellstone Plan

A comprehensive basic health benefits package should extend to such services as substance abuse treatment, mental health programs and long-term care.

McDermott/Wellstone Plan

SECTION 6

ORIGINAL TEXT

HEALTH CARE REFORM PLANS: ORIGINAL TEXT

This section contains original text material from documents which describe the twenty health care reform plans analyzed in this Atlas.

Page numbering continues uninterrupted through this section, but the Atlas page numbers appear in circles to differentiate them from page numbers reproduced as part of the original text.

Hawaii Plan **295**

Oregon Plan **305**

President Bush's Plan **339**

Heritage Plan **373**

Pauly Plan **389**

Reinhardt Plan **411**

American Nurses Association Plan . . . **421**

Health Insurance Association of America Plan . **437**

American Hospital Association Plan . . . **451**

Jackson Hole Group Plan **461**

Conservative Democratic Forum Plan . . 491

American Association of Retired Persons Plan . 505

President Clinton's Plan 515

Stark Plan 539

Shortell Plan 559

American College of Physicians Plan . . . 581

Aaron Plan 593

Catholic Health Association Plan . . . 609

Hagan Plan 619

McDermott/Wellstone Plan 637

HAWAII PLAN

Lewin JC. Reflections on National Health Care Reform Based on Hawai`i's Experience. Honolulu: Hawaii Department of Health; March 1992.

REFLECTIONS ON NATIONAL HEALTH CARE REFORM BASED ON HAWAI'I'S EXPERIENCE

JOHN C. LEWIN, M.D.,
DIRECTOR OF HEALTH
STATE OF HAWAI'I; AND
PRESIDENT, ASSOCIATION OF
STATE AND TERRITORIAL
HEALTH OFFICIALS
MARCH 1992

INTRODUCTION TO HAWAI'I'S HEALTH CARE SYSTEM

The 50th of the United States has become a focus of legitimate attention in America's health care reform debates of the 1990s. U.S. health expenditures have soared to levels 50-100% higher than those of our major economic competitors in Europe, Canada, and Asia. Americans are dismayed to learn that, despite these costs, our national health status in terms of longevity, infant mortality, and various chronic disease outcomes is diminishing when compared to other nations. Yet, in Hawai'i, where costs of just about everything are 30-40% higher than the rest of the country, health care costs are uncharacteristically low, and outcomes are among the best in the nation.

In 1990, more than 36 million Americans lacked public or private health insurance and decent access to care, and the numbers are increasing despite our runaway health expenditures.[*1] But Hawai'i has offered health insurance access to all its people and approximately 98% of the population have private or public health insurance.[*2]

To the nation's embarrassment, most of those in the access gap are minorities and poor, but 85% are either employed or are the dependents of an employed person, and 15% of America's children are uninsured.[*3] In Hawai'i the health care system is working much better, and the state, while continuing to address remaining obstacles to access, can focus more effectively on cost-containment strategies.

Despite endless clamoring about the virtues of prevention and primary care, our national system languishes in a mire of excessive use of emergency room, high technology, and institutional services for preventable conditions.

MORE PRIMARY CARE ACCESS

Meanwhile, Hawai'i has offered more of her people access to primary care than any other state, resulting in a one-third reduction in the use and costs of emergency room and inpatient care, when compared to national per capita use. This is a major factor in Hawai'i's lower health care costs.

Ironically, health care reform is fueled nationally NOT by moral indignation over gaps in access, but mostly by cost concerns of the the already insured businesses, unions, and consumer groups. In this respect, Hawai'i is focused with the nation on the priority to control costs.

HAWAI'I APPROACHES UNIVERSAL ACCESS

However, Hawai' i enjoys an enviable head start toward major system reform because it already approaches universal access, has overall the best health outcomes of the states, and has costs significantly below national norms. In fact, a recent analysis of Hawai'i's health care costs for the 1988 calendar year revealed some surprising numbers: Hawai' i spent approximately 8.1% of its Gross State Product on health care during that year, when the U.S. percent of GNP was well over 11.2%.[*4]

Since 1988 the state has experienced health costs inflation of more than 10% per year. This relates to increases in drugs, supplies and salaries, particularly in shortage areas such as nursing. It is also due to

1. The 1991 Current Population Survey; U.S. Census Bureau, Washington, D.C.
2. State of Hawai'i Department of Health data. HRA '91.
3. ERBI Issue Brief Number 123, Feb. 1991; Employee Benefit Research Institute, Washington, D.C.; ISSN:0887-137X
4. Stenson, Richard V. Comparison of Health Care Expenditures in U.S. and Hawai'i Economies. Hawai'i Medical Journal: Vol 51, No. 1—Jan 1992, pp.10-14

the state's determined expansion of access, in insuring the gap group, and in significantly expanding both Medicaid coverage and mental health services. However, compared to the rest of the nation, per capita spending on health care in Hawai'i continues to be lower [*5] and while 1991 numbers are not in yet, the amount of the Gross State Product Hawai'i residents spend on health care remains below 9%.

Until this most recent effort to directly calculate our state health product, Hawai'i had depended, as do other states, on various national predictions of state costs. These estimates are typically based on indirect measurements and analytical models using such things as costs of living, average family income, per capita numbers of physicians and specialists, hospital and technology related factors, Medicaid and Medicare estimated costs, and so on. Using these "models," Hawai'i would appear to be one of America's more costly health care states. Yet, the real numbers show Hawai'i has achieved near-universal access, in a typically American high-tech—let's face it, downright glitzy—health system at less than expected costs.

We have a system which meets the American expectation of high consumer choice, at costs and with outcomes consistent with or better than those of our major international competitors.

HAWAI'I COMPETES WELL WITH CANADA

Considering the attention the Canadian system is receiving in Washington, is it not surprising to learn that Hawai'i competes favorably with Canada in terms of health care costs, without Canada's perceived shortcomings—reduced access to high-tech services and long waiting periods for elective surgeries?

Several factors have blocked pertinent information relating to Hawai'i's health care experience from effectively reaching the mainstream of national health care reform discussions and into proposals before Congress and state legislatures. The major players and policy makers in Washington, D.C. consider Hawai'i to be too different demographically and geographically from the "contiguous 48" for relevant comparison.

MYTHS

There are the four "myths" of why Hawai'i's health system does so well:

- Great weather,
- Superior genetics,
- Healthy lifestyle, and
- Island-state geographic and economic isolation from the rest of the nation by a large expanse of Pacific Ocean.

These myths have lulled many valid observers, in Hawai'i and elsewhere, to assume that Hawai'i's accomplishments are not transportable. Of course, Hawai'i DOES have great weather and a big ocean separating it from California and Oregon. Superficially, these factors have some relevance, but, in reviewing Hawai'i's evolution and circumstances more carefully, they do not explain Hawai'i's present advantages satisfactorily.

Further, much of the debate being cited nationally about Hawai'i isn't accurate or comprehensive enough to arrive at relevant conclusions, resulting in misinformation and confusion about Hawai'i's present circumstances and conditions. Much of the lack of good data is Hawai'i's own fault. We missed tremendous opportunities to document the effects of eighteen years of Hawai'i's unique employer mandate health insurance law, and of the recently enacted state-financed insurance program for covering the remaining uninsured.

Until very recently, Hawai'i's leaders, businesses, and health care industry had little or no interest or incentive to share their innovations. However, *now* that the nation appears closer to instituting a national health program, Hawai'i recognizes it is at risk of mandatory participation *in a* national system, which, from the looks of what has been proposed, may well be inferior to our status quo. It now has become important for us, therefore, to become fully engaged in the national debate.

Finally, the relevance of Hawai'i's health care

5. Hawai'i Dept. of Business, Econ. Development & Tourism. Annual Report, 1991.

system to America is blurred to outside inspection both by the lack of general awareness in Hawai'i to the many advantages we enjoy, and also by the ever increasing expectations that we can and should be doing even better. While more citizens have recently become aware of our advantageous status, many were frankly surprised to learn, for example, that when the Northwest National Life Insurance Company released its "State Health Rankings, 1991", one of the best and most comprehensive state-by-state analysis of a population's health, Hawai'i ranked as the all-around healthiest state in the nation.[*6] And, our businesses are shocked to learn how much more their counterparts in other regions are paying for employees' health benefits.

But Hawai'i's costs are rising too, and faster than the consumer product index. That's why our small businesses, labor unions, and consumer groups increasingly demand that some action be taken to curb rising health care costs. After all, everything other than health insurance is more expensive in Hawai'i, and people are feeling the pinch.

RESIDENTS UNAWARE OF GOOD FORTUNE

National health policy experts visiting our fair state understandably expect local euphoria about our health care system. Instead they discover that most residents are unaware of their relative good fortune; they find that physicians and hospitals are outraged by low reimbursements and increasing paperwork associated with Medicare and Medicaid; they hear small businesses bemoaning government's *mandating* of employee health coverage as unfair and financially strapping. While these kinds of observations are certainly not universal, such comments are too often mistaken by outside policy analysts and observers as evidence that no real progress has been made in Hawai'i.

Hawai'i has made many significant and non-theoretical achievements in health care reform. Notwithstanding Hawai'i appropriate dissatisfaction with inefficiencies in the system, with remaining access issues for special populations, and with rising costs, there is nonetheless ample reason to apply Hawai'i's experience to the implementation of a health care reform strategy for the nation. In short, Hawai'i's example is real, relevant, and readily transportable.

HAWAI'I APPROACH TO UNIVERSAL ACCESS

America knows Hawai'i as a subtropical paradise, a jewel, a multi-cultural playground, a meeting place of East and West. What isn't commonly recognized is that Hawai'i has one of the best health care systems in the nation. Our system delivers high quality at low cost. Despite our high costs of living, we emphasize early intervention and outpatient treatment, but, without overt rationing, we enjoy high-tech tertiary care as advanced as any state or nation.

The key to Hawai'i's success, I submit, is both elegantly simple and at the same time profound: Hawai'i has committed itself to ensuring that basic and quality health care is a right of all our people. Despite the fear this commitment strikes in the minds of some national policy makers—based on the assumption that it will translate into yet higher costs—Hawai'i demonstrates that a commitment to universal access is the most effective way to reduce and control costs. No other point or message I can deliver in this paper will be as significant as this: The nation, learning from Hawai'i's example, must immediately make a similar commitment to basic and quality health care as a right of all citizens before we will be able to solve the problem of how to make such care affordable!

Committed to 100% access, Hawai'i has achieved about 98% coverage. Contributing heavily to that success is Hawai'i's innovative health care community, which experimented with short hospital

6. The NWNL State Health Rankings, 1991 Edition. T.E. Ekstein and Asso.., Inc. St Paul, Minn 55105

stays, outpatient surgery, and preventive programs some time before they became the norm on the mainland. And this tradition continues. Hawai'i's Healthy Start Program screens more than 60% of new mothers statewide, and then provides community outreach to high risk families in order to prevent child abuse, and promote well child care, immunization and early intervention. The program has nearly eliminated child abuse among those at-risk families it reaches. Hawai'i was the first state to set up HIV prevention and testing centers, HIV statewide school education programs, HIV early intervention and treatment programs, and even a state-sanctioned needle exchange program for IV drug users, linked to drug treatment and HIV testing and counselling. These and other similar efforts really pay *off*, but can only be effective when combined first with universal access to effective primary and basic health care for all.

Hawai'i is unique among the 50 states in that it has implemented a fairly comprehensive set of public and private programs to ensure universal access to health care for all citizens. The foundation of the system is the Hawai'i Prepaid Health Care Act of 1974, which requires that all employers provide health insurance to employees working more than 19 hours per week. The powerful triad of this employer mandate program, Medicaid, and finally the State Health Insurance Program (SHIP), the 1989-enacted state-subsidized "gap" insurance program for those NOT eligible for either the employer mandate program, Medicare, or Medicaid, has allowed Hawai'i to achieve near universal access.

While the success in achieving our access goals has been remarkable, we are concerned that some populations are in need of better public health outreach systems. However, the significant concern with our present system relates to controlling increasing costs. We need to address the fact that our three major systems of coverage, Prepaid Health Care, Medicaid, and SHIP all have different funding mechanisms, different benefit packages, different reporting forms and application processes.

These systems are both public and private, and are therefore very difficult to integrate and streamline together. Thus, we are very interested in advancing further reform as a state-federal partnership. We aim to bring these programs into a more consistent and efficient "seamless" system for all citizens, and in a health care marketplace capable of promoting provider and consumer incentives for cost-containment. We are further committed to developing a system based more on measurable health outcomes than on services delivered.

Emily Friedman, health policy analyst and consumer advocate, has eloquently expressed the view that America's approach to health care reform should proceed by building on what presently works well in our nation's system, rather than by a process of dismantling and starting over.[7] In what some feel has been a vacuum of federal leadership and resolve during the past decade, the fifty states have been attempting to patch the many defects in the American health care system. The SHIP program in Hawai'i is such a patch, not a complete solution. The states need federal leadership to move ahead, but the federal government must also allow sufficient flexibility in a national design to build on what already works well in the differing state infrastructures.

We in Hawai'i are certainly NOT interested in simply handing these problems over to the federal government to "fix" for us. In fact, as far as we're concerned,the greatest fixes are needed in the federal programs.

Hawai'i's infrastructure differs significantly from other states. We see parts of our model in various national proposals, but the time has come for us to suggest to the Administration and Congress that we have some ideas of proven merit which need to be considered seriously.

7. Friedman, Emily. The Uninsured—From Dilemma to Crisis. JAMA. Vol 265:19. May 15, 1991.

A STRATEGY FOR NATIONAL HEALTH CARE REFORM BASED ON THE HAWAI'I MODEL

The following ten steps represent a proposed action plan with which Congress might establish a system of national health care reform, based on Hawai'i's present and evolving system, and offer some unique features and potential advantages over other proposals.

1. FEDERALLY MANDATED STANDARD BENEFITS PACKAGE

As a first step, Congress must establish a standard benefit package for all citizens. The benefits must include a full spectrum of services, extending from clinical preventive services and primary care to hospital and catastrophic care, and including preventive dentistry, acute mental health and substance abuse care, and pharmaceutical drug coverage. The standard package should be periodically re-authorized by Congress, following thorough review of outcomes and costs, and state legislatures should be prohibited from mandating further benefits or reducing federal standards. The benefits in such a package would best be consistent with Medicare, but expanded to include prevention and the needs of the entire non-Medicare population.

2. FEDERAL HEALTH INSURANCE EMPLOYER MANDATE

A federal employer-mandate, similar to the ERISA exempted, "everybody plays" model of Hawai'i, should be the foundation of private coverage. It must be applied to all employees working more than 19 hours per week, and also require dependent coverage. The employee's contributions would increase on a sliding scale related to wages, but never exceeding a fixed percentage of gross income. The employer would pay at least 50% of premium cost. If more than one member of a household is employed, each would be covered by their respective employer, but the employer of the family member with the highest income would be required to add coverage of other dependents. Congress would delegate to states the responsibility to implement this provision, with an option to require hourly contributions by employers of part-time employees toward a state-sponsored insurance program for those not fully covered by virtue of employment.

3. FEDERALLY MANDATED INSURANCE REFORM

Insurers would be required to offer open enrollment and true community ratings; and, exclusions, restrictions, and waiting periods would be eliminated. Insurers would be required to accept the self-employed, students, and people generating income by contract or commission. These individuals would receive tax incentives to purchase premiums and would be included in the same risk pool with all other employed people.

Co-payments and deductions would be held within caps set progressively as a maximum percentage of gross income, and would be prohibited from being applied to clinical preventive services, prenatal care, well child care, immunizations, family planning services, and annual health assessments. In this scenario, there would be no further ability for insurers to "cherry-pick"; however, there would be no prohibition against insurers' offering supplemental coverage packages. For example, presumably coordinated and managed care packages will be favored by a competitive marketplace envisioned in this proposal, but for those consumers who still desire the privilege of self-referral to specialty care in a fee-for-service setting, insurers could offer "experientially-rated" supplemental options above the standard package.

With an appropriately designed standard benefits package covering essential benefits and services, supplemental coverage would only provide "amenities" , rather than creating a two-tiered system in which the affluent get better health outcomes through additional benefits. The design of the standard benefit package should ensure that such supplemental coverage be other than essential benefits or services.

4. A COST CONTAINMENT ORIENTED FEDERAL TAX INCENTIVE

Each year the federal government would establish a threshold of how much of insurance premiums would be tax deductible. This threshold would be based on the most cost-effective and quality premiums for employed people in each state. Those premiums below the threshold would be 100% tax deductible; those above, 100% taxable. This would serve as a strong incentive for both employers and employees to shop-around for lower cost, high quality coverage; and also encourage provider and insurer incentives for managed and coordinated care.

5. SEAMLESS COORDINATION OF PUBLIC ACCESS WITH PRIVATE COVERAGE THROUGH FEDERAL FLEXIBILITY

The federal funding to states for Medicaid, disproportionate share hospital subsidies, community health center funding, certain categorical public health funds, and any other federal health care funding to states, must be available in flexible blocks or grants to enable states to guarantee coverage to the unemployed, the poor, and other special populations not covered by private insurance through employment or retirement.

These funds would be applied to either contracting for private insurance for the beneficiaries, or to developing statewide special health delivery systems. All beneficiaries would receive the same standard benefits and services as provided through the employer mandate program.

Federal funds, available to states in formula blocks based on percent of population below federal poverty level, would be combined with the state contributions to Medicaid, primary care, and public hospitals. In states electing to contract for insurance coverage for public beneficiaries, HMO or managed care programs would likely be cost-favored, but, if fee for-service approaches were used, the reimbursement levels for services would need to be required to be at least 85-90% of average marketplace levels to ensure that public clients have equal access services.

6. STANDARDIZED CLAIMS & ENCOUNTER FORMS

The federal government would need to establish standardized and simple claims forms for use by all insurers, public and private. The same user-friendly forms would be used as "encounter forms" by HMOs and managed care providers as well.

In this manner, administrative costs would be greatly reduced, and better comparative data regarding costs and outcomes would be possible for all systems nationwide. The use of the forms as encounter forms in HMOs would allow better information regarding utilization by these kinds of providers and permit better analysis of cost comparisons with fee-for-service provider types.

7. CONSUMER EDUCATION THROUGH INFORMATION SHARING

The so-called proprietary information related to insurance, provider, hospital, and other costs of health care must be made public.

Legislation assuring that all health industry data relating to costs, outcomes, and consumer and provider satisfaction, must be annually compiled and published to encourage smarter shopping for health insurance, HMO care, and choices of providers on the parts of business, labor unions and consumers.

This is a key missing ingredient needed to create a cost-competitive health care "marketplace" in America.

8. COST CONTAINMENT COMMISSIONS AT THE FEDERAL AND STATE LEVELS.

A small amount of funds must be set aside at the federal and state level to develop and staff high-level appointed commissions charged to monitor and study health care costs, consumer and provider behavior and satisfaction, and health status and outcomes with respect to costs of care. These bodies would recommend state and national policy changes needed to meet global expenditure targets, and to improve the system, but would not need be rate-setting bodies.

9. TORT REFORM

The need to reduce defensive medicine and tort costs is well established. The federal government needs to establish a national policy and cost-containment strategy in this regard.

10. A FEDERAL MANDATE FOR PUBLIC HEALTH AND PREVENTION

If we truly expect to make strides in improving the health status of America, and cut health care costs at the same time, we clearly must devote resources and attention to public health, health promotion and education, and prevention through a Congressionally-legislated additional set-aside of at least 3% of all federal health care expenditures. Considering that the federal expenditures through Medicare and Medicaid already exceeds $300 billion, this would result in an additional $10 billion, or $40 per capita, to be available to states through the Department of Health and Human Services to change the context of personal responsibility for health for Americans, and support the ongoing need for population-specific safety-net services to supplement the national health plan.

10 STEPS LEAVE IMPORTANT STRATEGIES & IMPLEMENTATION TO STATES

These ten steps leave important cost containment options and implementation strategies to states to develop within the framework of their varying health care infrastructures and needs. The important need to explore delivery system innovation, with incentives for coordinated care, partnerships of physicians and other practitioners, and managed care options, would naturally occur in states in the cost-conscious marketplace envisioned here. The needs to combine health coverage issues with workers compensation costs and coverage and the health portion of auto insurance would be a state challenge. And long term care financing and universal insurance, a very critical concern to states, must also be developed in parallel to health care reform, although this will involve additional resources and special considerations worthy of separate and extensive discussion.

Regardless of the approach to health care reform the nation eventually chooses, nothing short of a commitment to universal access is worthy of our consideration. This is essential to re-establish our national vitality and integrity, but also to contain health care costs and to protect our international economic competitiveness.

States, including Hawai'i, are having the major influence on creative design and implementation of new strategies. The new federalism is not just a response to federal inaction and inability to arrive at consensus, it is an affirmation of the founding fathers' insights and intention. It is now time for the federal government to forge the necessary partnerships with states to move ahead, within a framework of a level playing field of guaranteed minimum standards and conditions, to achieve the long-awaited goal of universal health care access in America.

Considering the awesome agenda of domestic challenges our nation faces in education and literacy, housing and homelessness, substance abuse and crime, poverty and family disintegration, pollution and environmental protection, all in a circumstance of ever-increasing national debt and economic vulnerability, the health care crisis affords, by comparison, an opportunity. It lends itself to real, envisionable, and affordable solutions.

From the platform of a socially-just and effective national system of universal health care, associated with an commitment to public health, wellness, and prevention, America may just feel well enough to tackle the rest of our domestic woes.

OREGON PLAN

Garland MJ. (1991). Setting Health Care Priorities in Oregon. *Health Matrix.* 1(2):139-156.

Mason T. (1992). Sullivan Made the Right Choice in Rejecting the Oregon Plan. *Health Matrix.* 2(1) 85-88.

Congress of the United States. *Evaluation of the Oregon Medicaid Proposal.* Washington, D.C.: Office of Technology Assessment. 1992.

SETTING HEALTH CARE PRIORITIES IN OREGON

Michael J. Garland, D. Sc. Rel.†

THE PROBLEM OF THE "UNINSURED"

IN THE UNITED STATES some 31 million citizens (15% of the population under 65) do not have health insurance.[1] In Oregon, a state with a total population of 2.7 million, the number of uninsured persons has been determined to be approximately 400,000, most of whom are employed full or part time.[2] These facts are transformed into an ethical problem if health care is considered a common good and its distribution and financing matters of justice. The ethical challenge consists of finding a fair and compassionate way of responding to the fact that so many citizens are "uninsured for health care" at a time when health care costs are increasing at an unsustainable rate, when Medicaid programs are consistently straining their budgets and the usual patterns of employment based insurance are no longer serving to bring those "still left out" under the health insurance umbrella. The Oregon story is a microcosm of the national story.

The story originates in the closing years of the 1980s and its conclusion, yet to be written, will extend well into the 1990s. In the decade of the eighties, expenditures for health care continued in the growth pattern of the previous decade and placed increasing strains on public and private programs we Americans use to finance health services through collective means (taxes and insurance). With this social mechanism we seek to alleviate for one another the

† Associate Professor of Public Health and Preventive Medicine and the Associate Director of the Center for Ethics in Health Care, Oregon Health Sciences University, co-founder and President of Oregon Health Decisions. Portions of this paper were originally published as Garland & Hasnain, *Health Care in Common: Setting Priorities in Oregon*, HASTINGS CTR. REP. 16-18 (Sept. 1990).

1. P. SHORT, A. MONHEIT, Y. K. BEAUREGARD, UNINSURED AMERICANS: A 1987 PROFILE (1989) (report for Health Services Research and Health Care Technology Assessment, Department of Health and Human Services).

2. OREGON OFFICE OF HEALTH POLICY, GOVERNORS COMMISSION ON HEALTH CARE, REPORT TO GOVERNOR NEIL GOLDSCHMIDT ON IMPROVING ACCESS TO HEALTH CARE FOR ALL OREGONIANS, at 9 (1988).

economic burdens of health care when illness and injury strike. But the social value of solidarity can get lost in the confusing particulars of different programs and institutions, each trying to meet their own goals and budgets.

Medicaid, the tax-based program focused on certain categories of poor and disabled members of society, places serious demands on the state's human services budget. In the absence of new tax dollars (a chronic condition of the past decade), Medicaid budgets in Oregon and throughout the nation have consistently strained their states' resources for human services. When meager discretionary funds fail to meet projected needs, or when desirable new programs require reallocation of resources, administrators and legislators have habitually used four ways of altering budget outlays: they redefine eligibility requirements to reduce (or increase) the number of persons served; they change the list of specific services included in the current benefit package; they vary the reimbursement rates for providers of services; they seek to improve productivity at a given level of expenditure. Except for productivity improvements, the other three strategies save dollars by making health care less accessible for the poor while increasing cost shifting, a hidden tax, to pay for limited continued access for the poor. Because productivity improvements are the hardest to accomplish and the slowest to show effect on a budget, the three access-reducing strategies are the most frequently used when administrators face budget shortfalls.

The Oregon story about responding to the uninsured is profoundly affected by fiscal constraints on Medicaid that have characterized the decade of the eighties. A significant feature of the Oregon story is the existence of Oregon Health Decisions (OHD), a community oriented organization dedicated to encouraging public involvement in ethical aspects of health policy. Since 1982, this organization has been conducting community awareness projects focused on ethical issues such as autonomy in the face of terminal illness and allocation of health care resources. In 1987 and 1988, OHD organized a series of community discussions on the question of general priorities for health care.[3] State Senator John Kitzhaber, principal architect of the legislation to be discussed in this paper, chaired the Steering Committee for this project which held 19 meetings throughout the state and culminated with a "Citizen's Parliament" to focus the results of the community deliberations. The

3. Crawshaw, Garland, and Hines, *Organ Transplants, a Search for Health Policy at the State Level*, 150 W. J. MED. 361 (1988).

product of the Parliament was a statement of fifteen principles "intended to be guideposts for the state legislature, insurance companies, and others concerned with health care resource allocation."[4]

Another significant element of Oregon's story is the 1987 legislative decision to finance an expansion of Medicaid eligibility for many persons living below the Federal Poverty Level, especially pregnant women, with dollars saved by not funding most organ transplants for Medicaid eligible persons.[5] The tradeoff happened because both transplantation services and the "Poverty Level Medical Program" were optional programs available to states within federal Medicaid regulations.

The transplant issue became the center of a chaotic debate in Oregon and among many observers outside the state. The tragic case of a seven year old leukemia patient, whose family requested but was refused Medicaid assistance, became its symbolic focal point. Some objected violently to denying life-prolonging transplants to people just because they were poor. Despite the fact that private insurance policies marketed in the state were inconsistent about which, if any, transplants were covered, many advocates argued that the state Medicaid program was *morally* obliged to cover transplants on the grounds of equality. Others argued that certain health services, such as primary care for pregnant women, should be funded ahead of transplants—although there was no general list of priorities that would allow one to understand the reasons why any health services should come before any other.

The controversy revealed great ambiguity in public consciousness and made unmistakable the need for serious reform of the way Medicaid budget decisions are made. It also set the stage for thinking about how the state of Oregon might go about expanding third party coverage for persons currently uninsured for health care.

To make any progress toward universal third party coverage, whether in Oregon or at the national level, four component problems have to be worked on simultaneously. First, the strategy must aim at gaining effective access for all to adequate health care. Second, it must pay serious attention to controlling costs through delivery system reforms, administrative savings and efficiency in provider practices. Third, the plan must attend to maintaining quality of care. Fourth, it must be politically feasible, showing op-

---

4. *Quality of Life in Allocating Health Care Resources*, OREGON HEALTH DECISIONS, (Dec. 1988), at 1.

5. *Rising Cost of Medical Treatment Forces Oregon to Play God*, Washington Post, February 5, 1988, at A1, col. 1.

portunity for overcoming inertia, gaining interest group buy-in and having broad public acceptability.

Oregon's proposed solution is unique, but exhibits a general pattern also found in other state efforts to bring help to the uninsured: the state seeks to coordinate new developments in both Medicaid and private insurance in the effort to get all of the uninsured into some form of third party coverage.

THE LEGISLATIVE PACKAGE

The 1989 Oregon Legislature passed a package of three statutes intended to expand access to third party support for persons currently uninsured. One statute (Senate Bill 27[6]) expands Medicaid eligibility to 100% of the Federal Poverty Guideline; the second (Senate Bill 935[7]) sets up incentives for small businesses and their employees to purchase health insurance; and the third (Senate Bill 534[8]) provides requisite funding for a "high risk" insurance pool previously set up to help persons now considered "uninsurable" because of preexisting health conditions. These statutes will be referred to as "the Oregon Plan."

SUMMARY OF SENATE BILL 27

This law seeks to provide access to health services for persons with incomes at or below the Federal Poverty Level, to contain rising health services costs, to reduce cost shifting in the system and to promote the stability of the health care delivery system.

The basic provisions of Senate Bill 27 establish a program:

1. to provide Medicaid eligibility to all persons below the Federal Poverty Level;
2. to create a Health Services Commission (HSC) charged to prioritize services covered by Oregon Medicaid (with certain exemptions[9]);

---

6. S. Bill 27, (codified within OR. REV. STAT. §§ 414.025, 414.036, 414.042 (1989)).

7. S. Bill 935, (codified within OR. REV. STAT. §§ 316.096, 317.113, 353.725, 353.765, 353.775 (1989)).

8. S. Bill 534, (codified within OR. REV. STAT. §§ 735.605 - 735.650 (1989)).

9. Exemptions include: nursing facility services and home-based and community-based services funded through the Senior Services Division; medical assistance for the aged, the blind and the disabled or medical care provided to children under current Oregon Law; institutional home-based and community-based Medicaid programs special to Oregon; Community Mental Health Program care for mentally retarded or developmentally disabled, or chronically mentally ill, or emotionally disturbed, and substance abuse treatment programs; services to children who are wards of the Children Services Division by order of the juvenile court, and health and mental health services to children and families provided through the division.

3. to base priorities on comparative benefits of each service to the population being served;
4. to include with the priority report an estimate from an independent actuary stating the funding needed at each level to cover the costs of recommended services;
5. to conduct public hearings prior to submitting the report to the legislature;
6. to actively solicit public involvement in a community meeting process to build consensus on the values to be used to guide health resource allocation decisions.
7. to have the Joint Legislative Committee on Health Care determine whether or not to recommend the HSC report to the Legislative Assembly and to advise the Governor of its recommendation; and,
8. to leave to the Legislative Assembly the responsibility to fund the report to the extent that funds are available within the overall state budget. The legislature may not alter the priority list.

The Health Services Commission consists of 11 members appointed by the Governor to serve four year terms. The law requires that members of the HSC must include: 5 physicians (representing obstetrics, perinatal, pediatrics, adult medicine, geriatrics or public health, and including one Doctor of Osteopathy); 1 public health nurse; 1 social services worker; 4 consumers.

Waivers from certain requirements attached to the receipt of Federal Medicaid funding will be required for the implementation of new programs based on this law. The Oregon Medical Assistance Program (OMAP) is directed to seek such waivers after the Legislature has determined the Medicaid budget.

Prepaid managed care is proposed as the kind of health care system toward which OMAP is required to move under this law.

Whenever OMAP is required to reduce or permitted to expand its budget, the agency will eliminate or expand services in the order of priority established by the HSC. The population of eligible persons shall not be reduced, nor will the reimbursement rate in provider contracts be reduced.

Provider liability is safeguarded so that they shall not be subject to criminal prosecution, civil liability or professional disciplinary action for failing to provide a service which the Legislative Assembly has not funded or has eliminated from funding. Providers will be required, however, to advise a patient of any service, treatment or test that is medically necessary and would otherwise be provided but is not covered under the provider's contract with OMAP.

Mental health care and chemical dependency issues will be dealt with by having the HSC create a subcommittee charged to develop priorities for services to be presented by the HSC to the 1991 Legislative Assembly. These services are exempt from the first prioritization process.

SUMMARY OF SENATE BILL 935

The general purpose of the law is to extend access to health insurance to those with incomes above Federal Poverty but currently uninsured for health care.

Basic Provisions of the law establish a program:

1. to evaluate various alternatives for implementing a statewide insurance pool;
2. to assist small businesses (25 or fewer employees) to purchase health benefits;
3. to determine benefit packages to be offered by the insurance pool, based on a review of existing benefit plans and the recommendations of the Health Services Commission (HSC) established by Senate Bill 27;
4. to use the Medicaid package funded by the Legislature as the basic level for medical services that must be found in all Insurance Pool packages;
5. to establish guidelines for stepped increases in the proportion of the population covered by health insurance who were uninsured in 1989 (50,000 by October 1990; 100,000 by 1991; and 150,000 by 1992);
6. to use tax credits (for those employers who contribute to their employees' insurance premiums) to motivate voluntary employer participation in the program; and,
7. to levy a special additional payroll tax on employers who do not offer health insurance benefits by January 1, 1994.

The Insurance Pool Governing Board consists of seven members, six of whom are appointed by the Governor (including two employers and one representative of organized labor and two persons knowledgeable about insurance but who do not work in the insurance business) and one consumer representative appointed by the Director of the Department of Insurance and Finance.

The adequacy and effectiveness of health benefits in Insurance Pool packages and the effect of the plans on health care costs will be monitored by the Oregon Health Council, a sixteen member health policy advising council appointed by the Governor and representing the different geographic regions of the state.

SUMMARY OF SENATE BILL 534

This bill supplied needed funding to a High Risk Insurance Pool that had been created in the previous legislative session. Its basic provisions are:

1. provide coverage for those considered "uninsurable" in the market; and,
2. finance the pool by a combination of: state subsidy; assessment on insurers; and, premiums paid by subscribers or employers (with a ceiling set at 150% of standard premiums in the market).

POLITICAL ASPECTS

Senate President John Kitzhaber, the principal architect of the package, succeeded in gaining enough backing for the bills to win their passage. The essential motivating force behind the legislative success of the plan was the widespread belief that the system of dealing with Medicaid budgets needed to be reformed. The proposed instrument of reform was the prioritized list of services which could be used by the legislature and the agencies to guide the painful decisions of cutting back on the Medicaid budget or shifting resources from one category to another. This intuitive concept held the effort together throughout the legislative process.

The idea of the priority list was so central to this package that, in an innovative political move, Senator Kitzhaber convinced a private foundation to underwrite a demonstration project to give lawmakers an example of what the proposed priority setting process might yield.[10] In the demonstration, four provider panels each prepared a prioritized list of services they typically offered (pregnancy, pediatrics, adult, and geriatric care). The four lists were then blended into a single list by an executive group. Finally, an actuarial consulting firm (Milliman and Robertson) estimated the costs of funding different levels on the priority continuum. The project report became part of the information available to lawmakers as they prepared to vote.

The demonstration was useful in helping resolve some legislators' doubts, but has subsequently confused several commentators who mistakenly presumed that the demonstration had permanent standing and authority. In fact, the HSC examined it briefly and then set it aside and went about creating its own methodology for producing a priority list.

As the HSC has carried on its work, the prioritization concept has continued to enjoy the political support of a coalition of interest

10. J. Golenski, Oregon Medicaid Prioritization Project, (demonstration project conducted by Medical Research Foundation of Oregon, Dec. 1988-Feb. 1989).

groups such as consumer activists (the Oregon Health Action Campaign), organized labor (Oregon AFL/CIO), business (the Greater Portland Business Group on Health), and health providers (Oregon Medical Association, Oregon Hospital Association and Oregon Nurses Association). Each of these groups has a different primary reason for supporting the legislation, but the overlapping consensus remains functional. The process also maintains broad public acceptability due in large part to the openness and participatory nature of the HSC methodology. As in any real story, however, the outcome is never guaranteed either by the good will of the principal protagonists nor the general approval of less involved participants.

The continuing political development of the story will be profoundly affected by the impact of "Proposition Five," a property tax limitation passed by Oregon voters in November 1990. Proposition Five moves much of school funding from county property taxes to the state General Fund, putting tremendous strains on all state program budgets. Legislators in the 1991 Session were faced with a shifting revenue landscape while working out practical solutions to the challenges that threaten to overwhelm the Plan's goal of expanding access with equity and fairness.

PRIORITIES AND ETHICAL CONCERNS

The central moral premise of the Oregon Plan is the idea that, by using a prioritized list of health services to guide legislative budget decisions and agency administrative decisions, an ethically acceptable basic benefit package could be fashioned for Medicaid that would include those services considered most important and focus marginal decisions on services of lesser importance. The purpose of setting priorities is to define more rationally a basic benefit package for Medicaid and other third party programs directed toward the poor for whom the state has a primary responsibility.

Five areas of serious ethical concern have been raised by observers of the evolving Oregon Plan both inside and outside the state. First, because of its primary focus on Medicaid and the currently uninsured population, and because the legislative package makes no front end commitment of new dollars to pay for expanded access, the plan is at high risk of being grossly unfair to the poor,[11] and, in particular, to women and children who are major recipients of

11. Tom Higgins, *Oregon Plan Doesn't Merit a Medicaid Waiver,*" Healthweek, May 21, 1990, at 20.

Medicaid support.[12] This concern is heightened by the fact that the staging of the Oregon plan currently exempts from prioritization those Medicaid services now offered to the elderly, the blind and the disabled.[13] At the heart of this criticism is the view that, if allocation or explicit rationing of health services is ever to be considered ethical, it must include everyone, rich and poor alike, in the rationing scheme. It is fundamentally unfair, they say, to expand access for poor persons by rationing care only among the poorest members of society, in effect asking only other poor persons to bear the burden of expanding access.[14]

This concern is a fundamental challenge faced by Oregon as a community, namely, how to achieve greater *equity* in the distribution of benefits and *fairly* distribute the burden of producing improved equity. These criticisms come from the world of theory and seek to illumine real policy choices. In some cases the theoretical frame of reference describes an ideal order — rationing to all members of the society is preferable to rationing only among the poor — but the government now does not have the level of control over the whole range of third party systems needed to enact a universal rationing plan. On the other hand, the government does have control over health care systems aimed at providing access for the poor. Rationalizing that part of the system in pursuit of greater equity needs to be examined in terms of current policy dynamics and capacity to contribute to more ideal long term solutions.

Constructive ethical critique should explore whether proposed short term solutions are likely to contribute to or impede long term solutions to chronic problems. Fleck, for example, argues that persons now eligible for Medicaid would be making a rational choice to forego some lesser benefits in order to gain a greater assurance that they would have access to private health insurance even in low income employment circumstances—a situation they are likely to find themselves in as they move from Medicaid eligibility to greater financial independence.[15] The Oregon Plan can thus be a defensibly just solution under present circumstances. He goes on to argue that

12. CHILDREN DEFENSE FUND REPORTS, POOR CHILDREN AND WOMEN TARGETED FOR MEDICAID REDUCTIONS IN OREGON, 1, 6-7 (Aug. 1990); Morrell, *Oregon Puts Bold Health Plan on Ice*, 259 SCI. 468-71 (1990); Budetti, *Medicaid Rationing in Oregon: Political Wolf in a Philosopher's Sheepskin*, 1 HEALTH MATRIX CASE W. RES. J. L. MED. 205, 216-17 (1991).

13. *See supra* summary of Oregon Senate Bill 27 p. 142.

14. Daniels, *Is the Oregon Rationing Plan Fair?*, 265 J. A.M.A. 2232 (1991).

15. Fleck, *The Oregon Medicaid Experiment: Is It Just Enough?*, 19 BUS. & PROF. ETHICS J. 201 (1990).

it would indeed be more just, if circumstances permitted, to include all, rich and poor alike, in one grand health care rationing scheme.

A basic error in some of the criticisms described above results from assuming that the Oregon Plan is unethical, not because it is rationing, but because it is rationing in circumstances that are not ideal. This makes for clear and forceful theoretical argumentation, but in the end only dimly illuminates the policy decisions that have to be made now in less than ideal circumstances. Medicaid budgets, for example, have to be dealt with both in the long term and the short term, and the problems of persons without health insurance who need health care now need to be attended to in the less than ideal circumstances of today.

A second concern raised by critical observers is that the plan may seriously corrupt community spirit by legitimizing a mean spirited attitude toward the poor.[16] This criticism sees priority based allocations as ethically proper only if everyone in the community is at risk of having to live with the results of a priority system to be used to ration care. It is destructive of the moral basis of society to legitimize restrictions on health care for the poor while permitting the more well off to indulge in extravagant life styles, including excessive use of health services financed by collective resources such as private health insurance.

A third concern focuses on a subset of the community, namely health care providers, and urges that their basic ethic of patient advocacy will be corrupted if they play an active part in rationing health care.[17] The Oregon plan, these critics argue, is a rationing scheme and health care providers should never get into the business of rationing care either at the bedside or at the statehouse.

A fourth concern asserts that the Oregon Plan, which requires considerable societal effort, amounts to a futile tinkering with a fundamentally defective system.[18] For these critics the clear moral imperative is to get to a system of universal access to basic health care by the shortest possible path. Setting priorities is an intellectually and socially daunting exercise that merely postpones getting down

16. Caplan, *How Can We Deny Health Care to Poor While Others Get Face Lifts?* L.A. Times, April 25, 1989, at E6, col. 1.

17. R. Veatch, Deciding Levels of Care: The Case for Public Control (Oct. 1990) (unpublished manuscript presented at University of Minnesota Conference, "Drawing The Line: Defining a Basic Level of Health Care").

18. *See* Relman, *The Trouble with Rationing*, 323 NEW ENG. J. MED. 911 (1990); Himmelstein & Woolhandler, *A National Health Program for the United States*, 320 NEW ENG. J. MED. 102 (1989); Himmelstein & Woolhandler, *Cost Without Benefit: Administrative Waste in U.S. Health Care*, 314 NEW ENG. J. MED. 441 (1986).

to real business on the primary challenge: making a commitment to every citizen and seriously rooting out wasteful administrative and technical practices in the health care delivery system.

A fifth moral concern is rooted in the technical difficulty of constructing a prioritized list of health services. Critics argue that health care services are too complex to be prioritized with scientific validity.[19] Outcome research is too slow and cumbersome to offer any hope for a scientifically based prioritization. Expert opinion ultimately may not be reliable because health care providers, the relevant experts, have a monetary interest in arranging for their typical services to score high on any prioritized list. On the other hand, information about how people value specific services in the abstract as opposed to when they actually need them, raises serious methodologic problems. How these values can be validly and accurately discovered and then related to technical information about outcomes for specific services is thought by some to be an insurmountable obstacle. These circumstances, it is urged, cast grave doubt on the prudence of attempting to base social policy on such questionable data and inference.

These criticisms are an important feature of the moral story. They should cause a profound wariness in those playing responsible parts in the unfolding Oregon experiment. All of the above concerns deserve careful scrutiny by members of the Oregon community who hope that the Oregon Plan will create a higher justice and more secure common good. The criticisms identify important issues for ongoing strategic corrections as the plan unfolds.

Each criticism should be met, not with theoretical arguments, but with decisions that can keep the Oregon Plan moving in an ethically acceptable direction. It is important to note that each critique is particularly relevant to different moments in the story or steps in the process (see Figure 1 below). Some of the critics, for example, have failed to grasp the phased nature of the process and take issue, not with what is actually going on, but with a collapsed conception of the Oregon Plan. The result is usually to assume that certain steps are finished before they have begun. A glaring example is the assumption that there was no political play left in the Plan regarding new dollars for Medicaid, when, in fact, that issue did not become fully activated until the HSC delivered the priority list to the legislature (in May of 1991). The relationship of specific critical is-

19. Schwartz & Aaron, *The Achilles Heel of Health Care Rationing*, N.Y. Times, July 9, 1990, at F1, col. 1.

sues to steps in the prioritization process will be discussed below after the steps and their relationships with one another have been described.

PRIORITY SETTING AS A FOUR STEP PROCESS

The Oregon Plan creates a four step process for generating a list of health service priorities to be used as an instrument for budget decisions by the legislature and for program administration decisions by state agencies (See Figure 1). In the first step of the process,

Figure 1

Oregon Priority Setting Process

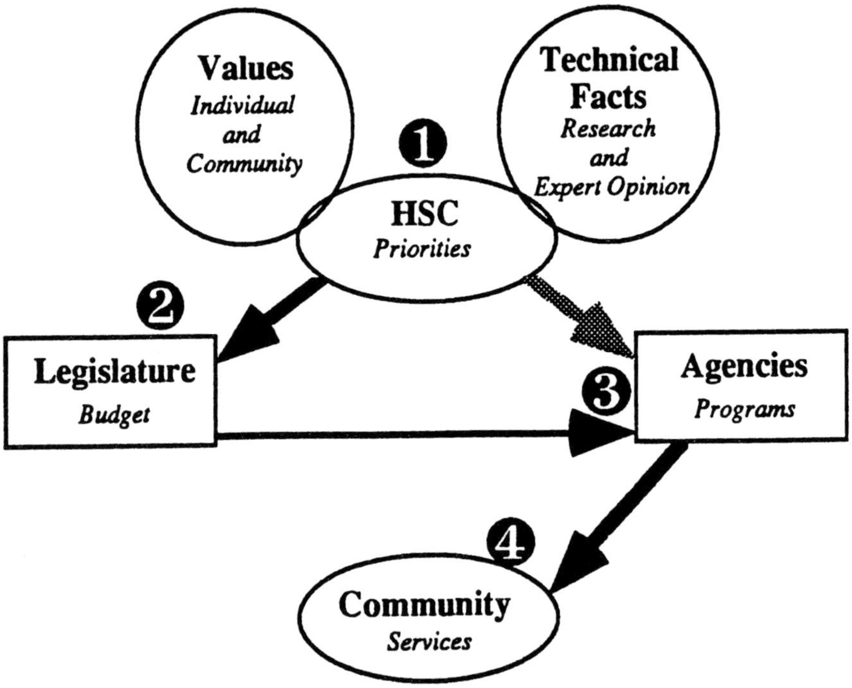

the Health Services Commission is required to develop a list of priorities based on community and individual values about health care and on technical information about the effectiveness of various health services relative to the needs of the population to be served. This list, together with actuarial estimates of the cost of funding different priority levels, is delivered to the Governor and the legislature in step two. The legislature's Joint Committee on Health Care must first consider the list and report its recommendations to both the Governor and the Legislative Assembly. Then the full legislature, using the list as a decision guide, has the task of setting budgets which will establish de facto the benefit package to be offered by Medicaid. This package will also become the basic minimum that must be contained in any private health insurance plan offered under the aegis of the small business (Senate Bill 935) and high risk (Senate Bill 534) insurance programs.

The third step in the process provides the relevant agencies (Medicaid, Oregon Medical Insurance Pool Board and High Risk Insurance Pool Governing Board) with the budget decision that creates the benefit package for Medicaid and associated private insurance packages. The first essential administrative task is for OMAP to request necessary waivers of several federal Medicaid regulations. Without approval from the Health Care Financing Administration (HCFA) in Washington, the Medicaid portion of the plan cannot be implemented. At this point the agencies must put in place all the administrative and evaluation elements that are necessary to run a complex social program. Figure 1 shows an arrow from the HSC to the agencies because part of the concept of the process is for the agencies to use the priority list to guide administrative decisions so that the new programs will be a consistent expression of the values on which the priorities are based.

The fourth step is the actual implementation of new service programs in the community. These services involve all persons at or below 100% of the Federal Poverty Level (e.g., an income of $880 per month for a family of three) who will be declared eligible for Medicaid. Those with incomes above 100% Federal Poverty Level (unless already included in a special categorical program for Medicaid) will be served through either of the two health insurance pools.

TIMELINE FOR THE PROCESS

The timeline for these steps is expected to be as follows. Community values and technical information have already been gathered and the HSC has completed the priorities list (step 1) and will deliver the list (with actuarial estimates of the costs of funding different levels) to the legislature on May 1, 1991. Step 2, the legislative budget decision, is expected to be completed by mid summer 1991. The request for waivers (initial stage of step 3) will be submitted only after the budget decision has established the basic benefit package (late summer 1991). The waiver decision is expected to take six months, so that should waivers be granted by January 1992, the new Medicaid program (step 4) would be implemented beginning in July 1992.

The process is temporally staged and cyclical. The HSC is a permanent Commission and is charged to review and revise the priority listing each biennium. For the 1993 legislative session, the HSC already has the task of bringing mental health and chemical dependency services into the priorities system, these two categories having been set aside from the first prioritization attempt.

The criticisms of the plan summarized above should be seen in relation to the several stages of the process. At step one, the priority generating stage, the issues of HSC methodology are paramount. The ethical challenge is to exercise wisdom in the selection of methods of gathering information and to maintain authenticity in combining value and technical information so as to produce a consistent list of priorities.

The Commission recruited 53 panels of provider experts to examine health conditions and associated treatments they commonly deal with. They were asked to describe probable outcomes of treating specific conditions in terms compatible with various states of well being. Data on preferences for certain states of well being were gathered from a random sample survey of Oregonians. This data and the outcome projections were combined in a net benefit formula used by the HSC to structure the priority list. In addition to the data on individual values about states of well being (the random sample survey data), the HSC, in collaboration with Oregon Health Decisions, developed a report on community oriented values about health care. Finally, the HSC held public hearings at seven sites throughout the state to give opportunity for special pleading by individuals and interest groups. All of these value information sources were being used by the HSC to shape the final priority listing that will go to the Legislature. Further information on the methodological questions and their results are available elsewhere.[20]

At step two the issues of justice and common good become paramount. Here the legislature must make policy judgments about the value of health care relative to other uses of public funds. The Legislature is always the primary locus of public policy efforts to do justice and promote the common good through public programs. Failures at this level in the past have produced the present circum-

20. THE OREGON HEALTH SERVICES COMMISSION. PRIORITIZATION OF HEALTH SERVICES: A REPORT TO THE GOVERNOR AND LEGISLATURE (1991). *See also*, H.D. Klevit, *Prioritization of Health Care Services*, ARCHIVES OF INTERNAL MED. 912 (1991).

stance in which Medicaid programs nationally serve less than half of those persons below the Federal Poverty Level while some 15% of the U.S. population remains without any form of third party coverage.

It is important for efforts at this step of the process to be critically examined in the light of ethical theory. But it is equally important for ethical theory to be critically examined in the light of real circumstances, needs and opportunities. A fundamental error made by several critics of the Oregon Plan is the assumption that there was no political play left in the process by the time the Legislature received the priority list. In fact, it is just that play that is required for justice and common good goals to be pursued and achieved, and the Oregon Plan is precisely designed for legislative choice to be determinative of the benefit package. The difference is that funding choices are to be made in terms of the priority list, not at random or arbitrarily or by jumping around an undifferentiated menu of services looking for just the right combination of program lines to achieve the bottom line needed to balance the budget.

Justice and common good issues continue to be primary at the third step the program design and implementation level for which state agencies have responsibility. The ethical issue of fidelity to the values and moral goals generated at the previous stages of the process is also essential here. The first element of the process at this stage will consist of applying for necessary Federal Medicaid waivers. It should be noted that the need for such waivers will certainly reach forward in time and affect the previous stage (step 2) i.e., the legislature's budget setting deliberations. It seems highly unlikely that the legislature will set the budget for Medicaid at a level doomed to be the basis of refusal of waivers needed to implement the Plan. The effort by the legislature to do justice at step two will, in part, be driven by the need to have a budget compatible with the sense of justice in the effective decision makers in Washington.

Some critics had prematurely begun lobbying the Health Care Financing Administration to reject the waiver request, but the decision they condemn had not yet been made. Advocates for organ transplantation coverage, for example, have made assumptions about how the priorities list would look before it had been created. On the other hand, advocates for child welfare, such as the Children's Defense Fund, which has declared itself unalterably opposed to a Medicaid waiver, made the assumption that there would be no new dollars added to the Medicaid budget before the legislature has had a chance to see the list and work with it as an instrument of budgetary decision making. These advocates were absolutely correct in their belief that the issue of new dollars was central to the question of justice in the Oregon Plan, but they mistakenly believed the question is closed before it had even been opened in earnest — namely, when the legislature had the list in hand as an instrument of decision making. In fact the Oregon legislature budgeted significant new dollars to Medicaid in the 1991 session. These critics' commitment to advocacy is admirable, but their understanding of stages in the priority setting process is surprisingly deficient and the distortions they have introduced into the ethical debate may unintentionally prolong present injustices rather than alleviate them.

REFLECTIONS ON COMMUNITY SOLIDARITY

At the heart of the ethical problem the Oregon Plan seeks to address is the historical fact that our current system of solidarity for health care assigns some citizens the invidious status of outsiders. The history of the growth of third party coverage since World War II reveals a public policy tending toward universal entitlement but lacking in clear public commitment to the value of social solidarity on which such an entitlement logically rests. Between 1940 and 1950, the proportion of the population with employment based hospital insurance rose from 9% to 57%.[21] By the early seventies, after the passage of Medicare and Medicaid, the proportion of the population with some form of third party support for health care reached approximately 80% and has hovered around that point to the present.[22] Those without insurance are simply left outside the circle of solidarity that the majority of us enjoy.

Michael Walzer in his analysis of the complex value pluralism of contemporary society offers instructive reflections on this point. He notes that the growth of communal provision of health care through both public and private third party systems gives a historical validation to the desire for health care, transforming the desire into a socially recognized need.[23] Once desire is transformed into need, the distributional logic for health care should relate to illness, not wealth. In such a society, to be deprived of access to health care is a double loss. Those left out of third party solidarity experience the

---

21. O. W. ANDERSON, HEALTH SERVICES IN THE UNITED STATES, A GROWTH ENTERPRISE SINCE 1875. 134, 142 (1985).

22. DEPARTMENT OF HEALTH AND HUMAN SERVICES, NATIONAL HEALTH INSURANCE RESOURCE BOOK, 86-91 (1974).

23. M. WALZER, SPHERES OF JUSTICE, A DEFENSE OF PLURALISM AND EQUALITY, 86-91 (1983).

adverse consequences of having unmet health needs and they are told that they do not have standing as full fledged members of their society. They suffer both the misfortune of illness and the insult of exclusion.

In Walzer's analysis, this failure of community solidarity results from the misplaced use of personal wealth (being insured or being eligible for a welfare benefit) instead of illness as the criterion for the distribution of health care. It is reasonable to extend Walzer's thought and argue that this mistaken use of wealth as the basis for health care distribution is perpetuated by society's failure to achieve full consciousness of the degree of solidarity implicit in all third party financing arrangements. The community meeting process built into the Oregon Plan, and conducted for the HSC by Oregon Health Decisions, is an effort to counteract society's lack of attentiveness to the structure and consequences of an unfinished commitment to third party financing for health care. The structure of the meetings called for participants to adopt the language perspective of the first person plural and to identify values that reveal why health care is important to us as members of a community.

The community meeting process functions as a vehicle for participatory social criticism, namely, the articulation of moral discomfort because an important aspect of social life contradicts fundamental values a society espouses. The meetings facilitate group participation in the public examination of values declared by participants themselves to be of major importance for defining the moral meaning of health care. At the meetings the participants collaborate to "hold a mirror up" to themselves in which they can glimpse their authentic longings for higher values and face up to their own and — through themselves — society's moral inconsistencies, hypocrisies, and quiet accommodations with injustice.

These are the essential tasks of the social critic described by Michael Walzer[24] in his study of that role as it is usually played by individual writers. Observations of the unfolding Oregon story make it evident that members of the community can, through the shared perspective of group dialogue, play a role analogous to Walzer's conception of the individual social critic. The community meetings opened up that role to ordinary people who participated in the process. Each participant in the context of group discussion be-

24. M. WALZER, THE COMPANY OF CRITICS: SOCIAL CRITICISM AND POLITICAL COMMITMENT IN THE TWENTIETH CENTURY, 229-240 (1988).

came a collaborator in the creation of a community owned and produced form of social criticism.

This participatory form of criticism fulfills Walzer's belief that the effective social critic must be psychologically "inside" the community being criticized, must feel connected to its successes and failures, must care passionately about the community's moral well-being, and remain attentive to the actually existing consciousness of the community. The capacity to generate this kind of participatory social criticism is essential to the exercise of meaningful community responsibility for the institution of health care at this point in its evolution when the unfinished agenda of universal access must be pursued with simultaneous concern for cost containment and rational allocation of resources.

Many critics of the Oregon plan have raised important moral concerns vital to the proper working out of the ethical story. Their contribution is extremely valuable. The critiques, however, of those who only view the story from the outside and point accusing fingers at "those people in Oregon" finally lack moral authenticity. They do not take responsibility for offering a better plan that can move the ethical agenda forward in a community to which they belong, in whose failures they are shamed and in whose good work they can take pride. These critics do not hold themselves accountable for the failure of their community to reach out in solidarity to those now uninsured for health care. Their criticisms provide the useful but limited benefit of a message from someone who looks on from a higher, but finally, too remote vantage point.

As the unfolding Oregon story continues and leaders at the state and national level struggle to extend the circle of solidarity and compassion to all citizens, the extent of direct community involvement in community forums will be critical. The health care system is now unfair in many ways. It also falls well short of an achievable level of common good. The possibility of change for the better is a challenge to the living ethics of the Oregon community—and the national community. On this point the unfolding Oregon story shows that we can reach a higher level of community responsibility for the fairness, prudence and common welfare generated by the health care system. The story also shows that improvements in fairness, prudence and common good are not guaranteed. They are always to be achieved.

Legislative Commentary

SULLIVAN MADE THE RIGHT CHOICE IN REJECTING THE OREGON PLAN

by Tom Mason†

HEALTH AND HUMAN Services Secretary Dr. Louis W. Sullivan's August 3 decision to withhold Federal approval of the controversial Oregon Medicaid rationing plan[1] has elicited a firestorm of comment. Medical ethicists, like Daniel Callahan have clucked their disapproval[2] and *The New York Times* has written two editorials criticizing the decision and accusing the Bush administration of engaging in election year politics.[3] As one of the Oregon law makers intimately involved the controversy I have been asked to share my perspective on the decision to reject the plan.

Let me start by saying that I haven't read a single evaluation of Secretary Sullivan's conclusion that even begins to understand, much less appreciate, the real issues raised by his rejection. Similarly, the outspoken supporters of the plan have never been willing to admit the real reasons for the "tough choices" the proposal requires between life for some and death for others.

Secretary Sullivan rejected the plan because it conflicted with the Americans with Disabilities Act ("ADA"), recently enacted, comprehensive and rigorous federal legislation designed to protect the rights of handicapped Americans. The Secretary decided that the prioritization process was legally flawed because the data derived from a telephone survey which was used to define "quality of

† Oregon State Representative, District 11.

1. For a full discussion of the Oregon Basic Health Services Act of 1989, *see* 1 HEALTH MATRIX 135-273 (1991) (Oregon Plan Symposium Issue). *See also* RATIONING AMERICA'S MEDICAL CARE: THE OREGON PLAN AND BEYOND (Martin A. Strosberg et al. eds., 1992) (available from the Brookings Institution, Washington, D.C.).

2. *See* Robert Pear, *Too-Bitter Medicine*, N.Y. TIMES, Aug. 5, 1992 at A8.

3. *See, e.g.*, *A Bold Medical Plan, Derailed*, N.Y. TIMES, Aug. 6, 1992 at A22; *see also* James E. Cottrell, *Finally, a Medical Plan That Faces Reality*, WASH. POST, Sept. 3, 1992 at A23; *Washington Prevails*, WALL ST. J., Aug. 5, 1992 at A14.

life" quantified "stereotypic assumptions" about disabled persons Respondents to the phone survey, which generated the numerical values eventually used in the prioritization formula, were generally not handicapped and therefore the Secretary concluded, would "systematically undervalue the quality of life of those with disabilities."

Secretary Sullivan was also concerned that other components of the ranking process reflected discrimination against disabled Americans as well:

> "According to the [the Oregon Health Services] Commission Report, the Commissioners ranked all categories and made hand adjustments to the list on the basis of certain community values, including 'quality of life' and 'ability to function.' These two values place importance on 'restored' and 'independence' and thus expressly value a person without a disability more highly than a person with a disability in the allocation of medical treatment. . .[A]ny methodology that would intentionally ration health care resources by associating quality of life considerations with disabilities does not comport with the mandate of the ADA."[4]

Finally, the Secretary points out that the plan's "refusal to cover life support" for some low birthweight babies may also conflict with the Child Abuse Amendments of 1984 which established standards for treatment of medically fragile infants, and presupposed the rendering of life support services to such infants.

The only surprising thing about the decision is that it took federal officials so long to see the obvious. His analysis is a bureaucratic version of the old fairy tale in which a forthright child points out what her elders have been afraid to say - - the emperor has no clothes! Of course the rationing plan discriminates, that is what it is all about. Decision makers in Oregon were so intent upon being the first to adopt an elitist health care rationing program that it never occurred to them that process involved discrimination. Discrimination almost always involves a benign act on the part of perpetrator - - a simple failure to comprehend that the act of discrimination requires a presumption upon the relative value of human sensibilities, human lives. That is what the Oregon plan does throughout, it values one person's life over another for subjective reasons, the ultimate act of discrimination.

Overall Sullivan's objections are extremely well taken, and in my opinion not the type of reservations which can be accommo-

4. Letter from Secretary of Health and Human Services Dr. Louis W. Sullivan to Governor Barbara Roberts and accompanying explanation, August 3, 1992 (on file with author).

dated by minor amendments to the plan. The rejection, however, along with almost all other commentaries on the plan, ignores the political motivation for the whole proposal.

Why is there so much interest in medical care in one of America's smallest states? As we confront the health care dilemma we search desperately for new solutions, new paradigms. It is fairly obvious that the Canadian health care system is seen by many as the most viable alternative to the American status quo. In Canada the government is the sole purchaser of health care and dictates what providers will receive for their services. The Oregon proposal, for expanding Medicaid but reducing services, is now looked upon by the American medical establishment as the alternative model to the Canadian system. Every major medical provider group in Oregon supported the new plan.

Effective health care availability in Canada is based upon paying less for services, i.e. real cost control or reduction. In Oregon the expansion of the availability of health care was based upon providing less services, literally one hundred and eighty degrees from Canada. The dirty little secret of the Oregon plan is that not only does it not control medical costs, but it actually mandates that providers get paid more! The law says that providers will get their actual costs and it has been estimated that this will increase Oregon Medicaid fees by more than thirty percent. This is why the Oregon plan is so attractive to medical industry. Not only does it offer a viable counter-proposal to Canada, but it preserves, if not increases, incomes. If this Oregon scheme is adopted it will give the opponents of a national health care system yet another excuse for postponing the inevitable.

There has been a woeful lack of appreciation of the political significance of the Oregon plan. Academics, and "medical ethicists" have been absolutely enamored with the proposal. It has given them a grand opportunity for discussion and a chance to make a hard "ethical" decision to approve the rationing of health care. Like so many young doctors with their first patients they can not wait to use their new found power. The discussion of health care rationing has turned into a modern day exercise in the selling of indulgences by a new priesthood.

It is probably well to conclude by revisiting the actual situation which produced the Oregon plan. The proposal was another chapter in a controversy over health care rationing which started several years ago in the state. During the 1987 legislature session, a joint appropriations sub-committee eliminated Medicaid funding for organ transplants. Funds saved by the elimination of the program were later used for the expansion of Oregon's juvenile detention center, MacClaren. The following dialog occurred at the end of the hearing:

> Senator Roberts: "I think that no one here likes the decisions we've made, but I guess I always think of that book *Sophie's Choice*, particularly when we are dealing with the situation (transplant funding) you are referring to, Tom, that you actually say to somebody, 'No, we can't save your life.'
>
> Representative Mason: "Mr. Chairman, I would buy that if I didn't see you pumping $680,000 into MacClaren. That sticks in my craw. I'm sorry. How you can put MacClaren on one side and soft organ transplants on the other side is totally beyond me. I just don't understand that. People need those transplants. Instead, you are beefing up a jail."
>
> Senator Roberts: "I know that."[5]

Seven months later this exercise in *real politic* took its first victim, seven year old Coby Howard, who died due to a lack of a bone marrow transplant.[6] Notwithstanding the policy questions, this is what health care rationing is about. Secretary Sullivan did the right thing in rejecting the Oregon plan. William Styron's heroine Sophie was forced to choose between the life of her son or her daughter by the ultimate embodiment of morally bankrupt government, a Nazi concentration camp officer. We owe it to our children, to our families and to ourselves not to be forced into making such choices.

---

5. *Hearing on HB-5027 Before the Human Resources Subcomm. of the Joint Committee on Ways and Means*, 64th Oregon Legislative Assembly, (May 15,1987), (Final action on Department of Human Resources budgets, Tape 148-B), HB-5027 Budget Report.

6. *See* Maxwell J. Mehlman, *The Oregon Medicaid Program: Is It Just?* 1 HEALTH MATRIX 175, 185 n.44 (1991).

SUMMARY

EVALUATION OF THE OREGON MEDICAID PROPOSAL

CONGRESS OF THE UNITED STATES
OFFICE OF TECHNOLOGY ASSESSMENT

Summary and Conclusions

INTRODUCTION

On August 16, 1991, Oregon petitioned the Federal Government for permission to use Federal funds in a novel health care financing program. The proposed program is premised on two basic assumptions:

1. all uninsured poor people should have publicly funded health care coverage, and
2. coverage for this population can be made affordable to the taxpayers through a combination of two mechanisms: the explicit prioritization of health care services, and the delivery of covered services through managed care systems.

Oregon's plan to revamp its system of health care coverage was motivated by the steadily increasing costs of health care to the public treasury and the large number of Oregonians who have no health insurance. The State has estimated that between 400,000 and 450,000 Oregonians, or about 16 percent of the State's population, are uninsured (33).

To address this latter problem, the Oregon legislature passed the Oregon Basic Health Services Act in 1989, which established three mechanisms for increasing access to health insurance (box A). For individuals who could not qualify for private insurance due to a "preexisting health condition," the State established a high-risk insurance pool with subsidized premiums. For individuals whose employers do not offer health insurance benefits, the State established a program that provides incentives for, and ultimately mandates, small businesses to provide such insurance to their employees. And for poor uninsured individuals, the Basic Health Services Act expanded the State Medicaid program to cover all residents with incomes up to 100 percent of the Federal poverty level (FPL).[1]

The last of these three measures has been the subject of particular controversy (4,5,8,12,16,19, 41,42). In part, the controversy stems from the need for the State to obtain permission from the Federal Government to implement its proposal as planned, since it wishes to receive Federal Medicaid matching funding for the program. The proposal is also controversial because of its explicit attention to determining how unfunded care should be denied, and because by design it encouraged public debate regarding the relative importance of different health care services (9,13,14,20,27,30,35).

Oregon's proposal is to make a sweeping change to its Medicaid program, the Federal/State funded, State-administered health care program for the poor. The proposed new program, if approved as it was submitted to the Federal Government, would continue for 5 years. The program was originally anticipated to begin by July 1, 1992, but the State now expects that implementation may be delayed because as of March 1992 the Federal Government had not yet decided whether to grant the waiver.

Under the proposed program, *the Medicaid-eligible population would be expanded to include all legal State residents*[2] *with incomes below the FPL.* In contrast, at present, most people in Oregon must fall into a federally specified need category (e.g., be eligible for the Aid to Families with Dependent Children (AFDC) program) to qualify for Medicaid. In addition, in most cases they must have incomes much lower than the FPL to qualify. Oregon residents who receive AFDC assistance, for example, generally must have incomes that are less than 50 percent of the FPL to be eligible for Medicaid.

According to the State of Oregon, the expansion in eligibility under the proposal would add approximately 120,600 people to the Medicaid rolls by the fifth year of the program. This number is predicted to be somewhat smaller (96,400) if the related employer-based health insurance mandate is in effect (table 1) (33).

Certain groups currently covered by the Oregon Medicaid program would not initially be affected by the proposed changes in the program. The waiver proposal does not cover Medicaid eligibles who are elderly, disabled, in institutions, in foster care, or in the custody of the State, because these groups were exempt from Oregon Senate Bill (SB) 27, the bill

[1] For 1992, the Federal poverty level is $11,570 per year for a family of three.

[2] Undocumented aliens do not qualify as legal residents and would not be eligible for the program.

Box A—The Oregon Basic Health Services Act

The Oregon Basic Health Services Act of 1989 consists of three separate bills to expand access to health insurance in the State. Each of the three bills targets a specific segment of the uninsured population.

The first bill, Senate Bill (SB) 27, expands the Oregon Medicaid program to include all legal residents with incomes up to the Federal poverty level. It also changes dramatically the method of defining benefits for the Medicaid population, greatly expands the use of prepaid managed care for this group, and makes other changes to the State Medicaid plan. To implement these changes and continue receiving Federal Medicaid matching funds, the State has proposed that its new plan be a Medicaid demonstration project, and it seeks Federal approval to carry out this project.

The second bill of the act, SB 534, establishes a State high-risk insurance pool. This pool sells subsidized health insurance to persons who are unable to purchase insurance on the market due to preexisting health conditions and anticipated future high health care costs. The premium charge for policies from this insurance pool is not to exceed 150 percent of the cost of an average private health insurance premium. Program costs not covered by the collection of premiums are financed through general State funds and through mandatory contributions by private insurers.

SB 935, the third bill of the act, addresses the problem of persons who are employed but have no employer-based health insurance. This law encourages, and ultimately requires, employers to provide health insurance to their employees that covers at least the level of services covered for the Medicaid population under SB 27. Businesses receive tax credits for providing insurance. They have the option of choosing private insurance plans or purchasing insurance from a State fund created for that purpose. The minimum benefits that must be covered are linked to the Medicaid benefits package. Employers who do not provide health insurance after 1994 will be required to make mandatory contributions to the fund, but that provision is repealed if at least 150,000 previously uninsured persons receive employer-based health insurance by January 1994.

Legislation passed in 1991 made some significant additions and changes to this three-part program. One particularly significant statute (SB 44) requires that the Medicaid-eligible elderly, disabled, and individuals in foster care or in the custody of the State be subject to the provisions of SB 27. These groups, originally exempt from the sweeping changes in the Medicaid program, are now intended to be included in 1993. Because the waiver proposal as submitted in August 1991 does not accommodate them, the State must submit an amendment to the waiver to do so if the waiver is approved in its current form.

The Health Insurance Reform Act (SB 1076), also passed in 1991, establishes some limits and safeguards on employer-based insurance. These limits would apply to the basic benefits package required under SB 935. The act establishes rate categories and limits rate increases in small group plans, provides for guaranteed issue and renewability of policies, and controls such factors as preexisting condition exclusions.

Finally, the Health Resources Commission Act of 1991 (SB 1077) "establishes a data and cost review commission designed to contain statewide health care costs as the above insurance expansions occur."

SOURCE: Office of Technology Assessment, 1992. Based on Oregon's SB 27, SB 44, SB 534, SB 935, SB 1076, SB 1077; and Oregon waiver application, August 1991.

authorizing the program changes. For the first year of the new program, these groups would continue to be eligible for all Medicaid benefits under the current rules and would continue to receive the same services as they would if the demonstration program were not in place. However, the State plans to file an amendment to the waiver permitting these groups to be covered under the new program beginning in October 1993 (33).[3]

Service delivery and payment would also change under the new plan. Most of the population receiving services under the demonstration program would be enrolled in some form of managed care reimbursed on a prepaid, per capita basis; the remainder would receive services on a case-managed, fee-for-service (FFS) basis. Payment to prepaid providers would no longer be linked to Medicaid FFS payment rates. Instead, payment rates to these providers would be

[3] The projected date for folding these groups into the program is apparently unchanged by the possibility that the program, if approved, would probably begin sometime after July 1992.

Table 1—Demonstration Enrollment Projections[a]

	Without employer mandate		With employer mandate	
Year of demonstration	Current eligibles	New eligibles	Current eligibles	New eligibles
Year 1 (FY 1993)[b]	150,700	46,800[c]	150,700	46,800
Year 2 (FY 1994)	156,000	81,100	156,000	81,100
Year 3 (FY 1995)	160,600	105,400	160,600	105,400
Year 4 (FY 1996)	165,400	120,000	159,600	96,000
Year 5 (FY 1997)	170,300	120,600	164,400	96,400

[a]Enrollment is expressed as average monthly caseload. It is lower than the actual number of eligibles who have benefits for some period of time during the course of a year.
[b]The Oregon State fiscal year begins in July.
[c]Of these new eligibles, 2,700 are currently covered under a State-only General Assistance (GA) program that covers the medically unemployable (unemployed for more than 60 days due to a medical condition). Oregon's general assistance program only covers outpatient care.
SOURCE: Oregon waiver application, August 1991.

based on the State's estimates of the average reasonable costs, across all providers, of rendering the given covered services.

Finally, *the covered services to which the Medicaid-eligible population is entitled would change*. For all Medicaid recipients subject to the program, the benefit package would be determined by a prioritized list of health services in which health conditions and their treatments are listed by importance from highest to lowest. The State legislature would then determine its budget for the program, and a line would be drawn where projected program costs equal the budgeted amount. All conditions and treatments at and above the line would then be covered; conditions and treatments below the line would not be covered. (Necessary diagnostic services are intended to be covered regardless of the condition and are not prioritized on the list.)

The prioritized list of services is limited to primary and acute health care services. Long-term care services would not be covered by the proposal and do not appear on the prioritized list; they would remain a separately covered set of Medicaid services. Mental health and chemical dependency services would initially be excluded from the prioritized list, but they are to be incorporated into the list in October 1993. Until that time, any of the group of Medicaid beneficiaries covered by the proposal, including newly eligible groups, would receive these services under current program rules.

Oregon has a 2-year budget cycle, and the State legislature would vote anew biennially on the threshold (i.e., the benefit package). An important provision of SB 27 is that if the Medicaid program should suffer a budget shortfall, the program may not cut people out of the program or reduce provider payments for covered services. Instead, the State must either allocate additional funds to the program or reduce covered services as necessary, with the lowest-ranked services being eliminated first.

Thus, as the program is designed, the benefit package could either expand or contract every 2 years, depending on the budget. In addition, benefits could be reduced in the middle of the biennial cycle if funds prove inadequate to meet projected costs. The need for Federal approval may inhibit this intended flexibility. Oregon's waiver application states that it will seek an amendment to the waiver if in fact benefits would change "significantly" during the 5 years of the program. Exactly what the Federal Government would regard as "significant" will not be known until (or unless) the waiver is approved.

Concern about the effects of Oregon's Medicaid proposal on program recipients, and the potential ramifications of the proposal for the ongoing national health care debate, prompted Congress to ask the Office of Technology Assessment to examine the proposal in detail.[4] The report was prepared in response to a request from Representative John Dingell, Chairman of the House Committee on Energy and Commerce, and Representative Henry Waxman, Chairman of the House Subcommittee on Health and the Environment. The request for the OTA study was endorsed by Senator Al Gore, Chairman of the Senate Subcommittee on Science, Technology, and Space, and by the Oregon delegation, including Senator Bob Packwood, Senator Mark Hatfield, Representative Les AuCoin, Representative Peter DeFazio, Representative Mike Kopetski, Representative Ron Wyden, and Representative Robert F. (Bob) Smith.

[4] Unless indicated otherwise, details of the proposal discussed within this summary are based on Oregon's Office of Medical Assistance Programs' August 16, 1991 waiver application.

322-105 0 - 92 - 2 QL 3

The goals of the OTA study were to describe and analyze the specifics of the proposed program and to discuss its most likely implications for the Federal Government, the State of Oregon, and Medicaid beneficiaries. The role of the report is not to critique the existing Medicaid program in detail. Rather, it is to examine the proposed program and especially its relevance to issues of particular interest to the Federal Government: the impact of the program on Medicaid beneficiaries, in whom the Federal Government (as a copayer) has a fiduciary interest; and the potential usefulness of Oregon's program if applied in other States and other contexts. This summary reviews the findings of the OTA report and draws overall conclusions regarding the technical merits of the proposal.

[SUBSEQUENT MATERIAL FROM THIS POINT TO MID-PAGE 18 OMITTED]

[PRECEDING MATERIAL

FROM MID-PAGE 4

TO THIS POINT OMITTED]

CONCLUSIONS

In designing its proposed Medicaid demonstration program and related changes to its health care system, the State of Oregon has achieved what few others have: a dramatic and comprehensive proposal to change the way health care is delivered that appears to be generally accepted by its residents and providers. The State has invested considerable resources into its unique Medicaid proposal. Many of the proposed changes have stimulated open public debate, and the lessons learned from the effort to develop a categorization of treatments and conditions are valuable ones. The State's explicit attempt to integrate and incorporate outcomes information and broad public input is especially notable.

The State believes that despite possible problems, the gains it anticipates from the proposal make the program worth trying. **The immediate issue for the Federal Government, however, is not only whether the proposed changes should take place but whether Federal revenues should be used to fund them.** Unlike the State, which is legitimately concerned primarily with the effects within Oregon, the Federal Government must consider the ways in which the information from the proposal might be useful to others. It must also consider the opportunity costs of funding Oregon's proposal relative to other possible uses for those funds.

Certain aspects of Oregon's proposal hold promise as a potential demonstration of ways that health care costs might be constrained or health care access improved. The proposal to include all Medicaid enrollees in some form of managed care, with an emphasis on various forms of prepaid care that grade the degree of financial risk to the size and experience of the provider, is intriguing. Many health care payers have looked to managed care to reduce costs without endangering health, and there would probably be considerable interest in the results of an experiment that tested comprehensive managed care for Medicaid beneficiaries. Oregon's past experience with managed care suggests that this State would be a reasonable location for such an experiment. The effect on provider participation of a changed method of payment likewise is of interest.

Expanding coverage to all poor persons is clearly a benefit of the proposal. This component of the proposal is both the most expensive and the most likely to yield positive results. Aside from the simple benefit to those involved, there are some solid reasons to test coverage expansion as an experiment; for example, such a study might shed additional light on the links between health insurance, health care access, and health status.

The move to simplify eligibility rules in conjunction with coverage expansion is also attractive, since it would be expected to increase program participation and reduce program expenditures relating to reviewing applications. However, **the possibility that some pregnant women and young children might be ineligible for benefits under the new rules is a significant drawback of the demonstration as proposed,** since it would almost certainly harm those affected. A simple remedy for this problem might be to increase the gross income eligibility level for pregnant women and children under age 6 applying to the program (e.g., to 150 or 185 percent of the Federal poverty level).

Despite the many positive aspects of these components of the program, **OTA has some serious reservations about the overall demonstration**

project as proposed. The most troublesome aspects are the prioritized list and the lack of any minimum level below which benefits may not fall.

OTA has made no attempt to decide whether open "rationing" of health care services is desirable, or unnecessary, or inevitable. However, OTA's analysis of Oregon's prioritization process and the resultant list of services suggests that if such a prioritization mechanism is adopted, **classifying health care by general service categories and CT pairs in order to prioritize services is not an especially promising approach.** The level of aggregation required by the CT pairs on Oregon's list means that treatments effective or ineffective for specific patients still cannot be adequately discriminated.

The prioritized list, while a potentially useful source of public opinion information to policymakers, would probably not be an effective internal cost-containment tool. The ranked list does enable overall program expenditures to be controlled by increasing or decreasing benefits. But the list itself does not necessarily encourage cost-efficient health care decisions to be made at the individual level. Diagnostic services, for example, are not prioritized; only existing review or management mechanisms (e.g., management practices of prepaid care providers) would limit their use. And despite the State's attempt to rank aggressive therapies for some diagnoses (e.g., cancer) low when patients are terminally ill, paradoxically the list does not preclude heroic procedures for these patients. A terminally ill patient would still be covered for last-minute life-saving therapies such as treatment for respiratory or cardiac arrest. This option would probably be desired by many patients, but it could not be expected to lower costs. **In fact, assuming Oregon's estimates of the cost savings that could be expected from managed care are correct, managed care might have a much larger effect on internal cost control than the prioritized list.**

A contribution of Oregon's extensive efforts is its demonstration that **outcomes and cost-effectiveness data, while extremely valuable for certain purposes, are inadequate for use as the building-blocks of a ranking system of all services.** More and better information on the outcomes of more health services would improve its usefulness, but it is unlikely that such information will ever be sufficiently comprehensive to enable all health care services to be objectively ranked. The value of such information lies in comparing the usefulness of particular sets of services on the margin—e.g., for use in guidelines, quality-of-care screens, or deciding whether specific individual services should be covered and under what circumstances.

In fact, any comprehensive ranking system would, like Oregon's, need to rely on judgment- and value-based decisionmaking. Because such a list cannot be derived from scientific evidence on effectiveness, outcomes, and cost, and because the replicability of the public meeting and survey information is still open to question, Oregon's list would probably not be exactly reproducible in another State even if the identical process was undertaken. Agreement between two ranked lists might be similar at the bottom (since many people would agree that certain services are ineffective or futile), but differences might be much more substantial further up the list.

Oregon's intensive efforts to make public input a basis for detailed priority-setting demonstrate both the possibilities and the limitations of this process. The State successfully involved providers and consumers in a process to inform public decisionmaking regarding health care priorities. However, the validity of public input in any quantitative ranking is still subject to challenge. The use of public preference data to weight health outcomes has promise, but Oregon's experience suggests that this method is not sufficiently developed to use as the basis for a detailed ranking system ready for implementation.

The information from hearings and public meetings was clearly informative and useful in a ranking process that proved to be unavoidably subjective, but the meetings were not representative of the community despite the efforts of organizers. In fact, the level of effort Oregon undertook implies that proportional representation is probably not a standard possible to achieve under any system.

Any attempt to change the way benefits are defined will involve tradeoffs of gains and losses, and Oregon's proposal cannot be legitimately criticized on the grounds that there is a clear net loss to current beneficiaries. Current beneficiaries lose some current benefits, and a few would almost certainly be harmed in some way by this loss. But beneficiaries would also gain some new services under the demonstration, and they could still receive some uncovered services as charity care. **At a benefit level set at line 587 on the prioritized list,**

the overall net effects of coverage changes on current Medicaid participants cannot be predicted with confidence.

If the benefit threshold changes and reduces the number of covered CT pairs, however, it would become more likely that the proposed program would result in net harm to the health of current beneficiaries. This finding is troubling because the related finding that demonstration costs may have been underestimated raises the likelihood that coverage would be cut during the course of the waiver. (Lower future funding itself would not necessarily mean that current beneficiaries would suffer net harm, because they might have lost some benefits under the current program as well. But lower future funding combined with relatively higher funding required to sustain the new proposal would increase the likelihood of net harm.)

In fact, **the lack of a guaranteed minimum set of benefits below which coverage would not be allowed to fall is the most disturbing aspect of Oregon's proposal.**[19] If program expenditures are higher than predicted, and if the passage of Ballot Measure 5 and internal budget priorities prohibit the State from making up the difference, the Federal Government would be faced with three possibilities. First, it could undertake to fund the difference out-of-pocket, covering Oregon's population at the expense of funding other health care experiments elsewhere in the Nation. Second, it could permit the benefit package to be cut, increasing the likelihood that Medicaid beneficiaries would be harmed by the demonstration. Third, it could withdraw or condition its continued approval and either modify the demonstration substantially or permit it to end, reducing the demonstration's usefulness for the purpose of research.

In summary:

1. Oregon's efforts to develop a proposal to make radical changes to its Medicaid program have yielded valuable information about the usefulness of outcomes data and public input in prioritizing services. The ranking process may also have value as a way to better inform policymakers and to enhance provider and patient awareness. Nonetheless, other States would not be well-advised at this time to rely on Oregon's particular CT-based prioritization method to categorize and rank services. The list itself cannot be applied in other settings with equivalent meaning. Also, the list discriminates poorly among effective services at the individual level, and it would probably not be an effective internal cost-containment mechanism in FFS practice settings.
2. At a coverage level set at line 587, health care access under the proposed program would be improved for newly eligible participants and would not be clearly either better or worse for most current beneficiaries. Current beneficiaries would be more likely to be harmed if the number of covered CT pairs was reduced.
3. If implemented as proposed, the demonstration program may yield relatively little useful information about the different effects of service prioritization, comprehensive managed care, and comprehensive insurance coverage for the poor. A somewhat more modest experiment testing the effects of the managed care and coverage expansions alone would yield more specific information while providing most of the benefits of the current proposal. (The Oregon proposal in its entirety might still be valued as a political experiment, however.)
4. If the full demonstration is approved, some specific components deserve attention to ensure that the program is fully ready to implement. Examples include:
   - The need for detailed instructions for providers on how to use the list;
   - The need to reconcile hospital DRG-based billing, CT pairs, and covered diagnostic services;
   - The need for more extensive baseline data for assessing program effects (particularly in the areas of utilization in the existing prepaid system, utilization and health status of the currently uninsured, and baseline health measures for specified subgroups of patients that could be significantly harmed if their treatments are not covered);
   - The difficulties that public health clinics may face as they try to become part of the managed care system; and
   - The possibility that some pregnant women and young children who would qualify for

[19] In contrast, at present the Federal Government requires that States cover at least some mandatory benefits and populations in order to receive Federal funding.

coverage under the current program would be ineligible under the proposed new eligibility rules.

5. Specifying a threshold below which coverage would not be allowed to drop and gaining greater confidence that Oregon could meet its financial responsibilities under the waiver would also improve the program's chances of success.

REFERENCES

1. Ammann, R., "A Critical Appraisal of Interventional Therapy in Chronic Pancreatitis," *Endoscopy* 23(3): 191-193, 1991.
2. Asch, D. and Patton, J., Philadelphia, PA, information prepared under contract to the Office of Technology Assessment, August 1991.
3. Behrman, R. and Vaughan, V., *Nelson Textbook of Pediatrics, 13th edition*, W.B. Saunders Company, Philadelphia, PA, 1987.
4. Brown, L., "The National Politics of Oregon's Rationing Plan," *Health Affairs* 10(2):28-51, 1991.
5. Callahan, D., "Ethics and Priority Setting in Oregon," *Health Affairs* 10(2):78-87, 1991.
6. Coffman, D., Researcher, Oregon Health Services Commission, Salem, OR, personal communication, Mar. 25, 1991.
7. Coopers & Lybrand, San Francisco, CA, *State of Oregon Cost Effectiveness Analysis for the PCO/HMO Program for the Period March 1985 Through September 1988*, May 19, 1989.
8. Daniels, N., "Is the Oregon Rationing Plan Fair?" *Journal of the American Medical Association* 265(17): 2232-2235, 1991.
9. Dixon, J. and Welch, H., "Priority Setting: Lessons From Oregon," *The Lancet* 337(8754):891-894, 1991.
10. Eddy, D., "Oregon's Plan: Should It Be Approved," *Journal of the American Medical Association* 266(17): 2439-2445, 1991.
11. Fisher, J. and Frost, J., "Epilepsy," *Journal of Nuclear Medicine* 32(4):651-659, 1991.
12. Fox, D. and Leichter, H., "Rationing Care in Oregon: The New Accountability," *Health Affairs* 10(2):7-27, 1991.
13. Granneman, T., "Priority Setting: A Sensible Approach to Medicaid Policy?" *Inquiry* 28(2):300-305, 1991.
14. Hadorn, D., "Setting Health Care Priorities in Oregon: Cost-effectiveness Meets the Rule of Rescue," *Journal of the American Medical Association* 265(17):2218-2225, 1991.
15. Health Insurance Association of America, *Source Book of Health Insurance Data* (Washington, DC: HIAA, 1991).
16. Heginbotham, C., "Rationing," *British Medical Journal* 304(6825):496-499, 1992.
17. Kessinger, A., Nademanee, A., Forman, S., et al. "Autologous Bone Marrow Transplantation for Hodgkin's and Non-Hodgkin's Lymphoma," *Hematology Oncology Clinics of North America* 4(3):577-87, 1990.
18. Kinney, S., Medicaid Coordinator, Public Health Service, Clackamas County Department of Human Services, Oregon City, OR, memoranda to OTA, Jan. 8, 1992, Jan. 21, 1992, and Mar. 13, 1992.
19. Kitzhaber, J., "A Healthier Approach to Health Care," *Issues in Science and Technology* 7(2):59-65, 1990-91.
20. Klein, R., "On the Oregon Trail: Rationing Health Care," *British Medical Journal* 302(6767):496-499, 1991.
21. Lotem, M., Katzenelson, V., Rotem, A., et al., "Impetigo Herpetiformis: A Variant of Pustular Psoriasis or a Separate Entity?" *Journal of the American Academy of Dermatology* 20 (2 pt. 2): 338-41, 1989.
22. National Legal Center for the Medically Dependent and Disabled, Indianapolis, IN, memorandum, Dec. 5, 1991.
23. Oregon Health Services Commission, list of proposed technical changes to the list, FAX to J. Eden, Mar. 30, 1992.
24. Oregon Medical Association, "Bridging the Gap: The Role of Oregon Physicians in Uncompensated Care," Portland, OR, 1989.
25. Physician Payment Review Commission, *Physician Payment Under Medicaid*, Report No. 91-4 (Washington, DC: PPRC, July 1991).
26. Read, L., Director, Prioritized Health Care Systems, Salem, OR, personal communication, Jan. 16, 1992.
27. Relman, A., "The Trouble With Rationing," *New England Journal of Medicine* 323(13):911-913, 1990.
28. Reynolds, J., Department of Pediatrics, Oregon Health Sciences University, Portland, OR, personal communication, July 10, 1991 (from Ehrenhaft contract).
29. Rosenbaum, S., Senior Research Staff Scientist, Center for Health Policy Research, George Washington University, Washington, DC, personal communication, Mar. 6, 1992.
30. Schwartz, W.B. and H.J. Aaron, "The Achilles Heel of Health Care Rationing, *New York Times*, July 7, 1991.
31. Shikles, J., General Accounting Office, testimony before House Energy and Commerce Committee, Subcommittee on Health and the Environment, Sept. 16, serial No. 102-49 (Washington, DC: U.S. Government Printing Office, 1991).

32. Sipes-Metzler, P., Executive Director, Oregon Health Services Commission, Salem, OR, personal communication, Feb. 25, 1991.
33. State of Oregon, Department of Human Resources, Office of Medical Assistance Programs, waiver application submitted to the Health Care Financing Administration, Aug. 16, 1991.
34. State of Oregon, Department of Human Resources, Office of Medical Assistance Programs, *The Oregon Medicaid Demonstration: Waiver Cost Estimate*, prepared by Coopers & Lybrand for the Health Care Financing Administration, Aug. 16, 1991.
35. Steinbrook, R. and Lo, B., "The Oregon Medicaid Demonstration Project—Will It Provide Adequate MedicalCare?" *New England Journal of Medicine* 326(5):340-344,1992.
36. Terhaar, B., Operations Project Manager, Prioritized Health Care, Oregon Medical Assistance Programs, Salem, OR, memorandum to OTA, Jan. 7, 1992.
37. Timm, I., Executive Director, Oregon Primary Care Association, Portland, OR, personal communication, Jan. 16, 1992.
38. U.S. Dept. of Health and Human Services, Public Health Service, Agency for Health Care Policy and Research, "Assessment of Liver Transplantation," Health Technology Assessment Reports, Number 1, Rockville, MD, March 1990.
39. U.S. Department of Health and Human Services, Food and Drug Administration, General and Plastic Surgery Devices Panel, Testimony, Nov. 12-14, 1991.
40. U.S. Department of Health and Human Services, Public Health Service, National Institutes of Health Consensus Development Conference. "Statement: Surgery for Epilepsy, March 19-21, 1990," *Epilepsia* 31(6):806-812, 1990.
41. Vladeck, B., "Unhealthy Rations," *The American Prospect*, summer: 25-33, 1991.
42. Wiener, J., "Oregon's Plan for Health Care Rationing," *The Brookings Review*, winter: 26-31, 1992.
43. Wilensky, G. and Rossitner, L., "Coordinated Care and Public Programs," *Health Affairs* 10(4):62-77, 1991.
44. Wilson, J. (ed.), *Harrison's Principles of Internal Medicine, 12th Edition* (Philadelphia, PA: WB Saunders, 1991).
45. World Health Organization, *International Classification of Diseases, 9th Edition, Clinical Modification* (Ann Arbor, MI: Edwards Brothers, Inc., 1980).
46. Wright, T. and Richart, R., "Role of Human Papillomavirus in the Pathogenesis of Genital Tract Warts and Cancer," *Gynecologic Oncology* 37(2): 151-164, 1990.

U.S. GOVERNMENT PRINTING OFFICE : 1992 O - 322-105 QL 3

PRESIDENT BUSH'S PLAN

The President's Comprehensive Health Reform Program. Washington, D.C.: February 6, 1992. [Pages 1-4, 17-30, and 89-94 are reprinted here.]

The President's Comprehensive Health Reform Program

February 6, 1992

Chapter 1

Overview

HIGHLIGHTS: The President's Plan For Comprehensive Health Care Reform

The President's Plan is a **comprehensive, market-based** reform that builds on the strengths of our current system to provide access to *affordable insurance* for all Americans.

- **The President's plan guarantees access to health insurance for *all* poor families** through a transferable health insurance tax credit (certificate)—available even to those too poor to file taxes—that is large enough to purchase a basic health package ($3,750 for a family).
- **The President's plan provides insurance security for all Americans.** The fear of "job lock"—where workers can't move to another job without losing access to insurance—is eliminated. Limits on the availability of insurance for those with "preexisting conditions" are eliminated.
- **The President's plan will *reduce the cost* of health insurance through major market reforms.** Smaller businesses and individuals would be pooled into larger groups—so they can receive the same favorable health coverage enjoyed by large employers. Millions of people who now can not find affordable insurance will be helped.
- **The President's plan provides new help to the middle class to pay for health care.** Up to $3,750 in health insurance costs can be deducted by families with incomes less than $80,000. Over 90 million Americans will receive new assistance for health costs.
- **The President's plan encourages the growth of coordinated care**—in private plans, Medicare and Medicaid. Laws limiting coordinated care would be prohibited—as would costly State mandated benefit laws. The comprehensive plan encourages individuals, employers and health providers to use coordinated care systems.
- **The President's plan will use the power of an informed marketplace to help control costs** by providing consumers with better information and by giving individuals the resources to choose the coverage that best meets their needs.
- **The President's plan would reduce administrative costs** through regulatory reforms that will streamline the current paperwork maze, and through market reforms that allow small employers to share—and thereby substantially reduce—administrative costs.
- **The President's plan includes major malpractice reform.** A comprehensive liability reform plan is proposed to reduce the costs of malpractice and the resulting defensive medicine that burdens the U.S. health system.
- **The President's plan would expand services in underserved areas.** Many inner city and rural areas have acute shortages of doctors and clinics. The President's budget expands funding for Community Health Centers, Migrant Health Centers and the National Health Service Corps to increase preventive care in these areas.

The President's Plan Does Not:

— include governmental price regulation or rationing of health care;

— burden small business with new and costly mandates that will stifle the creation of new jobs and be passed on in higher product costs and higher taxes for all Americans;

— require massive tax increases like "play or pay" and national health insurance;

— threaten poor older Americans with benefit reductions or premium increases.

The President's Plan builds on a system that provides the world's best health care. The plan provides all Americans access to affordable health care coverage through a transferrable health insurance credit (certificate)—available even to low-income Americans who do not file tax returns—that can be applied to the purchase of a basic health benefit package. To reduce the rapid growth of health spending, the plan makes radical reforms in the health insurance system and includes strong incentives for the development and expansion of coordinated care systems and other efficient arrangements for delivering high quality health care.

Summary Highlights

Expanding Access to Health Care (See Chapters 3 and 4)

Transferrable Health Insurance Credits (certificate) and Deductions—Benefitting Approximately 95 Million Americans—

- A transferrable health insurance credit (certificate) or tax deduction would be available to ensure access to affordable health care coverage for moderate and low-income families. About 95 million Americans would receive assistance. When fully implemented, families with incomes below the tax filing threshold, approximately the poverty line, would receive a credit of up to $3,750, sufficient to purchase basic health benefits. Similarly, individuals would receive $1,250 and two-person families $2,500. A health insurance credit (certificate) or deduction (also up to $3,750 per family) would be available to individuals, two-person, and larger families with annual incomes up to $50,000, $65,000 and $80,000, respectively.

Market Reform—

- *Basic Benefits.*—States would be required to develop a basic health insurance package equal to the value of the health insurance credit. This would enable low-income families to purchase adequate health care coverage.

- *Insurance Security.*—Workers changing jobs would no longer face concerns about "job lock"—the inability to change jobs for fear of losing access to insurance. Health insurers would be required to provide coverage to all employers requesting it. Coverage would be guaranteed, renewable, and preexisting condition limits would be eliminated.

- *Health Insurance Networks (HINs)—Pooled-Purchasing Power.*—When it comes to health insurance, small businesses do not have many of the advantages of large businesses. Large companies can self insure and avoid expensive benefit mandates and premium taxes. Large firms are sold coverage similar to that purchased by small firms, but at much lower prices. A new way of purchasing insurance, HINs would enable small firms to purchase low cost, high quality health insurance. HINs would enable small businesses to buy lower priced insurance by reducing administrative costs and by exempting insurance purchased from HINs from excessive State mandates, anti-managed care laws, and premium taxes. For the first time, groups like the National Federation of Independent Business, National Small Business United, and the U.S. Chamber of Commerce would be able to offer affordable health plans to their members nationwide or join with other groups to increase purchasing power in State or local markets.

- *Insurance Affordability.*—In the near term, premium costs for similar policies sold to firms in a single block of business could vary by no more than 50 percent. A health risk adjustment across insurers would be phased in—removing premium disparities and allowing for plan flexibility within a new insurance market driven by competition on quality and costs.

Containing Health Care Costs (See Chapter 5)

- *Malpractice Reform.*—The threat of malpractice litigation prompts physicians to order tests and perform procedures, enabling them to assert that every effort has been made to provide the best health care. These defensive practices are extremely costly to the system. To address this, the President's plan would provide incentives to States to: (i) eliminate joint and several liability for non-economic damages, (ii) cap non-economic damages, (iii) eliminate rules that permit double recovery, (iv) require structured awards, (v) promote pretrial alternatives, and (vi) implement new procedures to improve quality of care. Also, standards of care, developed in conjunction with the medical community, would be explored as a means to remove physician uncertainty over malpractice litigation.

- *Improving Consumer Information.*—To assist individuals and employers in evaluating various health insurance policies, consumers would have access to information, that would provide information like that in "blue books" on the average cost of services and the quality of care provided by physicians, hospitals, clinical laboratories, and other health care providers. This will help control costs by providing consumers with comparative value information that will enable them to make more informed choices.

- *Reducing Administrative Costs.*—The President's plan will reduce administrative costs, which now total $43 billion a year, by more than 25 percent through electronic billing for providers, electronic benefit cards for policyholders, simplified utilization review, and insurance market reforms.

  Insurance law changes and market reforms will cut back the paperwork blizzard that confronts all insured Americans—and costs billions of dollars. Standardized claims procedures and other reforms will reduce administrative costs. For small employers, administrative costs may account for as much as 40 percent of the cost of insurance purchased. Marketing to and servicing small employer policies is costly. HINs, which unite many purchasers, would reduce the cost of insurance administration and premiums. These costs are usually under 10 percent for large businesses. Federally certified HINs would also be required to adhere to uniform claims processing procedures, a source of additional administrative savings.

- *Expanded Use of Coordinated Care*—

  —In 1990, approximately 40 million Americans were enrolled in a coordinated care system—up from 10 million in 1980. The President's plan encourages broader use coordinated care including preferred provider organizations, point-of-service choice plans, case management, HMOs, and other forms of coordinated care.

  —States would be encouraged to develop coordinated care systems and would be prohibited from having laws that hinder effective operation of these systems. Excessive State-mandated benefits—that increase the cost of insurance—would be prohibited.

  —Medicare reforms would encourage increased coordinated care enrollment and increase incentives for coordinated care systems to contract with Medicare. The President's plan also would make it easier for beneficiaries of retiree group health benefit plans to be served by coordinated care systems.

- *Increased Flexibility for State Programs.*—States are encouraged to implement a coordinated care-based Medicaid program. They also would have the flexibility to redesign their entire health care systems.

  —States could choose to combine current Medicaid funding with the new benefits provided through the health insurance credit (certificate) to develop a single unified health plan for their low-income residents.

  —With the new Federal health insurance credit (certificate), all poor residents are guaranteed basic health coverage—without any further fiscal burden on the States. This will allow States to more effectively allocate their health resources for Medicaid and for the nonpoor population.

- *Cost-Effective Services are Expanded in Underserved Areas.*—The inner city and rural areas have acute shortages of doctors and clinics. The President's fiscal year 1993 Budget expands funding for Community Health Centers, Migrant Health Centers, and the National Health Service Corps to expand preventive care in these areas.

- *Prevention.*—The President's fiscal year 1993 Budget includes $26.4 billion, an increase of nearly $4 billion (18 percent), for preventive health activities. Prevention funding has increased by more than $11 billion (74 percent) since 1989. The President's fiscal year 1993 Budget proposes increases of 18 percent for childhood immunizations and infant mortality reduction, a 27 percent increase for Head Start and Early Childhood Development, a 24 percent increase for breast and cervical cancer mortality prevention, and a 90 percent increase for childhood lead poisoning prevention.

Alternative Approaches (See Chapter 6)

The two alternative approaches to health care reform have fundamental structural weaknesses:

- *Canadian Model.*—In Canada neither providers nor consumers have incentives for efficiency; health care costs are growing faster than in the U.S.; patients endure long lines and wait for surgery and access to advanced technology; and, high quality care is rationed. A Canadian-style plan would require from $250 billion to $500 billion a year in new taxes. For quality care, many Canadians go to the U.S.

- *Play-or-Pay Model.*—"Play-or-pay" would hurt workers by increasing unemployment and forcing employers to cut wages to offset mandated costs. One study indicates that under "play-or-pay" between 400,000 to 700,000 jobs would be lost in the short-run, and up to 2 million jobs could be lost in the long-run. The "play-or-pay" system is structurally unsound and guaranteed to degenerate into national health insurance. Upon enactment, 59 million privately-insured Americans would fall into the public plan and the plan's instability would quickly force universal public coverage. Play-or-pay is a tax on low-wage workers and would result in millions of lost jobs. Finally, at least $37 billion per year in new and additional taxpayer-financed subsidies would be required to adequately fund the public plan.

Chapter 2

Principles for Reform: Building on American Strengths

Overview

- The cost growth of the U.S. health care system is unsustainable, both for individual Americans and for the economy as a whole.
- Even with rapidly increasing health spending, 13 percent of Americans do not have access to health insurance.
- Most federal health care support goes to the non-poor, the segment of society that least needs government assistance.
- Despite the shortcomings of the American system, it delivers the world's best quality care, and the world's most sophisticated health technology.
- Reform should preserve the strengths of the U.S. system while addressing its weaknesses. Reforms should not destroy its incentives for choice, quality, and innovation.
- The President's Principles for Reform establish guidelines for a comprehensive restructuring of a market-based health system.

Americans need and deserve adequate access to affordable high quality medical care. Health care in the United States has evolved into the world's most sophisticated and advanced system.

Our health care system has strengths and weaknesses. A clear understanding of both is essential in guiding policy development.

Principles for Reform

The President has determined that several principles should guide the development of a comprehensive approach to health reform. The reform *should:*

- Build on the strengths of an American health system that provides the highest quality health care in the world;
- Assure access to basic health insurance for Americans, and increase the affordability of such coverage;
- Promote consumer choice to ensure that the health care system continues to respond to the needs and concerns of Americans;
- Strengthen market incentives for providers and health plans to improve quality while controlling costs;
- Emphasize prevention and personal responsibility;
- Reduce abuse and wasteful excess;
- Meet the requirements of fiscal responsibility and budget discipline.

The approach *should not:*

- Force the American people to give up the choice and diversity that makes the American health system unique;
- Lead to comprehensive governmental price controls and rationing health care by government;
- Create new spending mandates for States and employers;
- Require a net increase in taxes; or
- Threaten older Americans with the prospect of either benefit cuts or premium increases.

These tests cannot be met by either "Canadian-style" or "Play-or-Pay" approaches to reform. Such approaches necessarily involve major tax increases, comprehensive governmental price controls, or rationing.

Understanding the Cost and Access Problems

Health care costs are increasing too fast and too many Americans have inadequate access to health care. The causes of the cost and access problems are complex. Unfortunately, simplistic proposals, such as reducing administrative costs to fund a universal access program, are unrealistic (Doherty, 1991).

Moreover, the cost and access problems are not easily solved simultaneously. The political system tends to trade cost-control for access, and vice-versa. Addressing the access problem inescapably means re-allocating tens of billions of dollars each year. Addressing the cost problem requires correcting perverse incentives and market distortions—to encourage more efficient behavior by individuals, insurers, and health providers.

Unsustainable Cost Growth.—Currently, total health care expenditures are about 13 percent of the Gross Domestic Product (GDP)—up from less than 6 percent of GDP only three decades ago. If the current system continues unchanged, health care could consume over 16 percent of GDP by the year 2000, and between 27 and 43 percent of GDP by 2030 under mid-range and high-range projections (Sonnefeld et al., 1991).

These costs are shouldered by everyone—individuals, business and government. The federal government is spending increasing proportions of the federal budget on mandatory health outlays. Before the year 2000, health entitlement programs (Medicare and Medicaid) will surpass Social Security as the single largest component of federal spending. Federal Medicaid spending alone has grown from $14 billion in 1980 to $37 billion in 1989 to a projected $84 billion in 1993. These figures reflect a 43 percent increase for last year alone, an increase of 227 percent since 1989, and an increase of 600 percent since 1980.

Medicare spending will have grown from $34 billion in 1980 to about $131 billion by 1993—an increase of nearly 300 percent. Unrestrained, Medicare will grow at an average rate of 12 percent per year from 1993

Chart 1. HEALTH SPENDING IS PROJECTED TO REACH 16.4% OF GDP BY 2000 -- RISING FROM 5.3% IN 1960

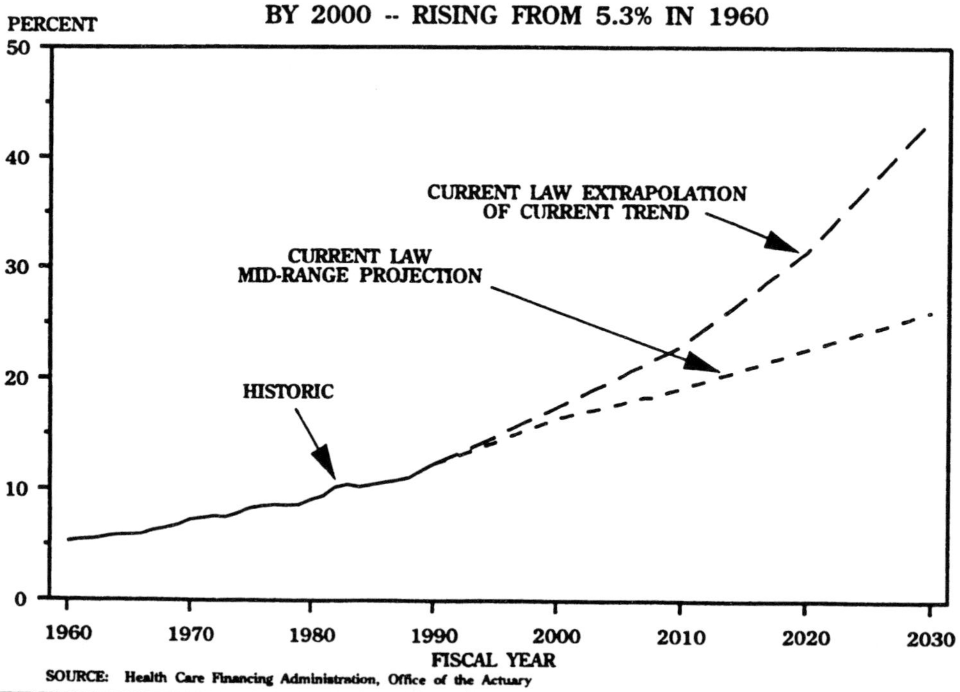

SOURCE: Health Care Financing Administration, Office of the Actuary

Chart 2. PROJECTED SOCIAL SECURITY AND HEALTH ENTITLEMENTS FOR 1990-2030

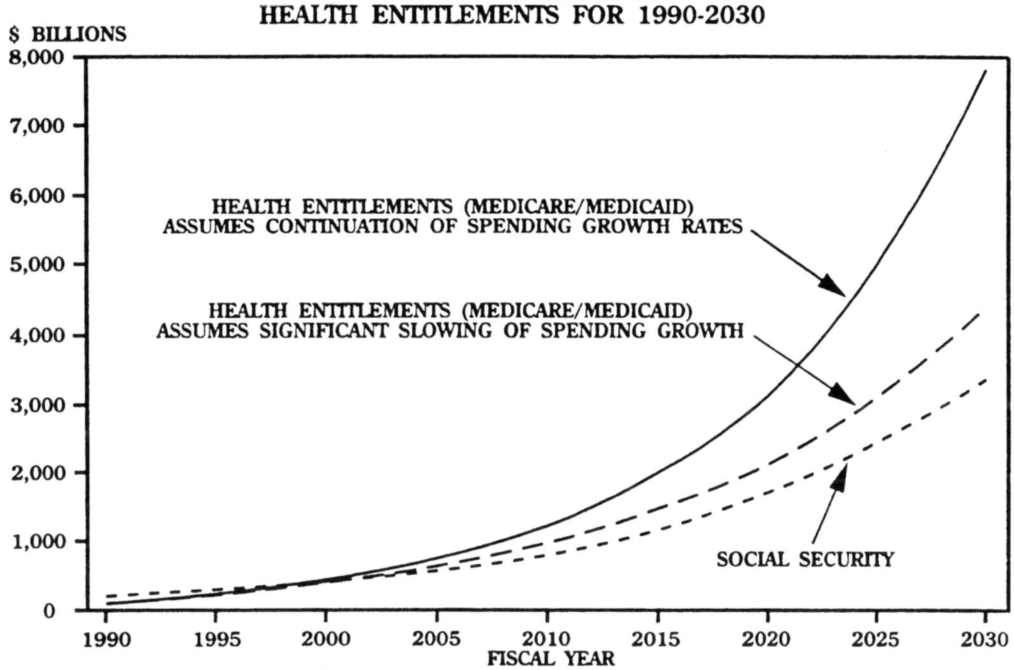

Note: Health entitlement projections based on data provided by Health Care Financing Administration, Office of the Actuary, October, 1991.

through 1997. By 2025, Medicare is expected to exceed 27 percent of the federal budget.

Even if it were possible to sustain health spending at nearly 30 cents of every dollar, it is difficult to imagine who would pay these enormous costs. Most individuals already feel that they are overburdened with health care costs. Businesses are spending increasing percentages of wages and other compensation on health care premiums—currently in excess of 100 percent of after-tax profits.

Clearly, health care costs must be contained, both in public programs and in the private sector. Neither individuals, business, nor government can afford to pay for the currently projected growth.

Inadequate Access Despite Increasing Spending.—Despite this rapid rise in health care spending, 13 percent of Americans—34.7 million—are without health care insurance.

Most of the uninsured are lower-income Americans—30 percent of the uninsured have incomes below the poverty level, and 32 percent have incomes between 100 and 200 percent of poverty (Needleman et al., 1990). Despite this, most of the massive federal spending on health care goes to the non-poor. In 1992, only 21 percent of total federal health care spending is estimated to be spent for the poor. Almost 90 percent of Medicare spending goes to individuals above the poverty level.

Uninsured Americans receive some health care, either by paying for it out-of-pocket, or in the form of "uncompensated" or "charity" care (Needleman et al., 1990). "Uncompensated" care is not free, in the sense that insured individuals must pay higher fees and thus higher premiums, and hospitals receive public (such as Medicare and Medicaid "disproportionate share" payments and non-profit tax treatment—now over $15 billion per year) and private (such as charitable contributions) subsidies to cover the costs.

The uninsured are more likely to receive health care in hospital emergency rooms, rather than in physicians' offices and clinics (NMES, 1987). This form of care can be harmful to the individual, who may only

Chart 3. BUSINESS SPENDING ON HEALTH PREMIUMS

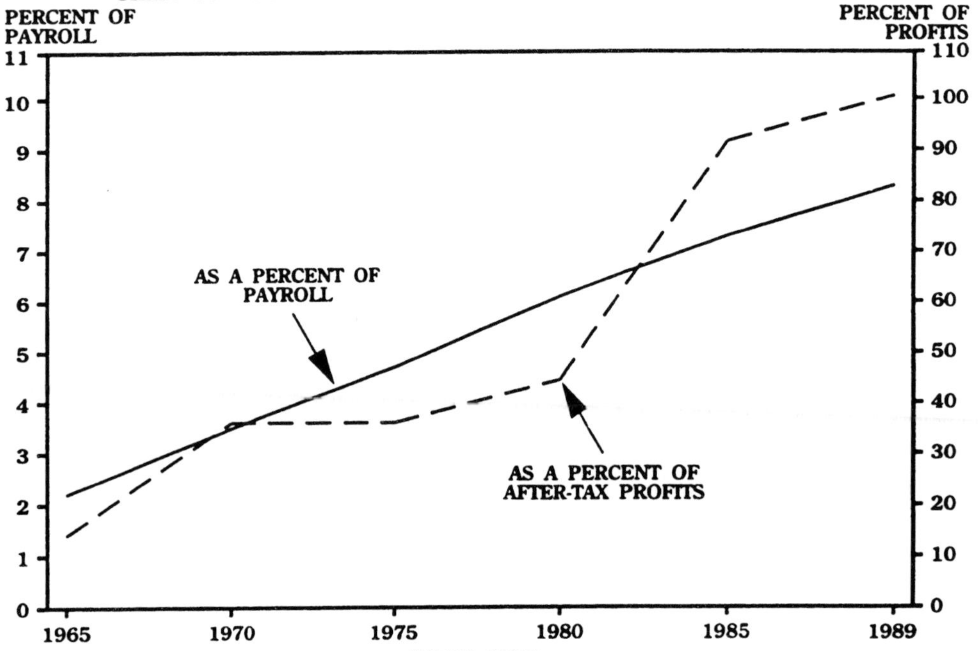

SOURCE: Health Care Financing Administration, Office of the Actuary

receive care for serious illnesses instead of coordinated, preventive care from a physician familiar with the patient. Emergency room care is also a more expensive and inefficient use of resources, since emergency room visits are much more costly than physician office visits.

No Easy Solution.—Rising health care expenditures are a function of many interrelated factors. These include: general inflation, population growth, relative aging of the population, growth in volume and intensity of medical care (HCFA, 1989), and "cost shifts" that re-allocate the costs of caring for the uninsured. The resulting medical inflation is consistently more than double the growth rate of the Consumer Price Index.

General inflation, population growth and relative aging necessarily occur. Other factors can be addressed, such as the growth in the intensity of medical services and of preventable illnesses. Despite increasing per capita U.S. costs, utilization as measured by hospital admissions, length of hospital stay, and medical visits per capita have been level or increased only slightly. This suggests that the intensity (e.g., more tests and procedures per hospital stay or per office visit) is the primary cause of spending growth. International comparisons confirm this conclusion (Schieber et al., 1991).

In addressing the growth in service intensity, it is difficult to know how much of the increase is due to advances in medical technology, and how much is attributable to excessive defensive medicine, poor health care management, and gaming of a public price-regulated system.

For preventable illnesses and conditions, though, the issues are more apparent. For example, at 13.8 per 100,000, the male homicide rate is more than 12 times that of Germany and 5 times that of Canada. More than 200,000 AIDS cases have been reported in the US. In 1989, the rate of incidence of AIDS was more than three times that of Canada and six times that of then-West Germany. And, there are about 375,000 drug-exposed babies in this country. This problem

Chart 4. MEDICARE FISCAL FINANCING GAP

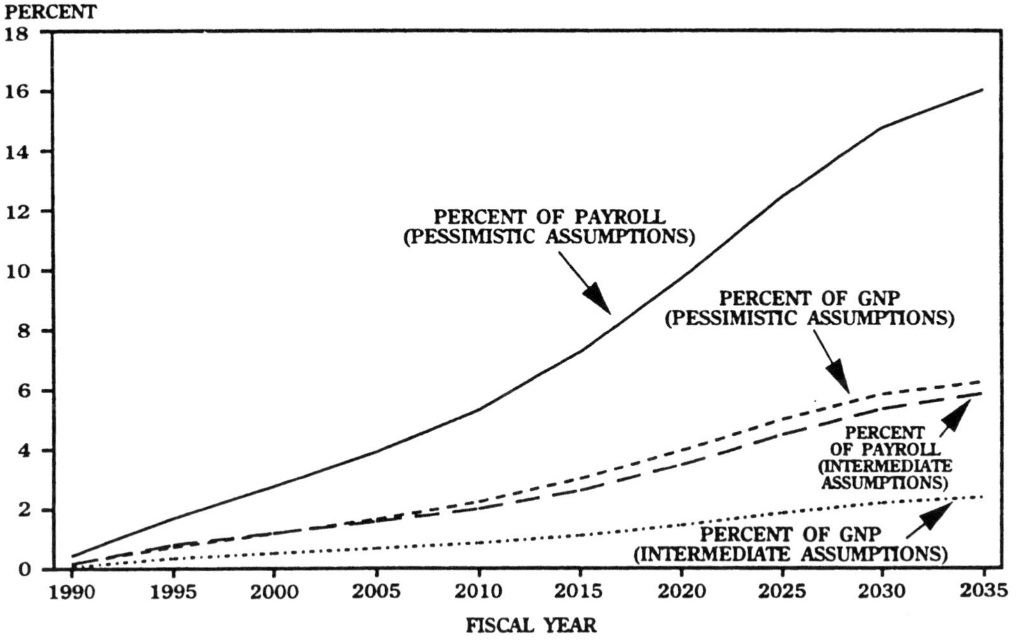

Note: The Medicare Fiscal Financing Gap is the projected HI trust fund deficit and SMI revenue requirements above 1987 levels.
Source: Holohan, J. and J. L. Palmer, Journal of Health Politics, Policy and Law, Spring 1988

is negligible in most other countries (Schwartz, 1991).

Rising costs are also the result of market distortions. Because medical treatment is largely in the hands of doctors and hospitals (who have financial and defensive incentives to provide more medical care) and not the consumer, consumer-based market discipline has been weak.

Under the current system, Americans with insurance are often overinsured and have few incentives to use medical care prudently. Instead, consumers tend to be risk-averse where health is concerned. Insulated from the real cost of medical treatment by employer and government subsidized insurance, Americans tend to over-consume health care. Moreover, because insurance itself is so highly subsidized for most Americans, they have little reason to prefer forms of coverage that are more efficient (e.g., coverage with higher cost sharing or coordinated care coverage)

The health care market is further distorted by limited consumer information about the treatments patients receive and the efficiency of their care. Consumers and large purchasers currently have few objective sources of information on which to base cost and quality comparisons.

The problems of access and cost are inextricably linked. Access ultimately is an issue of affordability. Many low-income Americans need help to be able to afford coverage. Cost growth needs to be slowed to assure continued affordability for others. Thus, the access and cost problems must be addressed together in a comprehensive series of reforms. Only then can all Americans begin to enjoy efficient health care at affordable prices.

[SUBSEQUENT MATERIAL FROM THIS POINT TO PAGE 16 OMITTED]

Chapter 3

Expanding Access and Increasing Affordability Through Market Reform

Overview

The President's proposal for reform of the health insurance market will make coverage more secure, available, and affordable for millions of Americans.

- Everyone—young and old, healthy and sick—will benefit from the assurance of the availability of affordable health insurance regardless of future changes in their health.
- Workers will be able to change jobs without fear that insurance coverage will be denied due to a preexisting illness.
- Premium costs will be reduced by as much as 20 percent for at least 70 million workers and their dependents affected by small group reforms.
- Five million Americans currently without health insurance will have insurance as a result of these market reforms.

The market reform proposal has four major components. These components will:

- Assure availability and security of coverage. Insurers would offer coverage without regard to health status. Coverage would be renewable, and preexisting condition limits would be eliminated. Employers would provide information and facilitate access to group coverage to all employees and dependents, but would not be required to administer or contribute to the cost of coverage. Further, colleges and universities would provide continued access to group coverage to recent graduates and other students for six months after leaving school.
- Assure affordability of coverage for individuals and small businesses through broad risk pooling. Insurers would participate in broad pooling arrangements to spread health risks evenly across insurers and thereby allow insurers to charge uniform premiums for the sick and the healthy. On an interim basis, pending phased implementation of this new system, insurers would be subject to limits on their ability to vary premiums.
- Encourage group purchasing of health insurance by small businesses to give them the same cost advantage enjoyed by larger businesses. Small businesses could pool their purchasing power through Health Insurance Networks (HINs). This will help small businesses negotiate discounts and save on overhead and marketing costs. Moreover, the Employee Retirement Income Security Act (ERISA) preemption that allows larger self-insured firms to avoid cost-increasing State laws will be extended to small businesses purchasing coverage through HINs. For the first time national and regional small business associations and other groups will also be able to establish inter- and intra-State HINs to better assist their membership.
- Give health plans increased flexibility to control costs. Health plans would be protected from mandated benefit and "anticooridnated care" laws that hinder designing cost-effective benefit packages to meet individual and family needs and drive up costs. Health plans would also be protected from laws and regulations that hinder innovative cost control measures, such as utilization review and selective contracting.

An important benefit of these reforms is strengthening significantly competition among health plans. In today's environment, health plans can gain a significant premium cost advantage by avoiding high risk individuals and groups. Under the Administration's reform proposal, such "risk avoidance" will be stopped. As a result, competition will focus on price, value, and quality, leading to long-term gains in efficiency and improvements in quality.

Strengths and Weaknesses of the Current System

153 million working age Americans and their dependents—62 percent of the total population—are covered primarily through private health insurance. Most of these are covered through employment. This system has worked well because employment can be a stable basis for risk-pooling, particularly for medium and large firms and because substantial administrative savings and economies of scale are possible through employment-based group coverage.

Special Problems for Small Business.—While generally successful, there are significant problems with the current system, especially for small group and individual coverage. Workers at small firms are much more likely to be uninsured than workers at medium and large firms.

This disparity in coverage reflects three main problems. First, many small businesses cannot afford to provide costly fringe benefits. Second, health insurance is more costly for small businesses due to (i) higher overhead and marketing costs and (ii) costs resulting from State mandated benefit laws and premium taxes which generally do not apply to self-insured coverage ("ERISA exempt" from State insurance laws) typically provided by larger businesses. Finally, the market for health insurance for small business is in turmoil due to risk selection.

Erosion of Risk Pooling.—For people with serious illness, the cost of medical care can easily consume a substantial share of family income. With broad risk pooling, through insurance, the costs of illness are spread across a broad pool of premium payers, making costs more uniform, thus more affordable. The value of risk pooling is particularly great because spending on health care is highly skewed. At any given time, most of the population is healthy, and has little need for medical care. However, a small percent of the population is

Chart 13. INSURANCE COVERAGE OF THE POPULATION UNDER 65

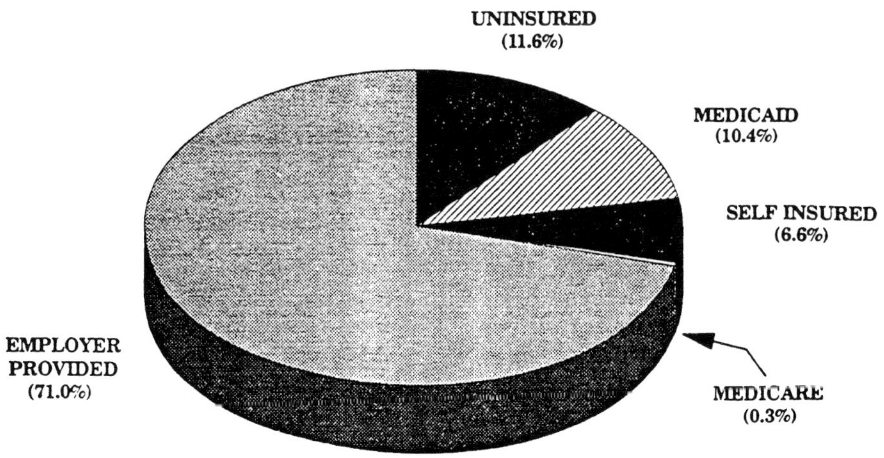

SOURCE: Agency for Health Care Policy and Research, NMES, 1987

Table 3–1. Number of Uninsured Workers and Dependents By Establishment Size—1987

(Source: AHCPR, 1991)

Establishment Size	Number of Workers and Dependents	Percent of Workers and Dependents	Number Uninsured	Percent Uninsured	Percent of All Working Uninsured
Less than 25	74.2 m	44	17.2 m	23.1	68
26–100	34.6 m	21	4.3 m	12.3	17
Greater than 100	59.2 m	35	3.9 m	6.6	15
Totals	168.0 m	100	25.4 m	15.1	100

Note: Interventions affecting groups below a threshold, such as a hundred workers, will generally affect all *firms* below the threshold, as well as workers in establishments below that threshold, where firms have establishments in one or more States that fall below the threshold. Even limiting to the strict "firm"-based definition of size it is estimated that about 70 million workers and their dependents fall below a size of 100.)

seriously ill, and requires extremely costly care. The top 5 percent of the population in terms of health care use (i.e., the 95th percentile) have per capita health expenditures ($7,100) 26 times greater than costs ($270) for people at the midpoint of the population in terms of health care use (i.e., the 50th percentile).

Insurance risk pooling is valuable for everyone because even those who are healthy today may develop a serious illness at some point in their life. However, *risk selection* can undermine insurance as a pooling mechanism. Risk selection occurs whenever a particular pool has a skewed selection of risks. Such a pool will have a higher or lower average per capita cost when compared with other pools.

Risk selection is extremely difficult to prevent. This is because healthy and sick people have different needs for health insurance and choose different health plans to meet these needs. Generally, healthy people are attracted to leaner benefit packages (higher cost sharing, fewer covered benefits) because they expect that they will not have a need for more extensive coverage. In contrast, sicker people prefer richer benefit packages because of their expected needs. Moreover, certain features of coordinated care, such as a greater emphasis on preventive care, could be more attractive to the healthy. As a result, sick and healthy people will

Table 3–2. Distribution of Per Capita Health Spending By Age and Within Age Categories, 1987

(Source: AHCPR, 1991)
(In dollars)

Age	Mean	25th Percentile	50th Percentile	75th Percentile	95th Percentile
0–6 years	1,133	50	180	600	3,800
7–18 years	643	15	120	400	2,500
19–24 years	839	0	150	550	4,000
25–54 years	1,238	50	260	860	5,500
55–64 years	2,469	160	570	1600	11,424
Greater than 65 years	4,551	330	960	3,500	22,528
Total	1,591	50	270	1,000	7,100

sort themselves into different plans, even without any effort at selective marketing by insurers. The result will be that sick people will face high premiums due to the non-random distribution of health risks.

Risk selection is especially likely in the market for small group because a single small business cannot serve as a stable risk pool. One or two sick workers can greatly increase average per employee health benefit costs. Insurers originally combined many small businesses into a single risk pool and charged all members of the insured group a uniform (or age-adjusted) premium that did not vary based on health risk. This approach helped to make coverage affordable for individuals with chronic illnesses.

However, in today's market, some insurers have developed strategies for attracting low risk groups, while leaving higher-risk groups without coverage or with unacceptably high premiums. Favorable risk selection provides an opportunity to make a profit by offering low premiums to attract healthy groups while discontinuing coverage (or increasing premiums to a prohibitive level) once a group becomes more costly. Some insurers are also using medical information (health screening) to exclude higher-risk groups or individuals from coverage. Some insurers exclude preexisting medical conditions from coverage. In some cases, even individuals with relatively mild health problems have been denied coverage.

As some insurers succeed in attracting low-risk groups and avoiding high-risk groups, other insurers face an upward premium spiral, and must risk select to keep up with competitive pressures. Similar—possibly even more severe—problems affect the market for individual non-group coverage.

These problems are increasingly common. Moreover, there appears to be no natural end to current trends. Thus, if left unchecked, broad risk pooling seems likely to unravel in the small group and individual coverage markets. If this were to happen, health insurance would become unaffordable for many Americans—especially those most in need of coverage.

Assuring Availability of Coverage

The President's reform proposal contains several initiatives to assure that health insurance coverage is readily available. These reforms apply broadly to all private health insurance coverage regardless of group size and to coverage provided by employers who self-insure.

Prohibition on Exclusion from Coverage Due to Health Status.—All insurers wishing to sell group health insurance in a State would be required as a condition of doing business to (i) accept every employer group in the State that applies for coverage and (ii) provide coverage to individuals within an employer group. In addition, all employers would be prohibited from excluding any individual from health insurance coverage for reasons of health status. Finally, any insurer selling coverage to individuals receiving health insurance tax credits would be prohibited from excluding any credit recipient from coverage.

Guaranteed Renewability.—Insurers wishing to sell group coverage in a State would be required to renew coverage for a group except in the case of nonpayment of premiums, fraud, or misrepresentation.

Portable Access.—Under the proposal, workers would be able to change jobs without loss of coverage due to a preexisting coverage exclusion. Currently, some health insurance does not cover costs related to any illness or disease diagnosed prior to the initial date of coverage. As a result, many working Americans with chronic illnesses have been afraid to change jobs for fear that the insurance provided at their new job would no longer cover their medical expenses.

The use of preexisting condition exclusions would be eliminated. This will assure that all workers can change jobs without losing access.

Access to Group Coverage for Workers and Dependents.—All employers would be required to provide information on affordable basic health insurance plans available in their respective States. This information is to be prepared and provided by State insurance commissioners. This will expand access to plans that provide individual and family coverage to all employees—but employers would not be required to administer a health plan or make any contribution towards the cost of health coverage. States would assist employers by making available information regarding the availability and cost of "basic" coverage from various health plans. Employers would be required only to arrange for deduction of premiums from paychecks if employees so requested, but would have no other administrative burden. Health insurance networks—group purchasing arrangements for small employers—would facilitate this process and it is anticipated that most small employers would join a HIN (see below).

Access to Group Coverage for College Graduates.—To help fill a significant uninsured gap for new work force entrants, all colleges and universities that provide group coverage to students would be required to offer extended group coverage for new graduates and other students for six months after they leave undergraduate and graduate programs. The college or university need not make any contribution toward the cost of coverage under such a plan.

Assuring Access to Coverage for Individuals and Families Receiving Health Insurance Tax Credits (certificates).—Each State would define a "basic" benefit package or a series of packages with an estimated actuarial value equal to the value of the health tax credit. A number of benefits packages are provided as illustrative examples (*See* Table 3–3).

Any health plan in a given State could offer the State-defined "basic" benefit package to credit recipients and to others. To ensure that credit recipients have a variety of plans available, if no insurers offer the "basic plan" the State insurance commissioner could require two or more health plans with a substantial market share to offer the "basic" benefit plan. Health plans could charge a market price for the "basic" benefit package.

The State and Federal Governments would implement outreach programs with the goal of securing 100 percent participation among credit eligibles. Broader participation would help prevent unnecessary and costly emergency care by encouraging primary and preventative care.

Table 3–3. **Basic Benefit Plan Examples for Approximate Amount of the Full Health Insurance Tax Credit in 1993**

(Plans are illustrative only—States will design benefits)

"Coordinated" Fee-For-Service Plans

Plan A—Unlimited inpatient hospital, inpatient physician care, prescription drug coverage, 3 ambulatory physician visits and associated diagnostic services with a $10 co-pay per visit.

Plan B—Unlimited inpatient hospital, inpatient physician care, and 5 ambulatory physician visits and associated diagnostic services with a $10 co-pay per visit.

Plan C—Unlimited inpatient hospital, inpatient physician care, 10 ambulatory physician visits and associated diagnostic services with a $10 co-pay per visit.

Plan D—Inpatient hospital up to 15 days, inpatient physician, lab, emergency room, and ambulatory physician visits and associated diagnostic services covered for $5 fee per visit for the first three physician visits, then a 10 percent co-pay up to a $500 out-of-pocket limit.

Plan E—Includes all services under Plan D, but with a 20 percent co-pay on physician visits after 3 visits.

Plan F—Includes all services and co-payment under Plan E, but would offer prescription drug coverage.

Model HMO Benefit Plan

Plan G—Unlimited inpatient hospital and inpatient physician services, emergency room, and unlimited ambulatory physician visits with associated diagnostic services (subject to a $10 copayment), prenatal care, and prescription drugs (subject to a $5 copayment).

In cases where a hospital emergency room is an individual's first point of contact with the system, rotating assignment would be used to enroll an uninsured credit-eligible individual to a specific health plan if the individual were unable to make a choice. So for example, a homeless person entering the hospital and having no preference for any carrier would be assigned to an insurer by rotation and the credit would automatically flow to the insurer.

Assuring Affordability of Coverage Through Risk-Pooling

As noted above, broad risk pooling is essential if health insurance is to be affordable for the sick as well as for the healthy. The President's market reform proposal provides both interim and longer-term solutions. Transition measures, including "premium bands" would be implemented immediately to stabilize the small group market pending full implementation of longer-term measures.

In the near term, premium bands will spread risks within an insurer's pool by limiting the difference in premiums that an insurer may charge to groups with different health risks. This will make coverage less costly in the near term for higher risk groups. However, premium bands may be unstable in the longer term. Because an insurer would be unable to vary premiums to reflect fully actual differences in expected health care costs, healthy enrollees would have incentives to shift to other insurers that have fewer sick people in their pools.

Health risk pooling would assure affordable coverage over the long term both for small groups (under 100 employees) and for individuals and families receiving health insurance tax credits. Under this approach, health plans insuring a sicker than average population would receive a net transfer from the risk pool while other insurers will be net payers into the pool. This will assure stable risk pooling over the long-term and will level the competitive playing field among insurers to focus competition on efficiency and quality.

The health risk pooling approach would be implemented immediately for tax credit recipients and would be phased-in over a five year period for small group coverage. Delayed implementation in the small group market is appropriate to permit an orderly transition and to avoid undue disruption of existing arrangements. Immediate implementation of health risk pooling would, however, be possible for credit recipients since this is a new market.

Transition Measures for Small Group Coverage.—These transition measures would apply to all insurance provided to small businesses employing fewer than 100 workers. The premium standards (or "bands") limit variation in premiums within each insurance company's overall set of offerings. They would not constrain premium variation between insurers. The premium standards would be temporary and would be phased-out with full implementation of a system to equalize risk among insurers.

- *Premium Standards Across and Within Demographic Categories.*—Insurers could vary premiums by age. This means that younger workers would not be forced to subsidize older workers (who typically have higher income and higher health risks). But, insurers would be limited in their ability to vary premiums based on health status or prior use of care. Premiums could not differ by more than 50 percent within age/sex categories in the first year decreasing to 35 percent by the third year.
- *Rate of Increase Standard for Renewal Premiums.*—Insurers could not increase premiums excessively for groups with deteriorating health status or claims experience. The maximum percent increase in renewal premiums would be set at 5 percent plus the percent change in the "base premium rate." The "base premium rate" is the lowest premium the insurer could have charged under the relevant block of business for a group with similar demographic characteristics, excluding factors related to health status, claims experience, industry, occupation, or duration of coverage.
- *Premium Standards Across "Blocks of Business".*—Premiums could vary by up to 20 percent across different blocks of business. A carrier may establish different blocks of business: (i) for business acquired

from another carrier, (ii) for business obtained through a distinct system of marketing (e.g., brokers vs. associations), and (iii) for business obtained through different associations (for example, HINS). Carriers could establish three different blocks of business for each of the three reasons, for a total of nine different blocks of business.

- *Enforcement.*—An independent actuary would certify compliance. Failure to have a valid certification would trigger a violation. The State enforcement agency could conduct an investigation to verify certifications.

States could also implement a prospective reinsurance or risk allocation system on an interim basis to pool risks among insurers.

- Under a *prospective reinsurance* model, an insurer could obtain optional reinsurance for any group or newly eligible group member. The primary insurer would be liable for an individual's health costs up to a threshold amount. Above the threshold, the reinsurance program would be responsible for most of the cost. The program would be funded by reinsurance premiums and an assessment on all small group insurers.
- Under *risk allocation*, each insurance carrier would have a quota of assigned risks based on the carrier's market share. Insurers could initially refuse to provide coverage based on health risk. However, the rejected group or individual would have a right to select any insurer from an assigned risk list maintained by the State provided that the insurer's allotment has not been filled.

Health Risk Pools.—Each State would implement two broad health risk pools: one for small group coverage and another for coverage provided to individuals and families receiving transferrable health insurance tax credits. These pools would spread risk broadly across all health plans providing such coverage within a State.

Under this system, health plans that cover a sicker than average population would receive a net payment from the pool, while other health plans would be net payers into the pool. Payments from and to the pool would be based on the difference between the expected health care costs for the entire covered population and the expected health care costs for the population covered by the insurer.

As a result, insurers would no longer have an incentive to deny coverage to individuals with chronic disease. Moreover, insurers would be able to provide coverage at a near uniform premium for the sick and the healthy. The health risk pool would have this effect because a health plan that enrolls an individual with a high-cost chronic illness will receive a transfer of funds from the pool equal to the difference between the expected health care costs for the individual involved and the average expected cost. This moves the system back toward a flexible community rate—where choice in plans is maintained, but risk is truly pooled.

A number of methods have been developed for measuring expected health care costs based on the health characteristics of the population involved. These methods include the Diagnostic Cost Group system developed at Boston University and the Ambulatory Care Group system developed at Johns Hopkins. Other systems are available for use by the States. The Department of Health and Human Services would fund research to refine these systems and to develop improved systems for adjusting for health risk. The Department would also provide technical support to assist States in establishing the risk pools.

As is true for any system that varies payment according to health status, some degree of overreporting is possible, but such overreporting would not have an adverse effect on the pooling system unless some insurers were more successful at it than others. If necessary, to prevent this outcome, a random sample audit of insurance claims and other records could be used to verify the accuracy of health risk assignments.

The health risk pools for small group coverage and for credit recipients would be similar in most respects. Participation would be required for all health plans providing coverage to small groups and to credit recipients. If an individual purchases the basic benefit package, the insurance company receives the credit plus or minus an amount related to the individual's age (and possibly gender). These adjustments mitigate the problem of adverse selection for the basic benefit packages.

Amounts received by an insurance company would also be subject to health status adjustments. On an annual basis, each credit recipient would be assigned to a health status category. Each health category would have a corresponding weight based on expected health care costs defined relative to the population average. Each insurer would calculate an average weight for all credit recipients covered by the insurer. Insurers with an average weight greater than the statewide average would receive net transfers from the pool, while insurers with an average weight less than the statewide average would be required to make contributions to the pool.

States would implement pools for credit recipients simultaneously with federal implementation of the transferable health tax credit system. Implementation of health risk pools for small group coverage would occur over a five-year period on a phased-in basis, starting in the third year after enactment of the reform proposal. Transition measures, including premium limits, would apply in the small group market in the interval.

Encouraging Group Purchasing For Small Employers: Health Insurance Networks

The President's reform proposal will help reduce insurance costs for small businesses by encouraging group purchasing. Group purchasing can reduce health insurance costs by as much as 16 percent through efficiencies of scale, lower administrative costs, and through pooling of purchasing power that helps small businesses negotiate better rates with insurers.

Cleveland's Council of Smaller Enterprises (COSE) operates a successful health insurance group purchasing program for small firms. While COSE has been successful, surprisingly little of this type of group purchasing is going on nationwide. The reforms described in the preceding sections will spur group purchasing by protecting against some of the abusive practices that have daunted some local purchasing groups. Additional assistance is provided as well to encourage rapid formation of group purchasing arrangements.

ERISA Reform/Incentives for Group Purchasing.—The federal preemption of State regulation of self-insured health benefit plans under ERISA that benefits virtually all large employers would be extended to small businesses that purchase coverage on a group basis through a Health Insurance Network (HIN). This would protect against (i) State mandated benefit laws that require firms to provide certain costly services, (ii) excessive State health insurance premium taxes, (iii) and State anti-coordinated care laws. These laws typically increase premium costs by 2 to 5 percent. HINs could also still self-insure, but in this case, enhanced insurance State solvency and increased Department of Labor standards would apply to ensure the economic stability of the plans.

Functions.—HINs could contract with insurers to provide coverage to members or could self-insure subject to enhanced State solvency

Table 3–4. **Savings From Small Market Reforms: Administrative and Bargaining Effects**

(Expressed as percent of total premium, by firm size)

Firm Size Claims	Total Savings
<4	15.9
5–9	13.1
10–19	10.9
20–49	8.5
50–99	6.0

regulation (if State solvency standards are insufficient, Department of Labor solvency standards would operate as a backup oversight system). All federally approved HINs would be required to offer at least one coordinated care option and to use a standard claims form.

Organization.—HINs would be structured as non-profit voluntary membership organizations with a board of directors elected by the membership. HINs would be registered and qualified, as applicable, by a State agency or by the Department of Labor. There would be no limit on the number of HINs that could be established in a given area. HINs could be established along the lines of professional societies, industry, or trade associations and would be subject to all of the market reforms listed in the preceding sections. By buying coverage through a HIN, small businesses would be able to achieve more effective purchasing power in the market, thereby helping reduce the cost of insurance to their employees.

HINs will provide the mechanism for pooling large numbers of individuals and employees of small firms, an advantage that is now only available to large companies. These plans have not grown in the past because of State laws. To allow for federal preemption, plans had to "self insure". Small groups have difficulty raising capital to self insure risk. This system allows "imputed ERISA exemptions"—small firms can join together without self-insuring, and have insurers carry the risk.

Intrastate and Regional Pooling.—The State or Federal government could certify an HIN. For example, Pennsylvania (or the Federal government) could certify an HIN of 1,000 small employers who pooled market power to negotiate with local providers in Philadelphia, or the Federal government could certify a similar HIN for the Philadelphia area (PA, NJ, and DE) that would pool market power in the entire region.

Multi State Pooling.—HINs would allow for the first time, multi State pooling of small firms. Groups like NFIB, National Small Business United and The Chamber of Commerce (or any other group) could offer the same basic plans to members nationwide. In the past, State barriers have prevented such plans. This will simplify marketing and administration and sharply reduce costs.

Increasing Flexibility for Health Plans

States would no longer be allowed to mandate benefits that unduly limit flexibility for health plans, thereby increasing health care costs and restrict coordinated care.

State Mandated Benefits.—Many State laws require insurers to cover certain optional or ancillary services. These mandated benefits drive up premium costs up by at least 3 to 5 percent.

Provisions that Restrict Coordinated Care.—Some State laws impose restrictions which prevent the development of coordinated care—and the competitive pressure it imposes on fee-for-service providers. Anti-managed care laws include:

- *Restrictions on reimbursement rates or selective contracting:* Laws that restrict the ability of a carrier to negotiate reimbursement rates with providers or contract selectively with a limited number of providers.
- *Restrictions on differential financial incentives:* Laws that limit the financial incentives that a health benefit plan may require a beneficiary to pay when a non-plan provider is used on a non-emergency basis.
- *Restrictions on utilization review:* Laws that (a) prohibit utilization review of any or all treatments and conditions, (b) require that such review be made by an in-State physician or by a physician in a particular specialty, (c) require the use of specified standards of health care practice in such reviews, or require the disclosure of the specific criteria used in such reviews, or (d) require payment to providers for the expense of responding to utilization review requests.

Federal/State Relationships

Most of the reforms described in the preceding section would be implemented by the States. Thus, the responsibility for regulating health insurance would remain primarily with the States. However, federal legislation would be amended to provide States with clear incentives to enact laws that will achieve national goals.In many cases, as with HIN certification and oversight, there would be backup federal certification and oversight procedures.

Under this approach, after an initial period to allow State action, if a State's health insurance laws do not meet prescribed federal guidelines, then insurance sold in-State would be certified through a federal back-up mechanism.

Other reforms would be implemented directly by Federal Government through amendment of the Federal Employee Retirement Income Security Act (ERISA) or through other appropriate legislation. Certification of HINs would fall into this category.

As stated above, federally certified HINs would be protected from State mandated benefit laws and State premium taxes in the same manner as an ERISA-qualified self-insured plan. Federally certified HINs would, however, be subject to additional State requirements to assure solvency. States could provide an alternative process for certification of HINs. If State laws and State premium taxes were excessive, a HIN could apply to the Department of Labor for federal certification—pre-empting State law. As a result, State would be encouraged to facilitate market pooling and access to coverage for small business—or risk losing their traditional insurance oversight and regulatory role to a federal backup system.

Chapter 4

Expanding Access Through Tax Measures to Help People Pay for Insurance: Health Insurance Tax Credit and Deduction

Overview

The cornerstone of the President's plan to increase access to health insurance is a new transferable tax credit and deduction designed to help most of the Nation's uninsured obtain health insurance. The plan places the highest priority on providing health insurance for low-income individuals, but also would provide substantial benefits to middle-income individuals who enjoy little or no employer contributions for health insurance and to self-employed individuals.

Policy Background

Current tax law provides substantial benefits to individuals whose employers contribute to their health care insurance costs. The entire amount of the employer's contribution is excluded from taxable income and from the FICA wage base.

Self-employed individuals are able to deduct 25 percent of their premium payments. And all taxpayers are able to deduct out-of-pocket medical expenses and premium payments to the extent that these expenses exceed 7.5 percent of adjusted gross income; however, this deduction is of limited value to most taxpayers because few have medical expenses significantly in excess of the AGI threshold.

Other federal programs—including Medicare and Medicaid—provide health insurance coverage directly to eligible groups including the elderly, disabled, and certain low-income individuals. However, many low income individuals—including many unemployed individuals and the working uninsured—do not qualify for any of these benefits and do not receive any direct or indirect Federal contribution to their health insurance.

Overall, there are estimated to be 34.7 million Americans without health insurance (CPS, March 1991). Lack of coverage has a number of adverse consequences. Health may be at risk because of reduced access to primary and preventive care. Moreover, uninsured people often seek medical care in hospital emergency rooms, which is costly and inefficient. The cost of providing care to the uninsured produces large cost-shifting within the health care system, increasing costs for the insured—by up to 15 percent for some services. For these and other reasons, expanding insurance coverage is an important goal for the Nation.

Analysts have suggested a variety of options as means of expanding insurance coverage. These options include national health insurance (see Chapter 6, section A), and a "play or pay" mandate to require employers

95 Million Americans Will Benefit

To make health insurance more affordable, the President's plan includes:

- A tax credit of up to $3,750 for low-income families;
- A tax deduction of up to $3,750 for middle-income families;
- An increase to 100 percent in the deduction for health insurance available to self-employed individuals.

to provide coverage or to pay a tax (see Chapter 6, section B). Both of these alternatives will lead to higher costs for American taxpayers, rationing of care, and inefficient delivery in an unstable system. The President's proposal instead relies on significant reforms of the health insurance market, a new transferable health insurance tax credit for low-income families, and a new health insurance tax deduction for middle-income families.

The President's plan will promote individual choice. With a system of health insurance tax credits and deductions, low- and middle-income families will be free to choose among a variety of health plans with increased availability due to the market reforms. This helps ensure that coverage meets individual and family needs.

Moreover, providing choice is a critical prerequisite of competition in any market system—and competition among health plans is the best way of assuring continuous improvements in quality of care, service, and cost-effectiveness. None of the alternative options for expanding insurance coverage promote choice or enhance competition. Indeed, they generally have the opposite effect. Other disadvantages are detailed more fully in Chapter 6.

Tax Credits and Deductions for Low-Income and Middle-Income Individuals

Low- and middle-income persons who are not covered by other federally subsidized health insurance programs will be eligible for a tax credit or deduction for the purchase of insurance.

Eligibility.—Eligibility for the credit or the deduction is related to income and extends up to a modified adjusted gross income of—

- $50,000 for single persons
- $65,000 for persons filing as heads of households, and
- $80,000 for married persons filing jointly.

These income levels will be increased to account for inflation.

Individuals who receive other federal support (e.g., covered by Medicare, Medicaid, CHAMPUS, and selected other federal health programs) would not be eligible for the credit. The transferable tax credit would replace the supplemental earned income tax credit available under current law for certain low-income taxpayers who contribute toward the purchase of health insurance coverage for their children.

Amount.—The maximum amount of the credit is $1,250 for single persons, $2,500 for married couples and other two-person families, and $3,750 for families of three or more. These credit amounts would be sufficient to purchase a basic health insurance benefits package (See Table 3–3). The amount of the credit would phase down to a minimum at increasing income levels.

Individuals, couples, and families may also elect to claim a deduction instead of the credit. The deduction will be available to persons without regard to whether they itemize or claim the standard deduction and will be equal to $1,250 for single persons, $2,500 for married couples and other two-person families, and $3,750 for families of three or more.

Both the credit and deduction amounts will be increased to account for inflation. Applicable credit and deduction amounts will be reduced by the amount of any contribution made by the employer to the employee's health plan. Individuals with employer contributions exceeding the applicable credit or deduction amount will receive neither the credit nor the deduction.

As noted above, the amount of the tax credit would vary based on modified adjusted gross income in relation to the tax filing threshold. The tax filing threshold is the sum of the standard and taxpayer and dependent exemptions and approximates the poverty level. Modified adjusted gross income equals the sum of adjusted gross income, plus nontaxable Social Security payments, Railroad Retirement payments, and tax-exempt interest.

The tax credit would be implemented over a five-year period. When fully implemented—

- All eligible individuals, married couples, or families with incomes below the tax threshold (100 percent of poverty) will receive the maximum credit (e.g., to $1,250, for individuals, $2,500 for married couples, and $3750 for families).

- All eligible individuals, married couples, or families with incomes above the tax threshold will receive a partial credit, decreasing to 10 percent of the maximum credit (e.g., to $125 for individuals, $250 for married couples, and $375 for families) at 150 percent of the tax threshold.
- All eligible individuals, married couples, or families with incomes above 150 percent of the tax threshold, will receive the greater of the minimum credit or the deduction of up to $3,750 as described above.

As noted previously, individuals, married couples, and families with incomes above $50,000, $65,000, and $80,000, respectively, would be ineligible for either the credit or the deduction. Also, as noted previously, individuals, couples and families could take the health insurance deduction instead of the credit. Moreover, the amount of the credit and the deduction would be phased out over the range of $40,000 to $50,000 for single persons, $55,000 to $65,000 for married couples and other two-person families, and $70,000 to $80,000 for families of three or more. The tax credit and deduction would cost about $35 billion in 1997 when fully phased-in.

Administration.—For filers, credits and deductions could be claimed on the tax return at the end of the year in the usual manner used for other credits and deductions.

Alternatively, low-income credit recipients could receive a transferable credit certificate during the year by applying to a governmental office. States may select a State agency, such as the Employment Service or contract with the Social Security Administration to certify applicants' eligibility and to notify the Internal Revenue Service of the issuance of the advance credit.

This mechanism would immediately qualify the individual or family for assistance in purchasing health insurance; people would not have to wait until they file their tax returns to benefit. Transferable credit holders would transfer the credit to an employer or insurer who provides health insurance in payment for coverage. The insurance provider will then reconcile the amount of the advance credit on their tax return.

Credits would be used to purchase a "basic" benefit package (or other health plans of their choice). States would ensure that insurance companies would make basic benefit plans available (See Chapter 3).

Tax Credits and Deductions for Self-Employed Individuals

The self-employed would be entitled to deduct 100 percent of the cost of their health insurance premiums or receive the applicable credit, whichever is greater.

Using the Tax Credit/Deduction to Purchase Insurance

The market reforms described in Chapter 3 would apply to help assure that coverage is both available and affordable for individuals and families receiving health insurance tax credits. Specifically, guaranteed issue, guaranteed renewability, and elimination of preexisting condition exclusions would all apply. Moreover, broad based health risk pooling would apply to insurance sold to credit recipients to ensure affordability of coverage for recipients with chronic illnesses. Finally, credit recipients would be able to buy low cost coverage through health insurance networks or HINs.

The initial credit amounts of $1,250, $2,500, and $3,750 for individuals, couples and families were selected to cover the cost of an efficiently-run health plan that provides "basic" services. Each State would define a basic benefit plan or plans that could be purchased for the approximate amount of the credit. Any insurer in the State could offer basic benefits to credit recipients. Credit recipients would be able to buy coverage other than the State-defined basic benefit package if such other coverage would better suits their needs.

Achieving the Goal of Expanded Access

The health insurance tax credit and deduction will help millions of low- and middle-income families afford health insurance. When fully implemented, approximately 86 percent of all individuals not receiving Federal medical support have income in the range of eligibility for a credit or deduction; the remaining 14 percent are higher-income individuals or families.

- Individuals who have employment based coverage, but who pay much of the cost themselves, would receive a substantial new deduction or credit.

A total of 95 million individuals would benefit from the health insurance tax credit and deduction when the President's program is fully phased in.

- About 25 million low-income individuals would receive the maximum credit (adjusted for any employer contributions).
- Approximately 13 million individuals with incomes between 100 percent and 150 percent of the tax filing threshold would receive a partial credit or deduction.
- Finally, about 57 million middle-income individuals would receive a partial credit or deduction. Of these, 51 million would receive a deduction.

Self-employed workers would also be helped. In 1993, 3.1 million self-employed taxpayers currently buying health insurance would benefit from the increase in the deduction available to the self-employed. Still more self-employed individuals will benefit because they qualify for the health insurance tax credit. And, the insurance market reforms discussed in Chapter 3 will reduce the cost of health insurance for self-employed individuals at all income levels.

After five years, 29 million Americans will become newly covered. The number of uninsured will be decreased from 34.1 million to 4.9 million—or less than 1.8 percent of the total population. Twenty-four million Americans will gain coverage primarily as a result of the new health insurance tax credits and deductions. And, by reducing premium costs substantially, the health insurance market reforms and other cost-containment reforms will encourage employers to expand coverage voluntarily to an additional five million Americans.

Table 4–1. **Effect of Overall Reform Proposal on the Number of Uninsured Americans**

(People in millions; projected to population)

Income Level	Below 100 Percent of Poverty [1]	Between 100 and 150 Percent of Poverty [1]	Totals	As Percent of Total Population
Current Law Uninsured	15.4	5.7	34.1	12.8%
Covered Through Tax Credits and Deductions	14.9	5.0	24.1	9.1%
Covered Through Market and Other Reforms	0.4	0.6	5.0	1.9%
Total Newly Covered	15.3	5.6	29.2	11.0%
Remaining Uninsured	0.1	0.2	[2] 4.9	1.8%

[1] Poverty here is the income level at which individuals, couples, and families must begin paying income taxes.
[2] Many of the 4.9 million remaining uninsured are eligible for a credit or deduction.

References

Agency for Health Care Policy and Research, National Medical Expenditures Survey, U.S. Public Health Service, Rockville, MD, 1987.

American Medical Association, Socioeconomic Monitoring System, 1983 and 1989, core surveys, Chicago, Illinois.

Anderson, G.M., Newhouse, J.P., Roos, L.L., "Hospital Care for Elderly Patients with Diseases of the Circulatory System: A Comparison of Hospital Use in the U.S. and Canada," *New England Journal of Medicine,* Vol 321, 1989, pp. 1443–1448.

Barer, M.L., Evans, R.G., and Labelle, R.J., "Fee Controls as Cost Controls: Tales from the Frozen North," *Milbank Mem Fund Q/Health & Society,* Volume 66, p.1–64, 1988.

Barer, M.L., Evans, R.G., and Stoddart, G.L., "Controlling Health Care Costs by Direct Charges to Patients: Snare of Delusion?" Occasional Paper 10 (Toronto: Ontario Economic Council, 1979).

Brennan, T.A., Leape, L.L., Laird, N.M., et al., "Incidence of Adverse Events and Negligence in Hospitalized Patients: Results of the Harvard Medical Practice Study I.," *New England Journal of Medicine,* Volume 324, pp. 370–376, 1991.

Brook, R.H., Ware, J.E., Rogers, W.H., Keeler, E.B., Davies, A.R., Donald, C.A., Goldberg, G.A., Lohr, K.N., Masthay, P.C., Newhouse, J.P., "Does Free Care Improve Adults' Health?," *New England Journal of Medicine, pp.* 1426–1434, December 8, 1983.

Chernick, H.A., Holmer, M.R., and Weinberg, D.H., "Tax Policy Toward Health Insurance and the Demand For Medical Services," *Journal of Health Economics,* pp. 1–25, 1987.

Congressional Research Service, Cost and Effect of Extending Health Insurance Coverage, Library of Congress, Washington, D.C., October, 1988.

Cunningham, F.C. and Williamson, J.W., "How Does Quality of Health Care in HMO's Compare to That in Other Settings? An Analytic Literature Review: 1958 to 1979," *Group Health Journal,* Volume 1, Number 4, 1980.

Current Population Survey, U.S. Department of Labor, Washington, D.C., 1988.

Current Population Survey, U.S. Department of Labor, Washington, D.C., 1991.

Darman, R., "Introductory Statement: The Problem of Rising Health Care Costs," Testimony before the Finance Committee, U.S. Senate, Washington, D.C., April 16, 1991.

Darman, R., "Comprehensive Health Reform: Observations About the Problem and Alternative Approaches to Solution," Testimony before the Ways and Means Committee, U.S. House of Representatives, Washington, D.C., October 10, 1991.

Danzon, P.M., "The Hidden Costs of Budget-Constrained Health Insurance Systems," American Enterprise Institute for Public Policy Research Conference, Washington, D.C., October 1991.

Deber, R.B. and Leatt, P., "Technology Acquisition in Ontario Hospitals: You Can Lead a Hospital to Policy, But Can You Make It Stick?" In: Home JM, (ed.) *Proceedings of the Third Canadian Conference on Health Economics,* Winnipeg: University of Manitoba, pp. 259–277, 1987.

Doherty, R.B., "Wishful Thinking and the Clamor Over Administrative Waste," The Internist, pp. 22–27, May 1991.

Dowd, B.E., "HMO's and Twin Cities Admission Rates," *Health Services Research,* Volume 21, pp. 177–188, Part I, June 1986.

Consumer Checkbook, *Washington Consumers' Checkbook Magazine,* Washington, D.C., 1982.

Employee Benefit Research Institute, "EBRI Issue Brief," Washington, D.C., February 1989.

Enthoven, A. "Competition of Alternative Delivery Systems," In *Competition in the Health Care Sector,* W. Greenberg, (ed.) Aspen Systems, Germantown, MD, 1978.

Enthoven, A.C., "Consumer-Choice Health Plan: A National-Health-Insurance Proposal Based on Regulated Competition in the Private Sector," *New England Journal of Medicine*, Volume 298, p. 709, 1978.

Enthoven, A.C., *Health Plan: The Only Practical Solution to the Soaring Cost of Medical Care*, Addison-Wesley Publication Co., Reading, Massachusetts, 1980.

Farley, P.J., Monheit, A.C., "Selectivity in the Demand for Health Insurance and Health Care," *Advances in Health Economics and Health Services Research*, R. Scheffler and L. Rossiter (ed.), JAI Press, Greenwich, CT., pp. 231–248, 1985.

Feeny, D., Guyatt, G., Tugwell, P., "Health Care Technology: Effectiveness, Efficiency and Public Policy," Institute for Research in Public Policy, Montreal, 1986.

Feldman, R.D. and Dowd, E.E., "Simulation of a Health Insurance Market with Adverse Selection," *Operations Research* Volume 30, pp. 1027–1042, Nov-Dec 1982.

Feldman, R., et al., "The Competitive Impact of Health Maintenance Organization on Hospital Finances: An Exploratory Study," *Journal of Health Politics, Policy and Law*, Volume 10, pp. 675–698, Winter 1986.

Feldstein, M.S., *Hospital Costs and Health Insurance*, Harvard University Press, Cambridge, Mass., 1981.

Feldstein, M.S. and Taylor, A., "The Rapid Rise of Hospital Costs," President's Council on Wage and Price Stability, Washington, D.C., 1977.

Feldstein, M.S. and Friedman, B., "Tax Subsides: The Rational Demand for Insurance and the Health Care Crises," *Journal of Public Economics*, Volume 7, pp. 155–78, April 1977.

Feldstein, P.J., *Health Care Economics*, A Wiley Medical Publication, John Wiley & Sons, 1988.

Florida Health Care Cost Containment Board, "Joint Ventures Among Health Care Providers in Florida," Tallahassee, Florida, September 1991.

Francis, W., and the editors of Washington Consumers' Checkbook, *Checkbook's Guide to 1982 Health Insurance Plans for Federal Employees*, Washington, D.C., 1982.

Freund, D. and Hurley, R., "Managed Care in Medicaid: Selected Issues in Program Origins, Design, and Research," *Annual Review of Public Health*, Volume 8 , pp. 137–163, 1987.

Fuchs, V.R. and Hahn, J.S., "How Does Canada Do It? A Comparison of Expenditures for Physicians Services in the United States and Canada," *New England Journal of Medicine*, Volume 323, pp. 884–890, 1990.

Fuchs, V.R., "Health Care and the United States Economic System,"*Milbank Mem. Fund Q/Health & Soc.*, Volume 1, Number 2 (Part I), p. 211, 1972.

Gabel, J., et al., "Trends in Managed Care," *Health Insurance Association of America*, Washington, D.C., 1989.

Ginsburg, R.B., "Altering the Tax Treatment of Employment-Based Plans," *Milbank Mem. Fund Q./Health & Soc.*, Volume 59, Number 2, p. 32, 1981.

Globerman, S., "Waiting Your Turn: Hospital Waiting Lists in Canada," Fraser Institute, Vancouver, May 1990.

Goodwin, C., "U.S. Miracle Workers Take Pay Cuts to Help Canadians," The Kirchner-Waterloo (Ontario) *Record*, February 15, 1990.

Greenspan, N. and Vogel, R., "Taxation and its Effect upon Public and Private Health Insurance and Medical Demand," *Health Care Financing Review*, Volume 1, pp. 39–45, Spring 1980.

Hadley, J. and Langwell, K., "Managed Care in the United States: Promises, Evidence to Date, and Future Directions," *Health Policy*, 1991.

Hahn, R.A., Teutsch, S.M., Rothenberg R.B., Marks, J.S., "Excess Deaths from Nine Chronic Diseases in the United States, 1986," *Journal of the American Medical Association*, Volume 264, pp. 2654–2659, Nov. 28, 1990.

Harvard Medical Practice Study, *Patients, Doctors, and Lawyers: Medical Injury, Malpractice Litigation, and Compensation in New*

York, President and Fellows of Harvard College, Cambridge, Mass, 1990.

Health Care Financing Administration, Medicare Hospital Mortality Information: 1986, 1987, 1988. U.S. Department of Health and Human Services, Baltimore, MD. 1989.

Health Care Financing Administration, *Hospital Data And Rehospitalization by Geographic Area for Aged Medicare Beneficiaries,* Volume 1–3, Health Care Financing Special Report, HCFA Publication Numbers 03300, 03301, 03303, U.S Government Printing Office, Washington, D.C., June 1990.

Health Care Financing Administration, *Report to Congress: Paying Physicians — Choices for Medicare,* Office of Research and Demonstrations, sent by the Secretary of Health and Human Services to the U.S. Congress, October 1989.

Health Insurance Association of America, *Canadian Health Care: The Implication of Public Health Insurance,* prepared by E. Neuschler, HIAA Research Bulletin, June 1990.

Hellinger, F., "Selection Bias in Health Maintenance Organizations: Analysis of Recent Evidence," *Health Care Financing Review,* Volume 9, Number 2, pp. 55–63, Winter 1987.

Hillman, B.J., Joseph, C.A., Mabrv, M.R., Sunshine, J.H., Kennedy, S.D., Noether, M., "Frequency and Costs of Diagnostic Imaging in Office Practice: A Comparison of Self-Referring and Radiologist-Referring Physicians," *New England Journal of Medicine,* Volume 323, Number 23, pp. 1604–1608, December 6, 1990.

Holmer, M., "Tax Policy And The Demand For Health Insurance" *Journal of Health Economics,* pp. 202–221, December 1984.

Hsiao, W., "Public Versus Private Administration of Health Insurance: A Study in Relative Economic Efficiency," *Inquiry,* Volume 15, p. 379, 1978.

Hurley, R. and Freund, D., "A Typology of Medicaid Managed Care," *Medical Care,* Volume 26, pp. 764–773, 1988.

Iglehart J.K., "Canada's Health Care System," *New England Journal of Medicine,* Volume 315, Number 3, p. 202–208, July 17, 1986.

Kim, H., "Canada Tabs Washington Hospital," *Modern Health Care,* March 26, 1990.

Langwell, K., "Structure and Performance of Health Maintenance Organizations: A Review," *Health Care Financing Review,* Volume 12, Number 1, pp. 71–79, Fall 1990.

Levit, K., Lazenby, H., Letsch, S., and Cowan, C., "National Health Spending, 1989," *Health Affairs,* Volume 10, Number 1, Spring 1989.

Luft, H., *Health Maintenance Organizations: Dimensions of Performance,* A Wiley InterScience Publication: John Wiley and Sons, New York, New York, 1981.

Luft, H.S., "HMOs and Medical Costs: The Rhetoric and the Evidence," *New England Journal of Medicine,* Volume 298, p. 1336, 1978.

Luft, H.S., "Health Maintenance Organizations: Competition, Costs Containment, and National Health Insurance," in *National Health Insurance: What Now, What Later, What Never?* M.V. Pauly (ed.) American Enterprise Institute, Washington, D.C., 1980.

Luft, H.S., "How Do Health Maintenance Organizations Achieve Their Savings?" *New England Journal of Medicine,* pp. 1336–1343, June 15, 1978.

Manning, W.G., Newhouse, J.P., Duan, N., Keeler, E.B., Leibowitz, A., and Marquis, M.S., "Health Insurance and the Demand for Medical Care," *The American Economics Review,* Volume 3, pp. 251–276, June 1987.

Manning, W.G., Leibowitz, A., Goldberg, F.A., Rogers, W.G., Newhouse, J.D., "A Controlled Trial of the Effect of a Prepaid Group Practice on Use of Service," *New England Journal of Medicine,* Volume 310, pp. 1506–1510, 1984.

Marquis, M.S., *Consumers' Knowledge About Their Health Insurance Coverage,* RAND Corporation, Santa Monica, California, July 1981.

McCaffree, K.M., Boscha, M.V., Drucker, W.L., et al., "Comparative Costs of Services," in *The Seattle Prepaid Health Care Project:*

Comparison of Health Services Delivery, NTIS No. PB–267 491, Springfield, Virginia, 1976.

Monheit, A., and P. Short, "Mandatory Health Coverage," *Health Affairs*, Volume 8, Number 1, Winter 1989.

Moser J.E. and Musacchio, R.A., "The Costs of Medical Professional Liability in the 1980's," *Medical Practice and Management*, pp. 6–9, Summer 1991.

Needleman, J., Sheils, J. and Lewin, L., *The Health Care Financing System and the Uninsured*, Lewin and Associates, Washington, D.C., under contract to the Health Care Financing Administration, April 1990.

Newhouse, J., et al., "Are Fee for Service Costs Increasing Faster than HMO Costs?," *Medical Care*, Volume 23, Number 8, pp. 960–966, August 1985.

Newhouse, J., Manning, W., Norris, C., et al., "Some Interim Results from a Controlled Trial of Cost-Sharing in Health Insurance," *New England Journal of Medicine*, Volume 305, pp. 1501–1507, 1981.

Newhouse, J.P., *The Economics of Medical Care: A Policy Perspective*, Addison-Wesley Publishing Co., Reading, Mass., 1978.

Newhouse, J.P., Anderson, G., Roos, L.L., "Hospital Spending in the United States and Canada: A Comparison," *Health Affairs*, pp. 6–16, Winter, 1988.

Organization for Economic and Cooperative Development (OECD), *Health Systems: Facts and Trends*, Paris, forthcoming 1992.

Pauly, M.V., "Taxation, Health Insurance, and Market Failure in the Medical Economy," *The Journal of Economic Literature*, Volume 2, pp. 629–675, June 1986.

Pauly, M.V., "The Economics of Moral Hazard: Comment," *American Economic Review*, Volume 58, Number 3, p. 531, 1968.

Pauly, M.V., "Future Research Needs: Competition in the Financing and Delivery of Health Services," presented to NCHSR Briefing, Washington, D.C., March 4, 1982.

Pauly, M.V., "Is Medical Care Different?" in *Competition in the Health Care Sector: Past, Present and Future*, W. Greenberg (ed.) Federal Trade Commission, Bureau of Economics, Washington, D.C., May 1978.

Pauly, M.V. "Overinsurance: The Conceptual Issues," in *National Health Insurance: What Now, What Later, What Never?* M.V. Pauly (ed.), American Enterprise Institute, Washington, D.C., 1980.

Pauly, M.V., "The Role of the Private Sector in National Health Insurance," Health Insurance Institute, Washington, D.C., 1979.

Pauly, M.V., "What is Unnecessary Surgery?" *Milbank Mem. Fund Q.* Volume 57, Number 1, p. 95, 1979.

Prospective Payment Assessment Commission, *Report and Recommendations to the Congress*, Washington, D.C., March 1990.

Reynolds, R.A., Rizzo, J.A., Gonzalez, M.L., "The Costs of Medical Professional Liability," *Journal of the American Medical Association*, Volume 257, Number 20, pp. 2776–2781, 1987.

Rice, T., "Containing Health Care Costs in the United States," Public Policy Institute, American Association of Retired Persons, Washington, D.C., May 1991.

Robinson, J.C., "HMO Market Penetration and Hospital Cost Inflation in California, *Journal of the American Medical Association*, Volume 266, Number 19, pp. 2719–2723, 1991.

Roemer, M.I., "Group Practice: A Medical Care Spectrum," in *Health Insurance Plans: Studies in Organization Diversity*, M.I. Roehmer, D.M. DuBois, and S.W. Rich (eds.), School of Public Health, University of California, Los Angeles, 1972.

Roemer, M.I. and Shonick, W., "HMO Performance: The Recent Evidence," *Milbank Mem. Fund Q.*, Volume 51, p. 271, 1973.

Roos, L.L., Fisher, E.S., Sharp, S.M., et al., "Postsurgical Mortality in Manitoba and New England," *Journal of the American Medical Association*, Volume 263, Number 18, pp. 2453–2458, May 9, 1990.

Roos, L.L., Wennberg, J.E., Malenka, D.J., et al., "Mortality and Reoperation after Prostatic Hyperplasia," *New England Journal of Medicine*, Volume 320, pp. 1120–1124, 1989.

Rossiter, L., et al., "Patient Satisfaction among Elderly Enrollees and Disenrollees in Medicare Health Maintenance Organizations," *Journal of the American Medical Association,* Volume 262, pp. 57–63, 1989.

Rublee, D., "Medical Technology in Canada, Germany, and the United States," *Health Affairs,* Volume 8, Number 3, p. 181, Fall 1989.

Scheffler, R.M., Gibbs, J.O., and Gurnick D.A., "The Impact of Medicare's Prospective Payment System and Private Sector Initiatives: Blue Cross Experience, 1980–1986," Blue Cross and Blue Shield Association and the Research Program in Health Economics, University of California, Berkeley, CA, 1988.

Schieber, G. and Poullier, J., "International Health Spending: Issues and Trends," *Health Affairs,* Volume 10, Number 1, pp. 106–116, Spring 1991.

Schieber, G., Poullier J., and Greenwald L.M., "Health Care Systems in Twenty-Four Countries," *Health Affairs,* pp. 23–38, Fall 1991.

Schwartz, L., "The Medical Costs of America's Social Ills," *Wall Street Journal,* June 24, 1991.

Sherlock, K., "Detroit Offers Short Wait For Health Surgery," *The Edmonton Journal,* January 6, 1990.

Sonnefeld, S.T., Waldo, D.R., Lemieux J.A., and McKusik, D.R., "Projections of National Health Expenditures Through the Year 2000," *Health Care Financing Review,* Volume 7, Number 3, pp. 1–27.

Advisory Council on Social Security, *Commitment to Change: Foundations for Reform,* Social Security Commission Survey, Washington, D.C., December 1991.

Taylor, C.R., *Universal Health Care in Maryland: A Consumer Choice Approach,* December 1991.

Taylor, A.M. and Wilensky, G.B., "The Effect of Tax Policies on Expenditures for Private Health Insurance," in *Market Reforms in Health Care,* pp. 163–184, Jack Meyer (ed.), American Enterprise Institute, Washington, D.C., 1983.

U.S. Department of Health and Human Services, *Health, United States, 1990,* National Center for Health Statistics, Public Health Service, Hyattsville, Maryland, March 1991.

U.S. Congress, *Health Care Resource Book,* Committee on Ways and Means, House of Representatives, U.S. Government Printing Office, Washington, D.C., April 16, 1990.

U.S. Congress, Congressional Budget Office, *Selected Options for Expanding Health Insurance Coverage,* U.S. Government Printing Office, Washington, D.C., July 1991.

U.S. General Accounting Office, *Canadian Health Insurance: Lessons for the United States,* GAO/HRD–91–90, Washington, D.C., June 1991.

U.S. General Accounting Office, *Medicare: Effect of Durable Medical Equipment Fee Schedules on Six Suppliers' Profits,* GAO/HR-92-22, Washington, D.C., November 1991.

Waldo, D.R., Sonnefeld, S.T., Lemieux, J.A., McKusik, D.R., "Health Spending Through 2030: Three Scenarios," *Health Affairs,* Volume 10, Number 4, pp. 231–242, 1991.

Washington State Hospital Association, *Weekly Report,* Volume 15, Number 8, February 23, 1989.

Welch, W.P., "HMO Market Share and its Effect on Local Medicare Costs," Urban Institute, Washington, D.C., report to the Health Care Financing Administration, under Cooperative Agreement #17-C-99223/3-01, December 1990.

Wennberg, J., Barnes, B., and Zubkoff, M., "Professional Uncertainty and the Problem of Supplier-Induced Demand," *Social Science and Medicine,* Volume 16, pp. 811–824, 1982.

Wilensky, G.R., "Government and the Financing of Health Care," *American Economic Review,* Volume 72, Number 2, p. 202, 1982.

Wilensky, G.R. and Rossiter, L.F., "Coordinated Care and Public Programs," *Health Affairs,* pp. 63–77, Winter 1991.

Wolinsky, F.D., "The Performance of Health Maintenance Organizations: An Analytic Review," *Milbank Mem Fund Q/Health & Society,* Volume 58, p. 537, 1980.

Woolhandler, S. and Himmelstein, D.U., "The Deteriorating Administrative Efficiency of the U.S. Health Care System," *New England Journal of Medicine,* Volume 324, pp. 1243–1258, 1991.

HERITAGE PLAN

Butler SM. A Policy Maker's Guide to the Health Care Crisis - Part II: The Heritage Consumer Choice Health Plan. In: Heritage Talking Points; Washington D.C.: March 5, 1992. [Pages 1-14 are reprinted here.]

March 5, 1992

A POLICY MAKER'S GUIDE TO THE HEALTH CARE CRISIS PART II: THE HERITAGE CONSUMER CHOICE HEALTH PLAN

By Stuart M. Butler, Ph.D.

INTRODUCTION

Part I of this *Talking Points* series on health care explained that proposals to reform America's health care system generally are based on one of three approaches. Each approach uses a different mechanism to allocate health care resources and to determine what services a family receives. These three methods are:

1) **The Single-Payer (or "Canadian") Approach.** The government becomes the monopoly provider of health care financing. It fixes a budget for health care and allocates money to hospitals, and it sets physician fees.

2) **The "Play or Pay" Approach.** The government gives employers a choice: either provide at least a specified health insurance plan to employees and their families, or pay a payroll tax to finance a public program for their health benefits, as well as for those Americans not currently insured. The government runs the public program and employers are responsible for financing and managing private insurance.

3) **The Consumer Choice Approach.** Americans are allowed to choose the health care plan they want. Unlike today, where government help to obtain a plan effectively is restricted to employer-sponsored plans, families would receive the same amount of government help wherever they obtained coverage. Further, there would be more help for the sick and the low-paid, less for the healthy and the high-paid. No national budget for health care would be set by the government, and efficient allocation and cost control would be determined by consumer choice and competition among providers.

Many of the key features of a consumer-based system already exist in the Federal Employee Health Benefits Program (FEHBP). This covers congressmen and their staff, agency heads and employees, and judicial branch employees—in all over nine million workers, their dependents, and retirees. Several proposals are versions of a consumer-based system. The Bush Administration's recent health proposal would establish such a system for today's uninsured.

A comprehensive proposal has been introduced in the Senate (S. 2095) by Steve Symms and Larry Craig, both Idaho Republicans, and elements of a consumer-choice model are included in a bill (S. 1936) introduced by Senator John Chafee, the Rhode Island Republican.

In addition, The Heritage Consumer Choice Health Plan has been developed by The Heritage Foundation.[1]

This *Talking Points* examines the Heritage plan in detail. It reviews the plan's features and implications. It also contains the findings of an analysis of the Heritage plan by Lewin/ICF, a leading Washington-based econometric firm specializing in health economics. The Lewin/ICF study was commissioned by Heritage. Lewin/ICF conducts similar analyses for the Administration, Congress, and the private sector.

HOW THE HERITAGE CONSUMER CHOICE HEALTH PLAN WORKS

The Heritage plan would create a health care system in America in which all families would have access to an affordable health plan and would choose the plan they wanted. Today a family normally must change its plan, or even lose coverage, when the head of household changes jobs or faces unemployment. Under the Heritage proposal, the family would keep the same insurance without interruption when changing jobs—much as families keep the same life insurance, car insurance, homeowner's insurance or mortgage. In addition, the tax code would be changed to give more help to lower-paid or sick families to afford health care. This change would not increase the federal deficit.

Reduced to its central elements, the Heritage plan involves two principal steps:

Step #1: Convert the tax exclusion for company-sponsored plans into a tax credit for plans from any source.

When a family is covered by an employer-sponsored health plan as part of the breadwinner's total compensation, the value of the benefits is not included in the family's taxable income. This is like a tax deduction for the family.[2] This is known as a "tax exclusion." For the vast majority of Americans, this is the only

1 See Stuart M. Butler and Edmund F. Haislmaier, eds., *A National Health System for America* (Washington, D.C.: The Heritage Foundation, 1989); Stuart M. Butler, "Using Tax Credits to Create an Affordable Health System," Heritage Foundation *Backgrounder* No. 777, July 20, 1990; Stuart M. Butler, "A Tax Reform Strategy to Deal With the Uninsured," *The Journal of the American Medical Association*, Volume 265, May 15, 1991.

2 It is actually more generous than a tax deduction for lower-paid families and many middle-income families, because Social Security taxes are not applied. Tax deductions by contrast are free of income tax, but not of Social Security taxes.

way they can obtain a tax break for health care costs (for the implications of this, see *Talking Points, Part I: The Debate Over Reform*, February 12, 1992).[3]

Under the Heritage plan, the current exclusion for company-provided plans, as well as other minor health tax deductions, would be replaced with a new tax credit available to all non-elderly and non-Medicaid families for the purchase of health insurance and out-of-pocket medical costs. The cost to the Treasury for the credit would exactly equal the cost of current tax breaks. In Washington jargon, this makes the plan "budget neutral."

Q: What does that mean for employees who have a company plan? Would they pay higher taxes?

A: **Generally no.** It just means families would gain tax relief in a different way. If they had a company-sponsored plan, the cash value of that plan now would appear as a taxable item on their end-of-year W-2 tax form from the employer. But the family then would be able to claim a credit for the cost of employer-sponsored plan and for out-of-pocket costs, such as deductibles. Further, if the family chose a plan from a source other than their employer, the employer would be required to "cash out" their current benefits by adding the value of those benefits to the worker's paycheck. As described below, the Lewin/ICF analysis of the proposal indicates that most families would pay slightly lower total taxes after this switch. And while some families would pay higher taxes, it would be because they had found ways to cut their medical insurance costs and thus gained more (taxable) income for other purposes.

Q: What about families without a company plan?

A: **They would receive a credit for buying insurance and out-of-pocket medical care.** Today these families normally receive no tax help or any other assistance, unless they go on welfare.

Q: What about the working poor, who pay little or no tax?

A: **The new credit would be refundable.** This means that if the family's credit exceeded its tax liability, it would receive the difference from the government, in the form of a voucher that could be used only for health care.

3 Three smaller tax breaks are available for some Americans. The self-employed can deduct 25 percent of the cost of insurance. Americans with high out-of-pocket medical costs can deduct the amount in excess of 7.5 percent of their adjusted gross income if they itemize their tax return. And low-income working Americans can obtain a credit for certain insurance to cover their children, through the earned income tax credit (EITC).

Step #2: Require all households to purchase at least a basic package of insurance, unless they are covered by Medicaid, Medicare, or other government health programs.

All heads of households would be required by law to obtain at least a basic health plan specified by Congress. The refundable credit system partially would offset the cost of such a plan for most Americans, as the exclusion does today for those with company-sponsored plans.

In addition to these core steps, the Heritage plan would institute reforms to smooth the transition to the consumer-based national system and to enable the market for health insurance and medical care to operate more effectively. Among these, the plan would:

- ✗ **Reform the insurance market:** The private insurance market would be reformed to make a standard basic package available to all at an acceptable price (see below).
- ✗ **End state insurance mandates:** Most states mandate that insurance sold within their borders must cover certain services. These mandates would in effect be preempted, to allow the basic plan to be marketed throughout the United States and to permit new types of group sponsors to sell plans. In addition, plans could not be made subject to state restrictions on managed care. These state mandates could be preempted by federal law, as they are for the Federal Employee Health Benefits Program. Or the federal government could widen current exemptions from state mandates for self-insured company plans to include any plan that complies with the insurance requirements of the Heritage proposal.[4]
- ✗ **Place requirements on employers:** In a system based on the Heritage proposal, employers would be required by law to do two things:

  1) **"Cash out" benefits during a one-year transition period.** Employers would have to add the cash value of their existing plan to the paychecks of any employee wishing to switch to an alternative plan or if the employer decided to terminate the plan. This means employees would be what economists call "held harmless" by the change. After

---

4 Heritage analysts believe that today's concerns about state mandates actually would decline or even disappear in a full-scale consumer based system. The reason is that voters would have a strong incentive to resist new insurance mandates since these would translate directly into higher insurance premiums they would pay. Today the higher costs due to mandates are buried in "free" company plans. Significantly Congress, which could mandate services in the federal employee system, chooses not to do so in large part because employees would face higher premiums if there were congressional mandates. See Robert E. Moffit, "Consumer Choice in Health: Learning from the Federal Employee Health Benefits Program," Heritage Foundation *Backgrounder* No. 878, February 6, 1992.

the transition, employers and employees would bargain for compensation packages as they do today.

2) **Introduce a payroll deduction for health insurance and adjust withholdings.** Employers would be required to make a payroll deduction each pay period, at the direction of each employee, and send the amount to the plan of the employee's choice. This would be like the payroll deduction that many employees instruct their employers to make for contributions to a 401(k) or similar savings plan. In the federal employee health system, a worker's agency or congressional office makes a similar payroll deduction to pay for premium costs.

Employers also would be required to adjust the employee's withholdings to reflect their estimated health credit, just as they do now when, say, an employee buys a house and becomes eligible for the mortgage deduction. This means that employees would not have to wait until the end of the year to claim the credit.

Q: What about a low-paid worker who does not have taxes withheld?

A: Actually even the low-paid normally have Social Security taxes withheld. In any case the employer would estimate the refundable credit available to the employee and send this, plus any contribution by the employee, to the employee's chosen plan. The employer would adjust the total withholdings sent to the IRS to reflect refundable credits for any employees.

Q: What about the unemployed?

A: If an individual became unemployed, normally he or she would become eligible for a larger credit, since family income would fall. For the unemployed, the government would send the value of the credit to the individual's plan. In addition, the unemployment check could be adjusted to reflect the contribution, if any, due to the plan by the individual. Further, since the paperwork for this change in the payment method would take time, health plans would not be permitted to drop coverage if a working family became unemployed. When the paperwork is complete, the plan would receive premium payments due during the interval.

ADVANTAGES OF THE HERITAGE PLAN

A consumer-based plan would have profound and beneficial effects on America's health care system. Among the most important:

✓ **Every American family would have access to affordable and adequate health care.**

Under the Heritage plan, all Americans—most important, all Americans now uninsured—would be enrolled in a health plan or covered by a public program (chiefly Medicaid or Medicare programs).

✓ Americans no longer would lose coverage when then they changed jobs.

American families would be able to obtain health coverage from any source, not just their employers, with exactly the same tax benefits. This means health insurance would be "portable." So when a worker changed jobs, he or she would take the family's health plan to the next job, just as they normally keep the same life insurance protection or mortgage company. For this reason, worries about "pre-existing condition" clauses in a new employer's plan would disappear, and families would keep the same doctor and benefits of their chosen plan.

✓ Americans could choose new kinds of group plans.

The fact that individuals will buy health plans does not mean that individuals must buy the kind of individual coverage typically sold today. Individual plans today tend to be more expensive for a number of reasons. Their administrative and marketing costs, for instance, are high because the insurer has to collect premiums from each individual. Group plans, such as those run by employers, cost less because the insurer is dealing in "bulk" and can negotiate with medical institutions.

Under the Heritage proposal, families could still gain the financial advantages of group purchasing. They could still join groups structured around their employer. More important, families could join plans organized by other groups and still receive tax benefits. Today, of course, if families are not part of an employer group plan, typically the families enjoy no tax benefits. Several new types of group probably would emerge. Among them:

Unions

Under the federal employee system, 35.5 percent of enrollees are covered in plans organized by a union or other employee organization. In many instances, these union plans are open to non-union members.[5] Sometimes the union health plan is much larger than the union itself. There are about 500,000 members of the Mail Handlers Plan, for instance, but only about 30,000 regular members of the union.

Union-sponsored plans likely would become a growth industry under the Heritage proposal. They would possess a marketing advantage because many workers would trust a union-sponsored plan rather than one from most other sources, particularly one promoted by management. Unions might also see a health plan as a good recruiting tool for attracting individuals as regular members. Further, many unions already have expert health benefits negotiators who could easily become the administrators of the union's own plan.

5 Technically, enrollees pay a small fee to become associate members of the union for the purposes of coverage, but are in no sense regular union members.

Churches

In many communities the church easily could sponsor a group health plan. This is especially true in the black community, where typically the church already functions as a social and economic development agency. Similarly, the Church of Jesus Christ of Latter Day Saints (that is, the Mormon church) carries out a sophisticated social welfare function for its members. Sponsoring a health plan for members would be a natural development.

Farm bureaus

Some state farm bureaus, such as Virginia's, already have a health plan for farm-based families. But often families receive limited or no tax breaks for joining such plans. With the Heritage proposal as law, farm bureaus and similar organizations would have a natural market niche in rural areas, especially for seasonal or casual workers.

Sickness groups

In some cases, a family might choose a plan offered by an organization of individuals suffering from a particular ailment. Many such organizations exist and give advice on obtaining treatment. Making a plan available to members would be a simple step. These plans, moreover, would structure medical services around the particular needs of the member, say a diabetic. Today, a diabetic typically has to take a standard company-sponsored plan containing items he or she does not use and then pay out-of-pocket for additional specialized services.

✓ Costs would be controlled effectively and efficiently.

The Heritage plan uses the best device ever found to hold down costs without sacrificing quality and efficiency: consumer choice within a competitive market. This works well and simply in the huge Federal Employee Health Benefit System, where cost increases are running at about one-third to one-half less than increases in company-sponsored plans.[6] It also works well in non-company insured markets, such as cosmetic surgery. It also works in every other private sector of the economy.

The Heritage plan would permit it to work in health care. Families would "shop around," comparing the premium prices and benefits of rival plans and making their choice accordingly, just as they do for life insurance, a car or a house, or college education for their children—and as federal workers do for health plans. Premium costs would be reduced by virtue of the tax credit, but families would still save money by choosing the least expensive plan that met their needs. In turn, plan organizers would have to compete aggressively for the family's dollars by developing plans that combined attractive benefits with a

6 See Moffit, *op. cit.*

good price—precisely the same imperative that keeps costs under control elsewhere in the economy.

✓ **The Heritage plan is budget neutral.**

The Heritage plan would not increase the federal deficit. This means that it is budget neutral. This is because the new credit system would cost the same as existing tax breaks for health care. As explained below, the plan also is budget neutral for states.

Q: Does a system based on the Heritage proposal have to be budget neutral?

A: No. But the basic plan could be made more generous to, say, the lower-paid by additional help from a state or the federal government. This, of course, would mean an extra cost to the budget.

DETAILS OF HOW THE HERITAGE CONSUMER CHOICE HEALTH PLAN WOULD WORK

The Heritage Foundation contracted with Lewin/ICF to construct a model of the plan within the framework of Lewin's econometric model of the health care economy. Lewin/ICF conducts econometric analysis for government and the private sector and is among the most highly respected companies in the field of health analysis. For purposes of this model, Lewin made small modifications, some to enhance the basic plan and others to simplify the modelling process. This required various assumptions and produced specific results.

✓ **How the tax credits would be structured**

Lewin/ICF modelled three versions of the basic Heritage plan. Other versions are of course possible. In each version, Lewin calculated the credit percentages that would result in budget neutrality for the federal government and the states. These are presented in Table 1. Minor adjustments could be made in the rates to produce more rounded numbers without departing significantly from budget neutrality.

Version #1 is a voucher plus a flat credit for remaining insurance and out-of-pocket costs. Each individual in a family would qualify for a refundable credit to help buy insurance. This "health insurance voucher" would be equal to a maximum of $220 per individual per year (80 percent of $275) or $880 for a family of four. In addition, the family could claim a flat 18 percent refundable credit for all insurance costs and out-of-pocket costs above $275 per year per individual (that is, above the amount subject to the voucher).

Version #2 is a sliding scale credit for all insurance costs and out-of-pocket costs. In this version, families would receive a sliding scale credit to help offset the cost of insurance and out-of-pocket costs. As these costs rise as a proportion

Table 1

Federal Tax Credit Alternatives

Tax Credit Version #1

- 80 of the cost of premiums up to $275 per family members, plus
- 18 percent of premiums over $275 per member, plus
- 18 percent of umreimbursed medical expenses.

Tax Credit Version #2

Premiums and Unreimbursed Expenses as a Percent of Gross Household Income	Percent Reimbursed Under the Credit
Below 10%	21%
10% - 20%	45%
20% or more	65%

Tax Credit Version #3

- 75 percent of premiums up to $275 per family member, plus
- 14 percent of premiums over $275, plus

Unreimbursed Expenses as a Percent of Gross Household Income	Percent Reimbursed Under the Credit
Below 10%	21%
10% - 20%	45%
20% or more	65%

Note: The credits are refundable.
This structure of credits is budget neutral at the state and federal levels.

Source: Lewin/ICF estimates using the Health Benefits Simulation Model.

of family income, the percentage credit also would rise. The structure of this sliding scale credit is much like the child care credit in today's tax code.

Version #3 is a combination of the first two. A voucher and flat rate credit would apply to insurance costs only, and a sliding scale credit to out-of-pocket costs. This version would encourage families to buy a basic plan, but give them a bigger incentive to accept higher deductibles and copayments.[7]

✓ **The minimum benefits package required by law**

Table 2 indicates the minimum benefits package that would be required by law under the Heritage proposal, as chosen by Heritage analysts and priced by Lewin/ICF. For a family of four this plan is estimated to cost $277.33 per month or $3,327.84 per year, so it is by no means a "bare bones" plan. It should be noted that the plan has been priced on a per capita basis. In practice family plans cost less than the total would be if each member bought a separate plan. So the cost for a family in the model is probably an overestimate in some cases. Equivalent coverage options would be permitted. For instance, instead of 75 percent coverage for physician services, a plan may have a higher percentage, but a

Table 2
Basic Plan Required by Law

Minimum standard coverage required for all Americans.

- $1,000 deductible ($2,000 per family).
- $5,000 cost-sharing maximum.

Benefit	Coinsurance
Inpatient Hospital Services (365-day per stay maximum)	80%
Outpatient Hospital Services	80%
Hospital Alternatives (extended or home health care)	Yes
Physician Services	75%
Prenatal/Well-Baby/ Well-Child Care	75%
Diagnostic Tests	75%
Prescription Drugs (inpatient)	75%
Emergency Services	100%
Mental Health Care	Not Covered
Dental Care	Not Covered
Vision Care	Not Covered

Average monthly cost of the plan is $69.33 per person.

Actuarial equivalent alternatives are permitted.

Note: Individuals covered by a government health program such as Medicare and Medicaid are exempt from those coverage requirements.

Actuarially equivalent plans are ones with different coverage or benefit levels than those specified here, but whose total cost is the same for individuals with the same actuarial characteristics such as age, sex, and geographic location.

7 A copayment, or coinsurance, is the percentage of an otherwise insured medical bill that must be paid by the patient.

lower percentage for inpatient prescription drugs. A prepaid managed health plan (such as a Health Maintenance Organization, or HMO) with at least the same basic coverage would be permitted.

The legally-required basic plan would limit deductibles for a family to no more than $2,000 and total unreimbursed costs (including the deductible) to no more than $5,000, often known as the "stop loss" amount or amount above which there is "catastrophic" protection. A family could choose a plan with a lower deductible or catastrophic protection, but normally that would mean a higher premium. These unreimbursed medical costs would be offset by a credit in each version of the Heritage plan (they are not normally given tax relief today) and so would be less costly to a family than the same amounts included in a company-sponsored plan today.

✓ The employer's responsibility

Table 3 summarizes the responsibility of employers. In essence employers act as bookkeepers for their employees, handling premium payments and tax adjustments on the employee's behalf. One important assumption is made about Social Security (FICA) tax. If employer-provided plans become subject to tax (offset, of course, by the new credit), the value of those benefits also would become subject to the "employer's share" of Social Security tax. Heritage analysts instructed Lewin/ICF to assume in modeling the plan that in con-

Table 3
The Employer's Responsibility

Employers have the option of:

- Continuing to provide health benefits; or
- Discontinuing the health plan.

For employers who continue to provide benefits:

- The average amount of the employer's contribution is counted as taxable income to the employee.*
- Employees may not take cash in lieu of coverage.

For employers who discontinue coverage:

- Employers must maintain their current level of effort by converting benefits to income.
- Employers must deduct premiums for workers.

Employers will hold workers harmless for the employer share of increased FICA tax payments due to taxation of benefits.

* Separate employer contribution amounts would be used for persons with single and family coverage.

verting current benefits to cash during the transition year, employers pay this extra tax (see below). Other than this small tax, there would be no change in taxes or total employee compensation costs for an employer.

✓ Changes in the insurance market.

Table 4 indicates the proposed reforms of the insurance market under the Heritage Consumer Choice Plan. The most important of these is that all health plans henceforth would be required to guarantee annual renewal for any enrollee who wished to do so, with a premium increase no greater than the average for all enrollees covered by the carrier. This means that insured individuals could not be dropped, or charged unduly high premiums, if they became sick. In addition, under the Heritage plan, three underwriting requirements would be placed on insurance companies—at least during a transitional period while the insurance market adjusted to the new financing system.

First Requirement: Uninsurable Americans (those for whom insurance is impossible in a free market except at prohibitive prices) who are currently uninsured would be randomly assigned to insurers and plans doing business in a state. This would spread the cost of insuring high-risk families among existing plans.

Second Requirement: If an insurer now covers a family, say through a employer-based plan, that insurer would be required to continue coverage if the employee wished it. This means a sick person now in a company-sponsored plan would not be dropped if the employer ended the plan or the employee moved. The insurer would be required to convert the group coverage to individual coverage, so the worker would not lose coverage if he or she changed jobs.

Table 4
Insurance Market Reforms

Reform of renewal practices.

- Guaranteed renewal.
- Renewal Premium updated by carrier-wide average increase.
- Changes in premium due to changes in health status are prohibited.

Current marketing/underwriting practices modified during at least the transition period.

- Uninsurable individuals who are currently uninsured are randomly assigned to carriers.
- Insurers must extend portable, individual coverage to all persons they now cover through employment-based group plans.
- In converting from group to individual coverage, premiums are permitted to vary by no more than 25 percent on the basis of age, sex, and geography-adjusted premiums.

State mandates are preempted by standard benefit package.

State Laws restricting selective contracting and managed care plans are preempted.

Third Requirement: Plans could not charge more than 25 percent above or below the average charged for new enrollees with similar characteristics. This means that sick families, who today often find the cost of coverage prohibitive, could not be charged premiums more than 25 percent above those for similar families of average health. If a family switched plans, moreover, the new carrier could not charge them more than 25 percent above the average premium charged for similar families.

✓ Modelling assumptions made by Lewin/ICF

Lewin/ICF had to make certain assumptions about consumer behavior and other features of the basic Heritage plan to "run the numbers." Some of these are crucial; others simply were to ease the process of modelling and could be changed in any final program. These are contained in Tables 5 and 6. Among the most important:

First Assumption: All employers are presumed to discontinue their existing plans and convert their value into additional cash income for employees. This makes the calculations easier and more reliable, but is not crucial to the plan. Some large companies might well continue to provide coverage.

Second Assumption: Healthy families buy a basic plan and pocket the savings, while currently insured Americans in poor or fair health either maintain their existing coverage or upgrade to better coverage. The model assumes all the uninsured buy the basic package, which includes catastrophic protection (although some doubtless would buy more elaborate plans).

Table 5
Key Assumptions

Employers who now offer insurance:

- All will discontinue coverage and convert benefits to wages.
- Firms with over 1,000 workers establish employee premium financed cafeteria plans, which will reduce administrative costs.

Workers now covered by employer insurance:

- Those in poor/fair health will select plans that at least maintain their existing level of coverage.
- Those in good/excellent health will downgrade to the standard package.
- Health services utilization for persons who downgrade coverage will decline based upon price elasticities reported in the literature (a price elasticity of -0.2 was selected).

Persons now covered by non-group insurance:

- Persons who now have coverage in excess of the minuimum standard will maintain that coverage.
- Others will upgrade to the minimum standard.

Currently uninsured persons:

- All will take the minimum standard package.
- Utilization will adjust to levels reported by insured persons with similar charactoeristics.

No change is assumed in the number of persons enrolled in Medicaid.

Third Assumption: Administrative costs are assumed to be lower than for today's individual health insurance plans. However, Lewin/ICF does not assume that all employers would make a payroll deduction for employees and send premiums to the chosen insurer. In fact, Heritage analysts make that a legal requirement. This might mean somewhat lower administrative costs than Lewin/ICF projects.

Table 6

Administrative Cost Assumptions

Administrative costs would be the same as under current policy for workers in firms where the employer arranges employee deductions.

Administrative costs for others purchasing individual insurance would be 21.9 percent of claims. This retention rate was estimated as follows:

Administrative Costs for Individual Coverage as a Percentage of Claims

	Current Policy[a]	Assumed level Under Tax Credit[b]
Claims Administration	9.3%	8.0%
General Administration	12.5	10.0
Interest Credit	-1.5	-1.5
Risk and Profit	8.5	2.7
Commissions	8.4	0.0
Premium Taxes	2.8	2.7
Total	**40.0%**	**21.9%**

a: Hay/Huggin estimates of administrative costs for groups with 1 to 4 members under current policy.

b: Hay/Huggin estimates of administrative costs for groups with 1 to 4 members under a voluntary risk pooling arrangement adjusted to assume that insurer profits as a percent of claims correspond to the national average observed in the current system.

Source: Congressional Research Service, "Cost and Effects of Extending Health Insurance Coverage," Washington, D.C. October 1988.

PAULY PLAN

Pauly MV, Danzon P, Feldstein PJ & Hoff J. *Responsible National Health Insurance.* Washington, D.C.:AEI Press; 1992. [Pages 3-21 are reprinted here.]

2
First Principles—Efficiency and Equity

Efficiency has two important dimensions: (1) minimizing the cost of whatever services are provided; and (2) choosing the level, quality, and mixture of health services, relative to other goods and services, that lead to the greatest excess of benefits over costs. Incorporating the need to balance quality and cost, efficiency reflects choices in which the resources used to furnish goods and services yield maximum value to consumers.

An efficient system does not necessarily have the lowest cost. The most cost-constraining system is the one that incurs no cost. This obviously is not desirable. Nor is a strategy that has contained costs in other countries necessarily either efficient or appropriate for the United States. "Failure" to achieve a zero rate of growth in real cost—to achieve a rate equal to the growth of gross national product (GNP), which would keep health care's share of GNP constant—or to achieve a rate as low as that achieved by a regulated system in some other country is not necessarily a deficiency. The appropriate objective is the right rate of growth in cost. That rate, in turn, depends in large part on the value that informed consumers, with both a quality and a cost stake in their decision, attach to new technology and to the use of health services. If a costly new technology is valuable in relieving pain or in reducing morbidity or mortality, a high rate of growth in cost—and the rising fraction of GNP that may result—is cause for cheer, not concern. The added cost reflects the greater benefits of higher quality. Whether rising expenditures are desirable depends on a comparison of value to cost. It is not appropriate to debate health reform within the limited framework of whether a proposal will hold cost increases to the rate of change in the GNP. The correct focus is on how to achieve a system that enables—and requires—consumers to balance value and cost as they do in other sectors.

Under proper incentives, a choice by informed consumers to spend more on health care and health insurance (including administration) and less on other goods and services is not to be decried.

Equity has a less precise meaning; neither economics nor logic can prove that one person's definition of fairness is necessarily superior to that of another. It is generally agreed, however, that horizontal equity is desirable: persons with the same real incomes should be treated equally. A person should not be able to pay lower taxes simply because his employer pays his health insurance premiums. It is also generally agreed that any income redistribution through the tax system should be made from those with higher incomes to those with less—vertical equity. But precisely how tax rates should rise and public benefits should decrease as real income increases is more debatable. We believe our current mildly progressive tax structure and highly progressive distribution of government welfare and transfer benefits should be maintained and that the current regressive system of tax subsidies to health insurance is an anomaly to be corrected.

3
Proposed Plan for National Health Insurance

To improve the efficiency and equity of the American health care system, we propose a plan that would guarantee coverage for all without unnecessary and unfair cross-subsidization, increase the efficiency of health care delivery and thus make more health care benefits available to more Americans, and provide the flexibility and freedom necessary to stimulate technological and administrative innovation. The plan we propose properly recognizes both the responsibilities of citizens to have adequate health insurance and the need of some for financial assistance to obtain this insurance. Our plan enhances and makes use of competitive markets; it avoids relying on the public tax and expenditure system whenever possible, to minimize tax-side distortions and to recognize the current constraints on government budgets. Our approach would permit informed individual preferences to determine the allocation of resources to health care, it would encourage the development of innovative and efficient forms of delivery, and it would advance the vitality and quality of the health care system. We call this plan Responsible National Health Insurance.

Underlying Assumptions

Our plan is based on eight assumptions.

1. Every person should be able to obtain health care on a timely and systematic basis. Society currently provides care to many of the low-income and privately uninsured families through a haphazard combination of uncompensated care, public insurance and programs, and public subsidies to some providers. It would be more effective and humane for recipients

and less costly for society if assistance came in the form of affordable insurance for all, rather than as grudging payment for care, often provided in the late stages of illness.

2. A monolithic, government-run or government-sponsored-and-controlled system is not necessary to provide universal health insurance. Such insurance can and should be effected instead through competitive markets, with government intervention only to make markets work and to give financial assistance to those who need it.

3. All citizens should be required to obtain a basic level of health insurance. Lack of health insurance imposes a risk that the individual will delay medical care, impairing his health and increasing costs for the rest of society, which then pays for his delayed care. Those who obtain insurance, usually by taking a job that comes with health insurance benefits in lieu of cash wages, subsidize those who remain uninsured, whether by choice or not. They receive lower cash wages to obtain insurance; the cost of that insurance and the taxes they pay are increased by the amount spent for the uninsured. Permitting individuals to remain uninsured results in inefficient use of medical care, inequity in the incidence of costs of uncompensated care, and tax-related distortions for the public subsidies they do receive. The risk of an individual's shifting costs to others has led many states to mandate that all drivers have liability insurance. The same logic applies to health insurance.

4. The ultimate obligation to obtain basic health insurance should be placed on the individual, not on the employer. This approach achieves universal coverage while satisfying individual preferences. It avoids interference with labor markets and employment contracts; it facilitates portability of coverage, employment mobility, and a competitive market; and it ensures coverage even when a person is not employed. An individual could take a job that does not carry health insurance, provided that he otherwise obtains the minimum level of insurance. Employment-based insurance is not necessarily the lowest-cost way to cover employees of small firms, which do not enjoy the scale economies of large groups; it can lead to excessive uniformity within a firm and to potential inequity. It also offers the misleading appearance that the employer pays for the insurance, whereas employees actually bear the cost by receiving lower money wages.

Placing the obligation to obtain coverage on the individual does not limit the freedom of employers or unions to offer group coverage as a fringe benefit to their employees, if they desire. Indeed, the great majority of the population would probably continue to obtain insurance through employment. There are substantial administrative cost advantages of employment-related group insurance in large firms. Moreover, group insurance may serve as a vehicle for helping individuals screen and choose among a variety of health plans; employee benefits managers develop specialized knowledge and have strong incentives to act as efficient agents for employees.

5. Government tax policy toward health insurance should be directed at making adequate insurance affordable for all, with minimum tax cost to the U.S. Treasury and minimum distortion in the choices made by individuals. This objective can best be met by requiring individuals to obtain appropriate coverage, while using predetermined tax credits, calculated on the basis of need, to achieve the desired degree of affordability, and equity. These tax credits would reduce income taxes and would be "refundable" in the sense that, if the credit exceeded an individual's tax liability, the excess would be refunded to the individual.

This assistance mechanism would replace the current system, which treats employer payments for health insurance as tax-exempt income to employees, without limit and without regard to need. The current system is horizontally inequitable, since only the employed are eligible for this tax subsidy. It is vertically inequitable, since the subsidy is higher for high-income individuals and for those who buy more comprehensive insurance. And it is contrary to the public interest; by permitting the purchase of insurance with pretax dollars, it encourages people to buy more insurance than they would otherwise purchase, thus fueling health care inflation. Because of the structure of the current tax subsidy, health care costs that an employee could pay out of pocket are covered by insurance, thus shifting a substantial proportion of the cost (equal to the individual's marginal tax bracket) to the government and hence to other taxpayers, some of whom do not have employer-paid insurance and consequently do not benefit from the same subsidy.

To extend the current tax treatment of insurance to subsidize almost everyone's purchase of insurance, as some have proposed, would perpetuate and worsen the present inequities and inefficiencies; it would also add to the already tremendous drain on the tax system (estimated at $60 billion in fiscal 1991), the real cost of which is the additional incentive distortion created by raising marginal tax rates to replace the tax revenues forgone by the tax exclusion for health insurance.

6. The required minimum level of insurance protection should be based on a family's income. Higher deductibles and out-of-pocket limits should be permitted for persons with higher incomes because they can absorb

more medical costs without risk of underusing care or generating bad debts. Allowing higher-income individuals to pay a larger percentage out of pocket would benefit everyone, since paying for care out of pocket results in more cost-conscious use, which in turn creates incentives for providers to keep fees and costs down. Individuals could, if they wished, purchase more complete coverage than the minimum required for their income, provided that they paid the cost of the additional coverage without government subsidy.[2]

7. Some modest increase in taxes may be needed to pay for the proposed expansion of coverage and tax credits. The amount would depend on choices about the level of required coverage and generosity of the structure of tax credits, in particular on the political will to cut back the current tax subsidies to middle- and high-income individuals. Our proposal relies on a visible and equitable source of financing in contrast with the hidden and inequitable system of financing that would result from mandating employer-paid coverage, as we discuss below.

Our proposal also contrasts with the present unfair and inefficient system. Now the amount of government assistance to those with employer-paid insurance is determined not by explicit government decision but by the amount and cost of insurance purchased and under which care for the uninsured and Medicaid beneficiaries is financed in part by a de facto excise tax on hospital charges paid by the privately insured, without regard to ability to pay.

8. A vigorous, competitive market in insurance and in health care delivery is more likely to create efficiency and high quality in health care and health insurance than is a system with one monopoly insurer operated or controlled by government. A market system, improved by purging open-ended subsidies, free riding, and cost shifting, is the most appropriate way to determine the allocation of resources to health care. A more efficient system would permit us to produce more real health benefits or more of other goods and services within our given resources. Placing the obligation to obtain insurance on the consumer would achieve universal coverage without distorting labor markets; it would encourage cost-conscious choices and a competitive market in which individuals (and employers on their behalf) have an economic interest in the selection of their insurance.

Elements of the Plan

Based on these assumptions, our plan addresses the problems of health care access and cost in the United States in the following way:

- It requires each citizen to obtain at least minimum adequate coverage against catastrophic medical expenses; because the costs that would be catastrophic necessarily depend on a family's income or wealth, the required coverage increases as family income declines. Poor people would have virtually complete coverage, and the well-to-do would not be required to buy more than basic protection that limits catastrophic out-of-pocket payments.
- The required coverage is made affordable by providing, to those families who need them, refundable fixed-dollar tax credits or adjustments in total federal taxes that are highest for those with the lowest incomes and decline at high income levels. Very poor families would receive a subsidy equal to the cost of coverage.
- The requirement to obtain coverage would be enforced through existing tax and welfare systems. The federal tax system would be used to collect the net premium (premium net of tax credit) for those persons who did not purchase insurance on their own. These premiums would be used to pay in full for coverage to be provided by private but federally or state contracted "fallback" insurers furnishing the minimum coverage for each income level.
- This system of tax credits would replace the tax treatment of health insurance, which subsidizes health insurance at the federal and state level by excluding from taxable income the health insurance premiums paid by employers. In our plan, such employer payments would be included in income subject to income tax and payroll tax.

These four features describe the qualitative nature of the basic plan. Any change in national health policy will require new administrative structures and additional payments by some citizens, and our plan is no exception. In what follows we will discuss in detail how the administrative and financing questions might be best addressed. We have no delusions of perfection in this process; there will have to be compromises among the goals of equity, efficiency, administrative simplicity, and political transparency. Many of our procedural and administrative suggestions are just suggestions and could be modified as part of the political process, based on experience gained in the transition stage. The purpose of providing detail is to show that what we propose is not only conceptually the best among imperfect alternatives but also practically feasible and that many apparent problems with the operation of this plan can be overcome.

4
Characteristics of Our Plan

Every person is required to obtain basic coverage, through either an individual or a family insurance plan. To satisfy this obligation and to be eligible for the tax credit, an individual must obtain coverage for specified health services; these should include basic acute care services and preventive services that are cost effective and beneficial.

Mandatory Catastrophic Coverage of Basic Services

The minimum services that must be covered are the same for everyone; plans could, however, offer more generous benefits or supplemental policies. The maximum amount of out-of-pocket expense (stop-loss) permitted is geared to income, with lower maximums required for lower-income people, to ensure that they do not face the risk of catastrophic out-of-pocket expenses, given their income.[3] A person would not satisfy his obligation if he obtained a plan with deductibles and copayments in excess of the income-related levels specified by the federal government. An individual could, if he wished, obtain coverage with lower required out-of-pocket expenses. All plans are also required to provide out-of-area coverage in emergency situations and to comply with possible requirements concerning selection, which are discussed below in connection with preferred-risk selection. The basic legislation would need to specify the core services, the conditions under which supplementation can occur, the extent of coverage, and the form of fallback coverage.

Core Services. National health insurance proposals require a definition of covered core services. Under public monopoly insurance, core services define what the government provides; under an employer or individual mandate, core services define the minimum list of services that must be covered by the mandated insurance.

The determination of core services will depend on the objectives for requiring insurance. One objective might be an intent to correct consumer misperceptions about the likelihood of incurring medical costs and the need for insurance. Another objective could be to encourage the use of care that individuals would not choose on their own but that will benefit others with altruistic concerns.

The first rationale arises from a belief that people may not recognize their risk of needing health care nor the cost that may be entailed should they become ill; they thus fail to obtain insurance. This is an often-cited reason for the high proportion of young adults who are uninsured. (Such myopia is often given as a rationale for compulsory social security.) Such poorly informed individuals may also underestimate the benefits of certain medical services. This behavior may therefore result in a lower demand for insurance and for some cost-justified services, such as preventive care with longer-term payoffs. There is little empirical evidence of such myopia, and good reason to expect that it may not be extensive. Since insurers are in business to sell insurance, it is not clear why they would not inform such potential purchasers of the value of insurance. If anything, one might fear an overselling, not underfunding. Some individuals, however, may be truly risk loving, while others may expect (usually correctly) that they will receive some care when they are severely ill, even if they cannot or will not pay. These free-riding individuals impose an external cost on others when they become ill and shift the costs of their care to others. They should be required to finance their care by obtaining the minimally required health insurance. If these misperceptions and free riding were the rationale for mandating coverage, the definition of core services would be based on the amount of insurance coverage typical persons would be willing to purchase if they had properly evaluated their risks and the benefits of medical services and insurance.

The second rationale for mandating insurance that suggests a second criterion for defining the minimum core benefits is based on the fact that medical care is a service whose use is of concern to others in the community; there are "altruistic consumption externalities." If the nonpoor want the poor to have more coverage and more use of services than the poor would obtain on their own, the nonpoor must pay for this change. This is one rationalc for the tax credit or subsidy that is a key component of our plan. The fact that the United States and all other developed societies attempt to ensure some minimum access to medical care for those who cannot afford to pay for themselves is strong evidence of a widespread demand for a minimum level of health care as an altruistic good.

This altruistic good rationale implies that core medical services should include all those that we as a society would be unwilling to deny others in need. This set may well differ from (and may be less than) what a typical middle-class person would choose for himself. Core services should then be defined to include all those that the taxpayers would be willing to pay for or partially subsidize for all.

As a practical matter, we assume, as we describe in the next section, that services for the poorest members of society will be fully subsidized and that subsidies will then decline and phase out at higher income levels. Accordingly, core services should be defined to include those that most taxpayers would be willing to subsidize for all, given the structure of financing.[4] Whether income taxes or some other tax base ought to be used depends, in theory, on which base is best attuned to variations in willingness to pay. In practice, we will probably have to use the roughly income-related federal income tax. Since social willingness to pay for others is likely to be more limited than private willingness to pay for one's own coverage, it seems reasonable to aim at defining the core services as the minimum required for everyone, based on social willingness to pay for those individuals who cannot afford to pay for themselves.

The definition of an ideal core set of services is primarily an exercise in exclusion. Services that are utterly useless or always harmful would be excluded. Most medical services, however, may sometimes offer both net positive health benefits and financial risk and therefore would *sometimes* be candidates for insurance coverage. Excluding services entirely from coverage is the bluntest of instruments; there are surely better ways to limit use to appropriate levels. We therefore generally prefer an inclusive definition of services that must be covered to some extent but rely on the proportion of costs covered, the circumstances in which benefits will be paid, and managed-care incentives to control excessive use.

In practice, the list of core services can be specified only by the political process, in which the interests of those who will be net recipients of benefits are balanced against those who will be net payers for those benefits. The lawmakers may decide to specify the benefits with some precision, or they may try to avoid disputes by stating the requirements in general terms and leaving the decision to other, less visible and less political forums. In either event, however, there will be disputes about the required coverage; if Congress provides a specific list of required benefits, there will still be issues of interpretation, aggravated by changing medical technology. Even if it is clear that an illness is covered, it is not clear what modalities of treatment are covered.

As an initially practical solution, we advocate a definition based on the services covered by a low-cost managed-care plan that has achieved a significant market share. Expanding the core services covered under RNHI requires either higher credits or higher premium payments by citizens. Under RNHI, in contrast to other proposals for health reform, taxpayers and citizens face the full marginal cost of more generous coverage. This factor should help control a tendency toward excessively generous coverage. The core services for which coverage is mandatory are only a minimum. No one is precluded from purchasing coverage of more comprehensive services; however, public funds do not subsidize these purchases.

Income-related Coverage. Our objective is to set the minimum required coverage at a level consistent with the proper purpose of insurance—namely, spreading the financial risk of events that are beyond the economic capacity of a particular family. Insurance should be encouraged for major expenses; first-dollar coverage of routine expenses for people who can afford to make copayments should not be encouraged. Since financial capacity is defined by the size of a family's aggregate medical bills relative to its income or wealth, we propose that the minimum required coverage vary with income. No copayment would be permitted at the lowest income levels, but sizable copayments would be permitted at higher incomes. Even for those with higher incomes, however, families would be required to have coverage against truly catastrophic financial events.

Varying the required coverage with income achieves several objectives. It ensures that the family has an adequate amount left over after paying for its health care. It also ensures that families are not required to buy coverage that is of little value to them but that consumes resources to pay for insurer administration and encourages the use of medical services that are worth less than their cost. For higher incomes, substantial deductibles or copayments would be appropriate. Many high-income households might want to buy more coverage than the required minimum. The minimum is selected, though, to reduce the risk that a family would be unable to pay its bills while allowing less risk-averse families to buy insurance with moderate deductibles in order to hold down their premiums.

Varying the level of coverage with income produces another benefit. If low-income families have a generous subsidy for coverage, the possibility that they will underconsume care is diminished. Greater out-of-pocket payments encourage higher-income families to economize. Although research on the subject is not definitive, it appears that there may be a modestly positive relationship between income and the level of use of medical care for people with the same insurance coverage and health status. If income does affect the level of use, it follows that providing uniform coverage with uniform cost sharing would reproduce the pattern in which the rich use more. In contrast, if all expenses are fully covered by insurance, we know that the use of higher-cost care of little medical benefit would be stimulated. If we seek to make medical care use more equal (at least by bringing up the lowest level of use), insurance coverage will need to be unequal. That is, insurance coverage that increases as income falls offsets the natural tendency of use and access to decline as income falls.

Finally, tying government assistance to income enables the poor to obtain the needed insurance and provides greater equity (although a political judgment would define the extent of that equity). Since income will need to be measured to award a credit in any case, there is little additional administrative cost to designing a plan in which coverage varies with income.

Fallback Coverage Negotiated by the Government

Although most people would be expected to obtain at least the minimum coverage in a timely fashion, particularly after one or two years of experience with the system, some individuals might, nevertheless, simply fail to obtain coverage. We therefore propose that a fallback insurer be established in each geographic market area. The government would solicit bids from insurers in each area to act as fallback insurers, offering one or more plans to provide the required minimum coverage. The bids would specify the premiums that would be charged for each rating category and for each level of maximum permitted out-of-pocket expenditures. The fallback plans could involve health maintenance organizations or managed care if such plans were able to offer a low bid. Consumers might be given a choice of fallback insurer, and both a conventional insurance and a managed-care option might be offered. The government would have to designate at least one insurer to serve as fallback insurer in each area and would thus have to accept whatever premium bid was necessary to do so.

In return for the franchise, the fallback insurer would agree to provide coverage for every applicant.

The fallback insurer would be expected to provide coverage in two situations. Some individuals might choose to obtain coverage from this insurer rather than from other private insurers; after all, the fallback insurer would provide government-approved reasonable insurance coverage at a reasonable premium. Those individuals who fail to choose an insurer would automatically be placed with the fallback insurer; their premiums would be collected through the federal tax system and through the welfare system. The very tiny minority who pay no federal income or payroll taxes and who receive no federal transfers would be enrolled by providers with the fallback insurer when they obtained care.

The process of determining benefits and specifications for the basic package is the same process as state governments must now go through to specify what their Medicaid plans will be. Offering the package for private bidding duplicates the process now used by some states (for instance, Arizona). There is no government regulation of premiums, only a decision by government of which bids it will accept for a small minority of the population. As is well known, competitive bidding processes (given a clear specification of the product being purchased) replicate the results of ideal competitive markets.[5] The winning bid for the basic plan for people below the poverty line then sets the amount of the maximum tax credit.

Since the government must specify coverage and obtain bids for the fallback insurer, especially for low-income persons, there is no way to avoid some government involvement in this sector. We believe that the approach we have described keeps the extent of government interference in the choices people make to the minimum. The government does not specify prices paid to providers, methods of cost containment, or providers to be included in a plan. Its only role is to provide a credit and make sure that people select plans that meet minimum guidelines. While no policy design can prevent politicians or bureaucrats with a taste for regulation and control from trying to meddle, the design we have suggested keeps opportunities for doing so to a minimum.

In a similar fashion, limiting the amount of the credit at any income to the amount needed so that the family can afford the required coverage and setting the required coverage as a minimum that declines with increasing income minimize the extent to which the government uses funds under its control to finance insurance and medical care.

Universal Tax Credits or Vouchers

Employer payments for health insurance premiums are currently tax-exempt compensation to employees. This exemption distorts insurance markets and offers larger tax subsidies to higher-income people. Our plan would eliminate the exclusion, replacing it with a system of refundable tax credits (which are in essence vouchers for persons with little or no tax liability) inversely related to a family's income. Very low income individuals would be entitled to a tax credit or voucher at least sufficient to cover the cost of the basic but comprehensive insurance policy with zero or minimal copayments. As incomes rise from the low cutoff level, the credit will fall below the cost of the policy, and the person will have to pay part of the policy premium as well as the out-of-pocket payments.

The "full cost" credit for the poor would depend on the cost of obtaining the required coverage. So that the lowest-income families can afford coverage, it may be necessary to tie the full cost credit they receive to the negotiated premium for fallback coverage. The credit also could be adjusted to reflect each individual's or family's actuarial category (age, gender, and family size) or its particular risk, depending on the design option selected to mitigate the effects of risk variation discussed below.

One policy issue is whether credits should vary across different geographic areas. If the tax credit at any income level were uniform—calculated, for instance, on a national average of insurance costs—people of a given income living in lower-cost areas who pay less for insurance would have more income left over to spend on other things.

Whether there should be a national rate (after a transition period) is a matter of policy design best left to Congress and the political process. The resolution will depend on perceptions of the reasons for the cost differentials between regions, particularly whether the differential is based upon unavoidable differences in medical costs, inefficient production or inappropriate use of health care resources, or differences in the quality of care.[6]

A similar question of whether area differences in health care costs should be reflected in the amount of federal assistance has arisen in connection with the Diagnostic Related Group (DRG) rates under the Medicare Prospective Payment System (PPS). The original differential in rates between urban and rural hospitals, which was based on the belief that there are valid differences in cost, is being phased out; but the rates may still vary between urban and rural hospitals as the standardized rate is adjusted by particular identified cost differentials such as wages and case mix. The decision is far more limiting under PPS than it would be under RNHI; the DRG rate set by the government constitutes the full amount of the hospital's reimbursement for treating a Medicare patient; the hospital cannot bill the patient for the difference. Under RNHI, however, except for the poorest individual who cannot and is not expected to supplement the government contribution, the tax credit does not have to be a perfect reflection of the cost of insurance. The federal tax credit is by definition an assistance to the individual to purchase insurance; the individual is expected to make his own contribution to the purchase of insurance. The government tax credit, unlike the DRG rate, does not set the price for the insurance.

We propose to replace the current exclusion of employment-related premiums from taxation with a fixed-dollar or closed-end tax credit because it is a way of improving both equity and efficiency. The current tax treatment of health insurance is horizontally inequitable because it depends on employment status and employer contribution. It is vertically inequitable because the subsidy per dollar of insurance premium is greater for persons paying higher marginal income and payroll tax rates. An open-ended tax exclusion implies larger subsidies for high-income workers and those who choose more generous coverage. Our plan would treat any employer premium payments (and premiums employees pay out of flexible benefit accounts) as part of taxable compensation, to be reported on the employee's W-2 form. Tax credits toward the purchase of the obligatory coverage would be provided to all, based on income, regardless of how the insurance is obtained.

The fundamental reason for the change is simple: "employer-paid" health insurance is part of compensation and should therefore be included in taxable compensation. The tax credit is then determined by the person's total income, without regard to the division between total income, wage income, and health insurance premiums. In the most fundamental sense, our proposed tax credits adjust the progressivity of the income tax, making it modestly more progressive. This modest increase in progressivity might be justified on the grounds that requiring purchase of insurance is, in itself, like a regressive tax (though one that the great majority of lower-income persons—who already have insurance—currently pay). The higher income-related credits offset this regressive payment.

Such a closed-end tax credit also gives proper incentives for efficiency. The amount of the credit is fixed for any family; it is based on the family's income, and the actuarial factors discussed below, and perhaps the cost of insurance in its geographic area. The credit is not calculated on the basis of the amount the family actually spends on health care or health insurance; buying more lavish insurance or using more medical care does not increase the amount of the credit received. A *fixed* tax credit does not distort incentives about how much insurance to buy, what type of insurance to buy, or where to buy that insurance. In contrast, because the amount of tax avoided grows as the current tax exclusion grows, the exclusion encourages the purchase of overly lavish and underaggressive health insurance.

The use of a tax credit of predetermined value, rather than one that is some proportion of the premium cost of the insurance policy the family chooses to buy, is a critical feature that makes our plan more efficient and less intrusive than that proposed by the Heritage Foundation. Not only is a fixed credit less distortive of the type or amount of insurance purchased than is such a variable credit, but it is much easier to administer—since the tax credit can generally be calculated without knowing what a person actually paid for insurance or medical care: we need to know only the person's income.[7] Combining a fixed tax credit with a requirement to buy insurance means that the credit does not change the individual's incentives; the credit only eases the financial consequences of the requirement to buy insurance.

Treatment of "Employer-paid" Group Insurance Premiums. While individuals will satisfy the requirement to buy coverage in various ways, we suspect that the great majority will continue to obtain their insurance in connection with employment, although we do anticipate that other groups, such as banks, schools, and credit unions or even insurance brokers and agents could become intermediaries for obtaining insurance, once the current tax bias in favor of the employment setting is eliminated.

Many employers will continue to contribute to employee insurance premiums. Since the employer's contribution is taxable income, the question is how this contribution should be distributed across workers. The most appropriate administrative structure is probably one in which the employer is free to designate how much of a total premium paid for group insurance is to be attributed to each employee; the only constraint is that the employer must allocate the entire group premium among employees if it is to be treated as employee compensation and therefore as an expense of doing business.

In the simplest case, in which the employer makes a fixed-dollar payment for all employees and then has them pay any additional premium, the administrative calculation would be easy: this fixed-dollar amount would be added to each employee's reported wage income. If all workers are of the same risk and the employer "paid" the entire net premium, it would likewise be obvious that the same dollar amount should be attributed to each worker and added to taxable compensation.[8]

But what happens if workers have somewhat different risk levels (for example, because of age) but the employer pays a single premium, as is the case for self-insured firms and large group purchasers? In this case, the most sensible strategy would be to permit the employer (or the union or employee group) to choose how it wishes to allocate the total premium expense across employees. Indirectly, the allocation method would be constrained by competition in the labor market, since workers evaluate job options on the basis of both money and fringe benefits. Our plan leaves it up to the employer or union to decide how to deal with differences among employees, such as family size and composition, when this is not determined by an insurer's premium calculation.

There is one potential complication. Suppose the employer or union does not vary the reported premium contribution for a group of workers who have the same skill level and cash wages but differ in expected health benefits because of differences in age or health status. By reporting a premium contribution that does not vary with employee risk class, the employer understates full compensation of higher-risk workers and overstates compensation of lower-risk workers. Here again there is a trade-off between administrative complexity and equity. Technically the premium attributable to a worker should be based on that worker's expected benefit, but ascertaining this would be extraordinarily complex. The amount of unfairness involved seems small relative to the administrative cost, since the only impact is a slight adjustment in taxable income.

Note that, with these adjustments, there would be subtle changes in the income categories of different individuals. Consider two workers who both currently receive $20,000 in money income, but one also gets a health insurance policy worth $2,000. Our plan would not classify these individuals in the same money income category, since the "before premium" income of the two workers would be $20,000 and $22,000, respectively. Since these individuals do not have equal consumption opportunities, it is appropriate to tax them differently, and that is what our plan would do. The person who formerly had to buy his own insurance policy would pay payroll and income taxes (if any) on an income of $20,000 and receive the tax credit appropriate to an income of $20,000. In contrast, the person who received health insurance as a fringe benefit would pay the taxes and receive the credits appropriate for an income of $22,000. This second employee would be regarded as a higher-cost employee in any labor market, and, if his skills justified receipt of total compensation worth $22,000, he should pay tax on that compensation.

Financial Impact. The net effect of RNHI on the after-tax cost of health insurance will differ across families, depending on their incomes and on the level of the tax credits adopted. In general, lower-income persons who currently obtain either individual or employment-based group insurance will enjoy a net reduction in taxes, since their tax credit under the proposal would probably exceed the value to them of the current tax exclusion. Indeed, at incomes below the poverty line, the tax credit would equal the premium; the insurance would be wholly financed by the government.

Higher-income employees, who benefit most from the current tax loophole, would pay higher taxes on balance; this would be an important revenue source for financing the new subsidies to the low-income families. The tax credit will phase out at zero for sufficiently high incomes; at the same time, the required level of coverage and hence the premium for the mandated plan would also decline with income, but expected out-of-pocket costs for those who buy only the minimum coverage would increase. On balance high-income families would pay a larger fraction of the cost of their health care than at present. Of course, over time the elimination of the tax loophole will increase efficiency and probably slow the rate of growth in health care costs, so that the real cost of health care may be lower than under the status quo even for higher-income families.

Setting the income threshold for eligibility for a full cost credit and the subsequent phasing down of credits and required coverage are basically political decisions. These decisions, together with the number of persons at each income level and the definition of core services, will determine the fiscal cost of the program. These choices will presumably depend on balancing the political cost of increasing taxes with the political gain of providing more generous subsidies and will be adjusted over time if the program proves to be more (or less) expensive than anticipated. Operationally, the size of the subsidy required to make the basic benefits package available to those with low incomes would be determined by the cost to insurers of providing the basic benefits, because the government would be required to pay enough to cover the cost of at least one fallback insurer in each area.

RNHI has a very strong advantage in encouraging rational democratic political choice—an advantage to voters, though not necessarily to politicians. The level and distribution of subsidies required, and the determination of who will be taxed to provide them, will be visible to voters as well as to legislators. It will be less possible than it is now for the political process to hide subsidies to middle- and high-income groups, while financing those benefits with regressive taxes. The trade-offs between beneficiaries and taxpayers will be obvious and subject to discussion and will likely be decided in open political debate. If the cost of subsidies increases over time, we would expect that Congress would consider the basic benefits package, the size of the subsidy in relation to different income groups, the necessary federal appropriations, and the required taxes. We would avoid useless and misleading discussions about "needed" care and about "giving" benefits, without facing up to the question of who will pay for them.

REINHARDT PLAN

Reinhardt UE. *An "All-American"™ Health Reform Proposal.* Princeton, NJ: Princeton University; August 1992.

AN "*ALL-AMERICAN*"™ HEALTH-REFORM PROPOSAL

Uwe E. Reinhardt, Ph.D.
James Madison Professor of Political Economy
Princeton University
609-924-7625 (tel)
609-924-6083 (fax)

August, 1992

If Americans are asked what they think of their *health system,* they now typically give it a very low rating. If, on the other hand, Americans are asked what they think of the quality of the *health care* available in their own community, they usually give that care a very high rating. The difference between *health system* and *health care*, of course, is the manner in which a nation *finances* that care. It is this nation's increasingly brittle *health insurance* system that gives the overall American *health system* its black eye in national and international opinion surveys.

DESIRABLE FEATURES OF A HEALTH-INSURANCE SYSTEM

The design of a superior health insurance system must begin with a specification of the ethical precepts that system is to obey. It seems reasonable to insist, for example, that the system should not exclude any individuals from insurance coverage--it should be *universal.* Second, most Americans probably believe that the premium levied on particular households should be divorced from the health status of its members--that families afflicted with illness should not be punished financially for their misfortune. One might even go so far as to say that the household's premium should be based strictly on the household's *ability to pay*, as is the case in most industrialized societies (save the United States).

The design of a superior health insurance system also should incorporate certain technical features. For example, most Americans probably would agree that health-insurance coverage should be *portable* between jobs, and from jobs into unemployment or retirement. Furthermore, the most Americans would probably agree that the system should be *administratively simple* from the perspective of both the insured and the providers of health care--as actually it is in the rest of the industrialized world. Next, the system should concentrate sufficient market power in the hands of patients and third-party payers to facilitate adequate *cost control.* Finally, many economists would argue that the system should not forcibly impose upon business tasks that are properly the government's, namely, to act as a tax collector for health insurance[1].

---

[1] A moment's thought should make it clear that "business" never pays any tax. It merely pays it in the first instance and then recoups it from either owners, customers or employees. In that sense, a government mandate upon business to provide employees health insurance merely appoints business firms as intermediary tax collectors.

SHORTCOMINGS OF THE CURRENT HEALTH-INSURANCE SYSTEM

The current American health-insurance system meets none of these design specs.

First, the system eclipses some 35 million Americans from coverage altogether and leaves an other 20 million or so underinsured. Many of these families are poor; one third of the uninsured are children. About two thirds of them are full-time workers and their dependents.

Second, the system ties the insurance protection of entire American families to particular jobs that are easily lost in the turbulent climate of the global market economy. Most Americans probably find it offensive that a family whose bread winner has lost his or her job should suffer the added burden of losing the family's health-insurance with it.

Third, our current system ties the health-insurance premiums paid by small business firms and individual families directly to the health status of their members through so-called *actuarially fair* pricing.

Fourth, our health-insurance system is administratively cumbersome. It absorbs a higher fraction of health spending in administration than does any other health system in the industrialized world. It also is a major irritant to physicians and other providers of health care.

Finally, by splintering the demand side of the health sector into literally thousands of small third-party payers, each lacking significant market clout vis a vis providers, the system has demonstrated its inability to control the annual growth of health spending. While some individual carriers may have had success with this or that cost-containment strategy, that success often has been ephemeral, and just as often has come at the expense of other payers through the mechanism of cost shifting. Overall, the much touted "pro-competitive" market strategy of the 1980s can hardly be said to have been a success.

The problem with our current health insurance system, of course, is not that the people working within it are either malicious or slovenly; they work hard and mean well. Rather, the system is so poorly configured that it literally brings out the worst in a basically decent group of citizens. A productive reform of the system must be one that channels the efforts of these hard-working people towards socially more desirable ends.

One approach that might achieve this goal would be the following private-public sector partnership that enlists the strengths of both sectors and that is rooted in the social ethic apparently preferred by Americans. Because the media insist that every proposal have a catchy name, I dub it the *All-American Deal*[2], to signify that it is not just some foreign import.

A REFORMED HEALTH-INSURANCE SYSTEM

Under the approach proposed here, employers would be left completely free to decide whether or not to make health insurance part of the total compensation package freely negotiated with workers in the labor market. Many firms probably would find that fringe benefit a good come-on in that competitive market. But employers would not be *forced* to make that offering.

A mandate on business to offer employees health insurance does not tax the mythical "fat-cat corporation." As already mentioned parenthetically in note 1 above, the cost of such a mandate is always shifted either to the owners (in the form of lower profits), to customers (in the form of higher prices) or to employees (in the form of lower wages or reductions in other fringe benefits).

In today's fluid, global capital markets, the owners of a firm's equity capital are unlikely to bear any of this cost shift, for they could easily take their capital offshore. In many markets, customers may resist price increases triggered by higher health costs. Probably the bulk of any employer-paid premium actually is borne by employees in the form of lower wages. In that case, a mandate upon business to pay for the health insurance of employees effectively becomes a highly regressive head tax on employment. It is a highly regressive tax, because the resulting wage cuts are likely to be roughly the same regardless of wage level; they will therefore constitute a higher percentage of low wages than of high wages[3].

Instead of mandating business to insure their workers, government should insist that every American family carry basic, comprehensive health-insurance coverage. Government should also make sure, however, that such coverage will be available to all families at

---

[2] My most preferred label is *The All-American, Public-Private, Judeo-Christian Health-care Partnership Plan.*

[3] See Uwe E. Reinhardt, "Are Mandated Benefits the Answer?" *Health Management Quarterly*, First Quarter, 1988; pp. 10-14, and "Health Care Spending and American Competitiveness," *Health Affairs*, Winter, 1989; pp. 6-21.

premiums they can afford. This requirement argues for a premium that is linked to a family's ability to pay.

Here's a thumbnail sketch of how such an approach might work. In that sketch, a clear distinction is made between the task of collection funds in an insurance pool, on the one hand, and disbursing these funds to the providers of health care, on the other. One should always treat these two facets separately when thinking about health-care reform.

Financing Health Insurance

On the 1040 tax forms, there would be two special lines pertaining to health insurance. On, say, line 31a, the taxpayer would be asked to enter X% of taxable income as a premium for a *Fail-Safe* health-insurance package that is automatically bestowed upon that taxpayer's household, unless that household attaches evidence of a private policy that is at least as comprehensive as the *Fail Safe* policy.

The premium rate "X" could be a flat rate or it could be made to increase progressively with income. For example, it might be set close to zero for very low-income households and might reach 10 to 12% for high-income households. At relatively high incomes, households would prefer to purchase private insurance policies, particularly if the industry figured out a way to make them available without the enormous administrative loading charges now added to premiums for individually sold health-insurance policies.

If written evidence of an adequate private policy were attached to the 1040, the household would be excused from the premium tax on line 31a. But it would be asked to pay, on line 31b, an small, progressive, earmarked *indigent-care* tax (perhaps an average 1% or so of taxable income). These funds would be needed to supplement the modest premiums collected from low-income families. Additional funds might be extracted from earmarked health taxes on alcohol, tobacco and gasoline, products known to contribute directly to the nation's health bill.

Finally, a case can be made on grounds of both horizontal equity and economic efficiency to include in am employee's taxable income part or all of the health-insurance premiums paid by an employer on behalf of that employee[4]. It has been estimated that the elimination of this tax-exclusion would yield an estimated $ 50 billion in additional federal taxes, and about $ 20 billion in additional Social Security taxes.[5]

The mechanisms described above, of course, deal only with one facet of a health-insurance system: the extraction of funds from individual households (who are always the ultimate payers in a health system) into an insurance fund. There remains the second facet, namely, the disbursement of these funds by the insurance funds to the providers of health care--the procurement and cost control facet of the system.

Procurement and Cost Control

A given *financing/insurance* mechanism can be coupled with a great variety of distinct *procurement/cost control* systems--an important point often lost in the debate on health policy when, for example, "managed care" or "managed competition"[6] is styled as a complete health-insurance program[7]. "Managed competition" per se is not a health insurance program; it is merely a particular form of procurement and cost control.

One can think of at least three distinct approaches to the procurement and cost-control facet of a health insurance system.

First, the Federal government could use its *Fail-Safe* fund simply to enroll all Americans who are not privately insured in the federal Medicare program. This would be a major move in the direction of the single-payer option proposed by some health reformers

---

[4] Although vehemently opposed by industry, labor and the insurance industry--for quite transparent reasons--economists have for years favored the elimination of this tax shelter as a matter of principle. For recent writings in the issue, see, for example, Stuart M. Butler, "A Policy Maker's Guide to the Health Care Crisis, Part I: The Debate Over Reform," *Heritage Talking Points*, Washington, D.C.: The Heritage Foundation, February 12, 1992, and Alain Enthoven and Richard Kronick, "A Consumer-Choice Health Plan for the 1990s," *The New England Journal of Medicine*, vol. 320, January 5, pp.29-37, and vol. 320, January 12, 1989, pp. 94-101.

[5] See Stuart M. Butler, *op. cit.*

[6] By "managed competition" is meant the arrangement by which competing "managed-care" systems are made to vie for enrollees. "Managed care" refers to the negotiation of prices by these systems with providers and the proctoring and controlling of the volume of services rendered patients providers. "Managed competition" implies "managed care," but not necessarily vice versa.

[7] *The New York Times*, an avid advocate of "managed competition," does this in its editorials with alarming regularity.

and one so often decried as "government medicine" by others. But this route is by no means the only procurement and cost control option one could couple with the *Fail-Safe* financing mechanism proposed above.

An alternative would be for the federal government to distribute its *Fail-Safe* fund to the states in the form of capitation payments that would be adjusted for age, sex and unavoidable regional cost variations. A fully operational mechanism for such capitation payments already exists for the current Medicare program. The individual state could then disburse these capitations (possibly supplemented with state funds) to the providers of care in a manner that suits local preferences.

Some states might prefer to enroll uninsured families in their own public, state-run program (for example, its own, modified Medicaid program). This would still be a government-run disbursement system, albeit a decentralized one.

Other states, however, may prefer to recycle the capitations into the private insurance sector by letting uninsured families choose one from a roster of competing, private "managed care" plans, an approach otherwise technically known as "managed competition" or, by the current Administration, as "coordinated care" and by Governor Clinton as "collaborative health networks."

If the *Fail-Safe* financing scheme outlined above were coupled with "managed competition" in this sense, one would not be operating what is so widely decried as "government medicine." Much of the current private insurance industry would survive health-care reform. But instead of spending its time seeking to exclude sick Americans from insurance coverage through expensive medical underwriting, the industry would be asked to turn its energy toward enhancing the value-to-cost ratio in health care through "managed competition" and "managed care." That would be a much more constructive role than the industry has hitherto played in American health care.

Adverse Risk Selection

In the absence of sanctions, the *Fail-Safe* component of the dual-track health insurance system outlined above would be subject to adverse-risk selection. Healthy people would tend to favor actuarially fairly priced private insurance; chronically ill persons would gravitate towards the *Fail-Safe* system, driving up its average cost. If such choices were feasible on an annual basis, they could destabilize the system over time.

Other nations that do operate dual-track insurance systems--for example, Germany--have dealt with that problem by making switches between the two systems cumbersome, slow and expensive. A German family that opts out of statutory semi-private health-insurance into the commercial, private system can return to the statutory system only under very rare circumstances (e.g., a lapse into extreme poverty)[8].

In the dynamic American economy, where a family's economic fortunes can fluctuate substantially over time, it would be difficult to outlaw returns to the *Fail Safe* system. Even so, it would probably be possible to make the process of switching sufficiently cumbersome and risky to avoid the clever and highly destabilizing cream skimming that has been the Achilles heel of any multiple track insurance system, notably the current one.

THE BEST AS THE ENEMY OF THE GOOD

Might the plan outlined above--private insurance alongside the *Fail-Safe* system--officially sanction a two- or multi-tiered health-care system in the United States? It might. Some tiering is inherent in the very idea of "choice" and "managed competition." But the system proposed here would be so much better than the multiple-tier system now in place, which literally offers "nothing" as its lowest tier.

Furthermore, Americans favor or at least tolerate a multi-tier approach in many other important human-services sectors, notably in education and in jurisprudence. For example, even otherwise egalitarian, Liberal thinkers who pledge allegiance to the idea of public schools nevertheless quite often rely on the upper-tier, private-school system for their own offspring, if they have the means to do so.

One should not evaluate proposed health-care reforms by ideal standards that are unlikely to be reached in practice. As Senator Moynihan has put it so aptly, in matters of social policy many well-meaning people too often have let the [hypothetical] *best* become the enemy of the [achievable] *good*. That approach may make well-meaning people feel good; but it usually ends up hurting the poor.

---

[8] In this connection, see U. E. Reinhardt, West Germany's Health-Care and Health-Insurance System: Combining Universal Access with Cost Control, in *A Call for Action*, Final Report of the U.S. Bipartisan Commission on Comprehensive Health Care, Vol. II; Washington, D.C.: U.S. Government Printing Office, September 1990, pp. 3-16.

AMERICAN NURSES ASSOCIATION PLAN

American Nurses Association. Nursing's Agenda For Health Care Reform. Washington, D.C.: ANA; 1991. [Pages 1-14, which constitute the Executive Summary, are reprinted here.]

NURSING'S AGENDA FOR HEALTH CARE REFORM

Nurses provide a unique perspective on the health care system. Our constant presence in a variety of settings places us in contact with individuals who reap the benefits of the system's most sophisticated services as well as those individuals seriously compromised by the system's inefficiencies.

More and more, nurses observe the effects of inadequate services and the declining quality of care on the nation's health. Firsthand experience tells us that the time has come for change. Patchwork approaches to health care reform have not worked. While preserving the best elements of the existing system, we must build a new foundation for health care in America. It is this realization that drives Nursing's Agenda For Health Care Reform.

Nursing's plan for reform converts a system that focuses on the costly treatment of illness to a system that emphasizes primary health care services and the promotion, restoration, and maintenance of health. It increases the consumer's responsibility and role in health care decision making and focuses on partnerships between consumers and providers. It sets forth new delivery arrangements that make health care a more vital part of individual and community life. And it ensures that health services are appropriate, effective, cost efficient, and focused on consumer needs.

A HEALTH CARE SYSTEM IN CRISIS

The strengths and weaknesses of our nation's health care system are well documented. Every day many Americans profit from the system's technological excellence, extensive medical research, well-educated health professionals, diverse range of providers, and myriad of facilities. Millions of people live longer lives because of the care they receive.

But America's health care system is also very costly, its quality inconsistent, and its benefits unequally distributed. Although the system provides highly sophisticated care to many, millions of Americans must overcome enormous obstacles to get even the most elementary services. In short, health care is neither fairly nor equitably delivered to all segments of the population.

As caregivers in a diversity of settings, responsible for providing care and coordinating health care services 24 hours a day, nurses clearly understand the implications of the system's failings. The more than 2 million nurses in America are at the front lines -- in hospitals, nursing homes, schools, home health agencies, workplaces, community clinics, and managed care programs. And what nurses see are the alarming effects of a system that has lost touch with the communities it is supposed to serve:

- More and more people must overcome major barriers to gain access to even the most elementary services.

- Too many Americans receive treatment too late because they live in inner cities or in urban or rural areas where service levels are inadequate.

- o People enter hospitals daily in advanced stages of illness suffering from problems that could have been treated in less costly settings or avoided altogether with adequate disease preventive and health promotion services.

- o The lack of access to prenatal care contributes to an alarming number of infant deaths and low birth weights each year.

- o Obstacles to obtaining fundamental services, such as childhood immunizations, are largely responsible for a resurgence in preventable diseases.

- o Disproportionate amounts of resources are used for expensive medical interventions which all too often provide neither comfort nor cure.

- o Every year expensive nursing home care impoverishes an alarming number of residents and their families.

Major changes in the health care system can no longer be put on hold. Further analysis and investigation will neither change the facts nor diminish the problems.

Today more than 60 million Americans are either uninsured or underinsured. This fact alone cries out for health care reform. Now the system's inability to contain costs is placing more and more Americans with 'adequate' insurance coverage at risk of hardship when major illnesses do occur. Employers and employees alike are desperately seeking solutions to the twin problems of rising health care costs and increased premium rates that threaten basic coverage for most American workers and their dependents.

Americans cannot afford to sit idly and do nothing. Health care costs are approaching 12 percent of the gross national product (GNP). Health care is expected to cost over $756 billion in 1991.(1) If nothing is done to control expenditures, spending is expected to reach $1.2 to $1.3 trillion by 1995 -- an increase of some $500 billion in less than five years. At this rate, if the system remains unchanged, spending will reach between $2.1 and $2.7 trillion by the year 2000.(2)

THE FRAMEWORK FOR CHANGE

Nurses strongly believe that the health care system must be restructured, reoriented, and decentralized in order to guarantee access to services, contain costs, and insure quality care. Our plan -- the product of consensus building within organized nursing -- is designed to achieve this goal. It provides central control in the form of federal minimum standards for essential services and federally defined eligibility requirements. At the same time, it makes allowances for decentralized decision making which will permit local areas to develop specific programs and arrangements best suited to consumer needs.

-3 change

Nursing's plan is built around several basic premises, including the following:

- All citizens and residents of the United States must have equitable access to essential health care services (a core of care).

- Primary health care services must play a very basic and prominent role in service delivery.

- Consumers must be the central focus of the health care system. Assessment of health care needs must be the determining factor in the ultimate structuring and delivery of programs and services.

- Consumers must be guaranteed direct access to a full range of qualified health care providers who offer their services in a variety of delivery arrangements at sites which are accessible, convenient, and familiar to the consumer.

- Consumers must assume more responsibility for their own care and become better informed about the range of providers and the potential options for services. Working in partnership with providers, consumers must actively participate in choices that best meet their needs.

- Health care services must be restructured to create a better balance between the prevailing orientation toward illness and cure and a new commitment to wellness and care.

- The health care system must assure that appropriate, effective care is delivered through the efficient use of resources.

- A standardized package of essential health care services must be provided and financed through an integration of public and private plans and sources.

- Mechanisms must be implemented to protect against catastrophic costs and impoverishment.

The cornerstone of nursing's plan for reform is the delivery of primary health care services to households and individuals in convenient, familiar places. If health is to be a true national priority, it is logical to provide services in the places where people work and live. Maximizing the use of these sites can help eliminate the fragmentation and lack of coordination which have come to characterize the existing health care system. It can also promote a more "consumer friendly" system where services, such as health education, screening, immunizations, well-child care, and prenatal care, would be readily accessible.

At the same time, consumers must be the focus of the health care system. Individuals must be given incentives to assume more responsibility for their health. They must develop both the motivation and capability to be more prudent buyers of health services. Promotion of healthy lifestyles and better informed consumer decisions can contribute to effective and economical health care delivery.

Finally, in implementing reforms, attention must be directed to the unique needs of special population groups whose health care needs have been neglected. These individuals include children, pregnant women, and vulnerable groups, such as the poor, minorities, AIDS victims, and those who have difficulty securing insurance because of pre-existing conditions. Lack of preventive and primary care for this sector has cost the nation enormously -- both in terms of lives lost or impaired and dollars spent to treat problems that could have been avoided or treated less expensively through appropriate intervention.

Access to care alone may not be sufficient to resolve the problems of these vulnerable groups. For those individuals whose health has been seriously compromised, a "catch up" program characterized by enriched services is justified. Coverage of pregnant women and children is critical. This first step represents a cost effective investment in the future health and prosperity of the nation.

It is this set of values that distinguishes nursing's plan from other proposals and offers a realistic approach to health care reform.

A PLAN FOR REFORM

Nursing's plan for health care reform builds a new foundation for health care in America. It shifts the emphasis of the health care system from illness and cure to wellness and care. While preserving key components of the existing system, it sets forth new strategies for guaranteeing universal coverage; making health care a more vital part of community life; and insuring that the health care services provided are appropriate, effective, and cost efficient.

The following pages provide a general overview of nursing's vision for a better health care system.

Universal Access To A Standard Package Of Essential Services

Nursing's plan envisions a new and bold approach to universal access to a standard package of essential health care services and the manner in which these services are delivered.

The federal government will delineate the essential services (core of care) which must be provided to all U.S. citizens and residents. This standard package will include defined levels of:

- o Primary health care services, hospital care, emergency treatment, inpatient and outpatient professional services, and home care services

- o Prevention services, including prenatal and perinatal care; infant and well-child care; school-based disease prevention programs; speech therapy, hearing, dental and eye care for children up to age 18; screening procedures; and other preventive services with proven effectiveness

- o Prescription drugs, medical supplies and equipment, and laboratory and radiology services

- o Mental health services and substance abuse treatment and rehabilitation

- o Hospice care

- o Long-term care services of relatively short duration

- o Restorative services determined to be essential to the prevention of long-term institutionalization

By taking this approach, traditional illness services are balanced with provisions for health maintenance services which prevent illness, reduce cost, and avoid institutionalization. Thus, hospital coverage and emergency care are covered, as are such services as immunizations, physical examinations, and prenatal and perinatal care.

The creation of federal minimum standards for essential services will necessitate modifications in existing public programs. The ultimate goal will be, over time, to merge all government-sponsored health programs into a single public program.

<u>Coverage Options</u>
Universal coverage for the federally defined package of essential services will be accessed through an integration of public and private plans and resources.

- o A public plan, administered by the states, will provide coverage for the poor (those below 200% of the federal poverty level), high-risk populations, and the potentially medically indigent. Any employer or individual will also have the option of buying into this plan as their source of coverage.

- o Private plans (employment-based health benefit programs and commercial health insurance) will be required to offer, at a minimum, the nationally standardized package of essential services. This package could be enriched as a benefit of employment or individuals could purchase additional services from commercial insurers if they so choose.

All citizens and residents will be required to be covered by one of these options. Under both the public plan and private plans, no one will be denied insurance because of pre-existing conditions. If employers do not offer private coverage, they will be required to pay into the public plan for their employees. Employer payments will be actuarially equivalent to the costs of employee and dependent coverage. Financial relief will be made available to small businesses (25 employees or less) for whom this provision would not be feasible. Individuals with no source of private coverage could also buy into the public plan. To assure universal access to essential services, systems will be developed to identify the insurance option through which each individual's needs are met.

Premiums and Payment Rates
Access to health care services will be enhanced by offering insurance premiums that the public can afford and payment rates to providers that are equitable and inclusive.

Both the public and private plans will utilize deductibles and co-payments to ensure that beneficiaries continue to pay for a portion of their own care and, therefore, have financial incentives to be economical in their use of services. Deductible amounts and co-payment rates, however, will never serve as barriers to care. Provisions will be made to waive or subsidize deductions and co-payments for households with incomes below 200% of the federal poverty level. Deductibles for certain types of programs and services (e.g. health promotion, such as well child care, immunizations, and mammograms; managed care plans) will be held to a minimum to encourage wider use of cost efficient wellness-oriented options.

Public and private payers will be required to offer fair and consistent rates of payment to providers. To protect access to care, providers will not seek payment at the point of service; nor will they be permitted to engage in balance billing. Because providers will be reimbursed fairly through insurance and the problems of uncompensated care will be largely eliminated, there will be no need for providers to charge consumers amounts above the established rate. Consequently, consumers' financial responsibility for health care services will be more predictable.

To make insurance more affordable to individuals and to reduce costs to insurers and employers, nursing's plan calls for reforms in the private insurance market. These reforms may encompass a variety of strategies, including:

- o Community rating for all insurers.

- o A cap on the out-of-pocket expenses individuals must pay for catastrophic care, including nursing home and other long-term care.

- o State reinsurance pools to protect insurers and consumers against the high costs of insuring a broader range of patients.

Special Programs for Vulnerable Groups

Countless individuals suffer from long-term health problems associated with inadequate access to basic health services over time. Often the poor and many members of minority groups are in this category. Special programs will provide services and outreach to vulnerable populations in order to compensate for formerly inadequate care and its consequences.

For infants and children (e.g. low birthweight babies, battered and neglected children, pregnant teenagers, children who abuse drugs, and young victims of violence and homelessness) such programing could be viewed as a health service (Healthstart) equivalent to the Headstart Program for those who are educationally disadvantaged. An expanded version of the Women's, Infants and Children (WIC) Program may be needed to produce quality outcomes in maternal-child health for poor and minority populations. Other special population groups may also warrant compensatory health programs beyond the scope of essential health benefits and services.

It is important to note that the ultimate goal of improved health is not achievable exclusively within the confines of the health sector. Social failures have serious health consequences. Improvements in the broader environment have a major impact on health status and health care costs. While the focus of this plan is on the health care system, nursing's long-term policy agenda for the nation is much broader. National health reform must also consider the interrelationships between health and such factors as education, behavior, income, housing and sanitation, social support networks, and attitudes about health. Better health cannot be the nation's only goal when hunger, crime, drugs, and other social problems remain. Consequently, nursing is committed to pursuing reform in other areas affecting health. Discussion of such reform, however, is beyond the scope of this paper.

Long-Term Care

High costs of long-term care often threaten to impoverish patients and their families. Nursing's plan seeks to prevent impoverishment and the potential loss of dignity by recognizing both public responsibility for long-term care and continued personal commitment to planning for such care. Financing arrangements will provide "front-end" coverage for chronic care and long-term care services of short duration through a variety of public and private options.

Beyond addressing short-term needs, individuals will be expected to assume personal responsibility for long-term care through strengthened private insurance programs and a variety of innovative financing arrangements. Such strategies will include privately purchased long-term care insurance, new savings and tax incentives, and home equity conversion opportunities. Such steps are essential to prevent individuals and their families from becoming impoverished by necessary care that can be anticipated and planned for. Emphasis on personal responsibility, however, does not ignore the fact that there will always be some individuals who will be left without resources who must reach out for public assistance.

Catastrophic Expenses
Length and/or intensity of illness may generate catastrophic costs. Given this fact, limits will be placed on individuals' out-of-pocket payments for catastrophic health care expenses. Costs to insurers or individuals that exceed preset limits will be covered through a state reinsurance pool, to which all insurers must contribute. Under nursing's plan, insurers will tap into the pool when their total costs or costs per patient exceed preset limits. When costs decline, they will resume normal financing.

Decentralized Delivery System
Although standards for essential health services and eligibility requirements are to be mandated at the federal level, delivery mechanisms for health services will be decentralized in terms of planning and administration to foster greater consumer orientation. Because local needs differ, states will have the authority to modify implementation to reflect geographical diversity.

To promote greater use of disease prevention and primary health care, services will be delivered, whenever possible, in convenient, familiar sites readily accessible to households and individuals. Maximizing the use of local settings, including schools, homes, places of work, and other community facilities, will help reduce the fragmentation of primary health care delivery and promote a more consumer-friendly system.

Cost Effective, Quality Care

By properly balancing individual health needs and self-care responsibilities with provider capabilities, care can be provided in a more efficient and coordinated manner. It can be more effectively directed at health promotion activities that will ultimately improve outcomes and reduce costs. Nursing's plan for reform is designed to achieve such balance.

Provider Availability
Financial and regulatory obstacles, as well as institutional barriers, that deny consumer access to all qualified health professionals will be removed. The wider use of a range of qualified health professionals will increase access to care, particularly in understaffed specialties, such as primary health care, and in underserved urban and rural geographical areas. It will also facilitate selection of the most cost effective option for care.

Under this arrangement, health providers must be reasonably and fairly compensated for their services. Where fee-for-service payment arrangements continue, payments for patient services must be made directly to providers.

Consumer Involvement
Consumers will be encouraged to assume more responsibility for their own health. Health professionals will work in partnership with consumers to evaluate the full range of their needs and the available services. Together the consumer and the health professional will determine a course of action that is based on an understanding of the effectiveness of treatment.

Outcome and Effectiveness Measures
Development of multi-disciplinary clinical practice guidelines is essential to the proper functioning of the health care system. These guidelines will be used to sensitize providers and others to the proven effectiveness of practices and technologies. With clear-cut information on the value of various procedures, payers, providers, and consumers can work together to eliminate wasteful and unnecessary services. Moreover, increased dissemination of research findings regarding health care outcomes will enhance provider and consumer involvement in making the most effective choices about care and treatment. By taking this approach, the likelihood of serious disputes or litigation over appropriateness of care will be minimized. Likewise, the need for defensive practices designed to protect providers against malpractice suits will be greatly reduced.

Practice guidelines and directives derived from research, while providing an element of control, will be supportive of innovation. Coverage will be extended to procedures shown to be significantly more effective, less costly than existing approaches, and/or useful in improving patient outcomes and quality of life. At the same time, an effort will be made to carefully weigh new therapeutic approaches with high start-up costs that may ultimately be less expensive than present methods.

Use of advancements in clinical practice and technology will be conditioned on satisfying criteria related to cost efficiency and therapeutic effectiveness. Such an approach will not deny people essential services. It will, however, assess carefully the appropriateness of providing high-tech curative medical care to those who simply require comfort, relief from pain, supportive care, or a peaceful death.

Review Mechanisms
State and local review bodies, representative of the public and private sectors and composed of payers, providers, and consumers, will be established. These groups, operating under federal guidelines, will determine resource allocation, cost reduction approaches, allowable insurance premiums, and fair and consistent reimbursement levels for providers. Such review will be sensitive to ethical issues.

Managed Care
Managed care will be instituted both to reduce costs and assure consumer access to the most effective treatments. Nursing's plan envisions managed care as organized delivery systems which link the financing of health care to the delivery of services, serving to maximize the quality of care while minimizing costs. To promote the use of managed care, enrollment in approved provider networks will be a requirement for those covered by the public plan. Managed care will also be encouraged for recipients of private coverage through reductions in deductibles and co-payments.

In the past, managed care has been used, in many instances, to protect the pocketbooks of insurers rather than the rights of consumers. Managed care must be restructured to retain the maximum possible consumer choice and to place a premium on services that address the health of consumers.

Case Management
In contrast to managed care systems, case management is rooted in the client-provider relationship. Case management services will be used to integrate, coordinate, and advocate for people requiring extensive services. The aim of case management is to make health care less fragmented and more holistic for those individuals with complex health care needs. A variety of health care professionals are qualified to provide this service. The first allegiance of these providers will be to their clients. Acting as advocates, they will provide both direct care and negotiate with systems on behalf of their clients. They will be authorized to access services for a given client.

Both case management (provider) and managed care (delivery systems) models are important to the smooth functioning of the health care system.

A Realistic Plan Of Action

Under nursing's plan, universal coverage will be achieved through implementation of both the public plan and private plan options. Employers will be motivated to collaborate with employees in shaping private plans which best satisfy their needs. At the same time, as larger numbers of more diverse groups participate in the public plan, the attractiveness of this option in terms of cost, quality, and image will be enhanced.

While the public and private sector plans can move forward simultaneously, it may be necessary to expand coverage to segments of the population in sequential steps. These steps would be introduced at an acceptable and financially reasonable rate until the ultimate goal of universal coverage is achieved. This approach would avoid excessive shocks to the health care system and allow the public to adjust to changing patterns of service.

Given this perspective, the first targeted population would include all pregnant women, children under age 6, and those individuals who demonstrate health status seriously compromised by a history of inadequate care. Improvements in coverage and benefits for these groups will have the greatest impact on the nation's future health and productivity.

As expeditiously as possible, other segments of the population would be covered. These groups might be approached as outlined below. This sequence, however, is not necessarily intended as a rigid order.

- o All children and young people, ages 6-18
- o All those above age 18 with incomes below 100% of the federal poverty level
- o All employees and dependents
- o All those with incomes below 200% of the federal poverty level

The process will culminate with the merger of all entitlement plans into a single public program to provide coverage to all citizens and residents who do not have or cannot obtain coverage through a private plan.

The Fiscal Implications Of Reform

It is impossible to predict the dollar amount which will be associated with the expansion of services or the efficiencies in nursing's plan. It is predictable that additional funding will be necessary to support start-up costs and transition. It is also possible that such expenditures will be recaptured over time.

A number of proposals for reform have been introduced. Among those proposals with cost estimates, additional health care costs range from $60-$90 billion. (3)(4) While nursing's plan for expanded coverage is similar in a number of ways to some of these proposals, offsetting proposed efficiencies integral to the plan will create significant dollars for real location. These resources will be directed to areas currently underfunded or excluded, including long-term care and primary care services.

While precise financial estimates are impossible at this time, several general observations can be made.

Cost Impact

Extension of coverage for essential services to the uninsured and underinsured will result in the dedication of more dollars. One source estimated that such coverage, if provided in 1990, would have added approximately $12 billion to health spending.(5)

It will also be necessary to dedicate more dollars to the expansion of long-term care services. Cost estimates for improved long-term care coverage vary. One 1990 study suggests that provision of comprehensive long-term care services, if implemented in 1990, would have cost $45 billion, $34 billion of which would have been new costs.(6) Nursing's plan, however, calls for more limited coverage supported through a combination of public dollars and enhanced personal responsibility.

In the initial phases of nursing's health care reform, the emphasis on preventive services will require dollars. Over time, however, improved health resulting from the availability of comprehensive primary care services will produce a cost-reducing "health dividend." By placing greater emphasis on health promotion and disease prevention in community-based settings, the system will reach out aggressively to individuals and households to foster an increased commitment to healthy lifestyles, prevention of disease, periodic screening for early detection of illness, and earlier treatment and promote informed decision making by the consumer. All of this will contribute to cost-effective, early interventions which, over time, will reduce the need for more costly care.

<u>Cost Savings</u>
New costs associated with nursing's plan will be offset to a considerable degree by the following cost saving initiatives:

- o Required usage of managed care in the public plan and encouraged use in private plans.

- o Incentives for consumers and providers to utilize managed care arrangements.

- o Controlled growth of the health care system through planning and prudent resource allocation.

- o Assurance of direct assess to a full range of qualified providers.

- o Development of health care policies based on effectiveness and outcome research.

- o Incentives for consumers and providers to be more cost efficient in selecting health care options.

- o Elimination of unnecessary bureaucratic controls and administrative procedures through such measures as standardized billing, simplified utilization review, streamlined administrative procedures, regulatory reforms, and consolidation of plans.

Sources of Revenue
To the extent that any additional dollars are needed, sources can be found. Responsibility for financing health care reform must be distributed equitably among individuals, employers, and government.

Individuals will continue to pay a portion of health costs through co-payments by households and individuals with incomes above 200% of the poverty level, and through reduced co-payments for those whose incomes are 100-200% of the poverty level.

Employers will provide private health insurance that meets or exceeds minimum federal standards for their employees and dependents or provide coverage through the public plan. Accommodations will be made to provide small businesses with the necessary financial relief to meet this obligation.

State governments currently pay a portion of health care expenses for the poor and fund certain other health programs. Nursing's health reform plan calls for consolidation of existing government health plans into a single public program. When this occurs, all states will contribute revenues to the program through maintenance of effort arrangements.

Revenues to pay for any increased costs could be derived from some combination of higher tobacco and alcohol taxes, additional payroll taxes, higher marginal income tax rates, and the increase or elimination of the income ceiling for FICA tax collection. A value-added tax (similar to a national sales tax) could also be considered.

A LOOK TOWARD THE FUTURE

The existing health care system stands as evidence of the futility of patchwork approaches to health care reform. America's nurses say it is time to frame a new vision for reform -- time for a bold departure from the present. Reform of any single component of the system will not do the job. Insurance reform alone will not guarantee access to care if the health care delivery system is not restructured. Conversely, many people will remain unserved or underserved if health care services are so costly that millions of Americans cannot afford to purchase care. To be most effective, a health care system must do more than provide equipment, supplies, facilities, and manpower. It must guarantee universal access to an assured standard of care. It must use health resources effectively and efficiently -- balancing efforts to promote health with the capacity to cure disease. It must provide care in convenient, familiar locations. And it must make full use of the range of qualified health professionals and diverse settings for care. It is this insight that underlies nursing's plan for reform, making it the most viable solution to the health care crisis.

-14 sources

SOURCES

1. U.S. Department of Commerce, U.S. Industrial Outlook 1991, Chapter 44, Health and Medical Services, 1-6.

2. National Leadership Coalition for Health Care Reform, A Comprehensive Reform Plan For The Health Care System, 2.

3. The Pepper Commission, A Call For Action; Final Report, September 1990, 137.

4. Mark G. Battle, National Association of Social Workers, Remarks During NASW's National Health Care Press Conference, January 8, 1991.

5. Lewin/ICF estimates in To The Rescue: Toward Solving America's Health Care Crisis, Families USA Foundation, November, 1990, 13.

6. Pepper Commission, 151.

LF:021
4-24-91

HEALTH INSURANCE ASSOCIATION OF AMERICA PLAN

Health Insurance Association of America. Health Care Reform Proposal, Washington, D.C.: HIAA; February 1993.

HIAA

Health Insurance Association of America

VISION STATEMENT

Our vision is a society of healthy individuals and communities. Our nation, through systemic change, will build upon our employer-based system to create a consumer-responsive, prevention-focused, affordable and cost-effective health system which fosters individual responsibility, human dignity, improved health status, and enhanced quality of life for all.

VISION GOALS

- *Promote a healthy and productive existence for all Americans, maximizing the dignity and quality of life for each individual.*
- *Recognize, as a society, that heroic efforts to extend life are not always appropriate or desirable. Dignity, quality of life, and the potential of returning to a healthy existence must be considered in treatment decisions and in the allocation of resources.*
- *Provide compassionate care to all people, especially to those who are chronically or terminally ill and cannot recover from their illnesses.*
- *Encourage Americans to take personal responsibility for maintaining good health regarding lifestyle factors within their ability to control.*
- *Stabilize health care costs as a percentage of individual financial capacity--earned income and other sources.*
- *Harmonize health care spending with other essential national requirements--the environment, education, the economy and security.*

February 18, 1993

1025 Connecticut Avenue, NW Washington, DC 20036-3998 202/223-7780 Telecopier 202/828-4511

GUIDING PRINCIPLES

Reform of our health care system requires comprehensive change. Change must include a shift in emphasis away from sickness and repair and toward health and wellness. The principles below comprise a unified whole, not a cafeteria menu. All elements integral to universal coverage and cost containment must be implemented together, not piece-meal nor staged over time one state at a time. HIAA believes that reform of our system must be guided by the following principles:

1. Reform must rely on competitive, pluralistic, and flexible delivery and financing systems in which all players--public and private alike--abide by the same rules. Government should not anoint winners; winners should be determined by the marketplace--a marketplace free to abandon failures and embrace promising new ideas.

2. Universal, "cradle to grave" coverage must be achieved by requiring all employers and individuals to pay for an essential package of benefits which should include primary, preventive and catastrophic coverage. Government cannot shirk its role; it must help subsidize those employers and individuals who cannot afford to purchase an essential package.

3. Insurers and other private payors must issue and renew coverage for all. To protect insurer solvency and maintain employer incentives to control costs and promote employee wellness, insurers can, within limits, establish premium rates which reflect risk. Coverage must be portable; there must be no pre-existing condition limits once in the system; and the problem of "job lock" must be eliminated.

4. Reform must build on our employment-based system. Employers' active participation in financing, selecting, and administering an essential package of coverage is critical to maintaining an open, flexible, and innovative health care system. Given their significant financial commitment, employers must retain control over their employees' health care coverage. Therefore, requiring employers to participate solely through group purchasing pools would invalidate the cornerstone of our employer-based system.

5. Changing the delivery system is fundamental. Managed care should be the primary vehicle for achieving sustained systemwide cost savings; we must allow it to evolve and develop into its next generation, including full participation of Medicare and Medicaid beneficiaries in managed care systems. A defining element of managed care systems will be their ability to collect and publish data which allow purchasers to compare outcome and price information. Employers and managed care systems will also provide incentives that promote healthy lifestyles and

personal responsibility. Managed care alone may not sufficiently control systemic health care costs. Therefore, alternative approaches (such as expenditure targets and provider rate regulation) should be explored as an additional means of controlling health care costs.

6. Government's role must be one of an enabler, not of a "doer". A primary and essential function must be to eliminate cost-shifting to private payors. Self-regulatory bodies will develop, implement and enforce rules of conduct for all players. These include rules of market behavior for all private and public payors, rules for providers to follow to ensure consistent payment levels which eliminate cost-shifting, and standards for electronic data interchange and for reporting outcome and cost information. Government-sanctioned self-regulatory bodies will also define essential package(s) of care, evaluate technologies for their cost-effectiveness, and establish a mechanism for pooling certain cost and utilization data. In addition, government must enact legislation reforming the malpractice adjudication system.

7. Tax preferences should be limited to the essential package of care, thereby motivating the public to seek the best value and providing additional revenue to finance expanded health care coverage.

CREATING A WORKING HEALTH CARE SYSTEM

We Americans have shorter life spans, higher infant mortality rates, and higher rates of violent death than do the citizens of other industrialized countries. Yet we pay more for health care per capita and more in total health costs--close to $900 billion a year--than does any other country in the world. Furthermore, an estimated 37 million people in the United States do not have health care coverage; if we as a society continue "business as usual," that number is expected to reach 40 million by the year 2000.

To make matters worse, the private sector has had to shoulder more than its fair share of the costs. The Prospective Payment Assessment Commission estimates that, in 1990, private payors paid $22.5 billion more than the costs incurred by their hospital patients to make up for losses hospitals experienced from the uninsured as well as Medicaid and Medicare patients. Put another way, private payors paid an average of 128 percent of actual provider costs; this amounts to almost a 30 percent "tax" on hospital costs paid by the nation's employers.

Clearly, these trends must be reversed. Over the last year, the Vision Committee of the Board of Directors of the Health Insurance Association of America (HIAA) met to discuss health care reform. The Committee members approached their task as

Americans who happen to know about health insurance rather than as health insurance executives who happen to be Americans.

HIAA's vision is a framework for comprehensive reform. Its underlying premise is that everyone with a stake in the success of American health care, including insurers, will have to do what it takes to create a working health care system. It reflects the conviction that the nation's health care needs can best be met by a competitive and pluralistic system, not a monolithic one, and that the private sector will continue to play a dominant role in financing health care. It calls for universal coverage for all and changes in the behavior of providers, payors, including insurers, and the public. It advocates that government be an "enabler," not a "doer," that it eliminate cost-shifting, and that it establish guidelines for everyone to follow. Our vision is premised on comprehensive reform; all initiatives central to its goal of universal coverage and cost containment must be implemented together, and in coordination with one another, to ensure maximum success.

Taken together, these reforms will lead to a sustainable reduction in the growth of health care costs and improve the health of the American people. We recognize, however, that these reforms will require significant new government spending. We have identified one possible revenue source--a limit to the tax preference employer-sponsored health insurance currently enjoys--but we recognize that other sources will be needed as well. It is critical that these newly generated tax dollars be applied only to building a health care system that will produce long-term sustainable savings; new revenues should not be wasted perpetuating the status quo.

The health insurance industry anticipates further discussion on many aspects of the system it proposes. Some areas need more thought, and some gaps need to be filled. As areas of uncertainty are clarified, this paper, which is not final, will be modified to reflect these changes. Some lack of specificity will have to be tolerated while we struggle to find solutions to difficult issues. (For purposes of this discussion, "health care" refers to services to prevent, diagnose or treat medical conditions. The reforms proposed here do not apply to coverage outside of the essential package, such as disability income, supplemental hospital indemnity, specified disease, Medicare supplement or long-term care insurance.)

COMPONENTS OF THE NEW SYSTEM

1. *Based on Pluralistic Financing and Delivery Systems*

Reform must rely on market-based pluralistic and competitive financing and delivery systems. Pluralism and choice are what engender competition--competition among ideas, among companies, among plans, and among values such as cost, quality and convenience. Only true competition can assure that our health care system remains flexible and open to innovation, so that it will continue to evolve to better meet consumers' needs in the future. A system with many buyers and sellers will assure breadth and depth of services and responsiveness to consumers. Market forces must be allowed to determine which systems shall succeed.

Comprehensive health care reform will require an expanded federal role to eliminate costly variations in state regulation and assure uniform standards--a level playing field--for all public and private payors. It will also require that government remove barriers to the growth of pluralistic, competitive systems.

2. *Builds on an Employer-Based Foundation*

Employers have a unique interest in maintaining employee health--as it affects productivity. Therefore, employers must provide coverage for all their employees and dependents. Employers will pay for at least part of this coverage. Some employers will receive government assistance to help cover their employees.

All employers, regardless of their size, will select plans based on the performance of competing managed care systems. A system built on an employer base is categorically inconsistent with the concept of exclusive group purchasing that bypasses employers altogether, thus relieving them of their responsibilities. Purchasing pools, such as group association and multiple employer plans, are common methods of obtaining coverage. We have no objection to a variety of demonstrations and experimentation with other forms of purchasing pools provided employer participation is voluntary. In no case should employers be required to buy health insurance solely through group purchasing arrangements.

A competitive and pluralistic system should allow purchasing pools to exist side by side with other methods of arranging coverage. **Insurance reform measures will prevent any one entity from bearing an inequitable share of risk because all payors will follow the same market rules to guarantee coverage.**

In addition, employers should:

- be free to experiment with and invest in a variety of approaches in providing an essential package of coverage;
- provide incentives to promote healthy behavior; and
- have incentives to help restrain costs because some element of their experience is considered.

3. *Achieves Universal Coverage for an Essential Package*

All Americans will have continuous coverage for an essential package of primary, preventive, and catastrophic care. Achieving universal coverage will require a series of mandates--on government, employers, insurers and individuals. How to divide these responsibilities will probably be the most difficult and controversial aspect of health care reform. Ultimately, it will be a political decision, not a health care decision. Clearly governments--federal and possibly state--will bear the cost of covering low-income people. Employers, in our view, should at the very least be required to incur the costs of offering health insurance to their employees.

HIAA supports a requirement that employers help pay for coverage for their employees and dependents. Even a modest employer payment would heighten employer cost consciousness and help restrain health care inflation. So-called employer mandates, however, are in effect a mandate on employees as well as employers, since employee premium contributions are envisioned in virtually all employer mandate plans. We are reserving judgment on how the costs should be shared between employer and employee, recognizing that there are practical limits on the ability of both employers and employees to shoulder the financial costs of a health care mandate. It may be necessary--however the cost is divided--to phase in the mandates over a period of years, taking account of any other employer mandates--such as increases in the minimum wage--that may be imposed at the same time. If an employer mandate is phased in, it will be necessary to coordinate it with other aspects of health care reform. For example, certain aspects of insurance market reform are not feasible absent a mandate; the two reform measures must be synchronized.

To achieve universal coverage, the following steps must be taken:

- Government must require all employers to arrange and help pay for an essential package of coverage for their employees and dependents. All individuals--those employed and those not connected to the work force--are required to obtain such coverage.

- Government must help employers and individuals who cannot afford to purchase an essential package. (Certain employers receive financial help, but they cannot "opt out" by paying a tax instead.)

- All individuals--those employed and those not connected to the work force--must receive the same tax incentives to purchase an essential package.

- The essential package covers primary, preventive, and catastrophic care. Government will authorize an independent body of providers, payors, employers and consumers to define the essential package of coverage. The design of this package must be flexible to encourage cost-conscious behavior; it must have inherent limits to prevent continuous expansion, recognizing that people's wants and desires may exceed society's resources; and it must not overlap or duplicate medical care coverage available elsewhere such as under workers' compensation and automobile insurance.

- There should be no difference in the essential package of coverage received by the poor and the non-poor. Government will finance coverage for low income individuals, but there will no longer be the need for a separate Medicaid program.

4. *Ensures Universal Coverage Through Market Reform*

Market reform must be premised on a government requirement that all individuals and employers purchase coverage. In this environment, all health plans will be subject to national rules of market behavior to guarantee universal and continuous coverage. The same rules will apply to all health plans, whether offered by commercial insurers, Blue Cross/Blue Shield plans, HMOs, self-insured employers, government, or any other entity. Problems such as "job lock" and lack of coverage for pre-existing conditions will be resolved. The rules of market behavior will:

- require that coverage be made available to every employee in an employment-based group;
- assure that every individual will be able to purchase the essential package, regardless of their health, financial or employment status;
- guarantee that coverage will not be cancelled, terminated or not renewed based on the health status or claims experience of any individual or group;
- prohibit insurer rating practices that create large rate differentials for groups of similar age, sex and geographic composition;
- maintain, at the same time, insurers' ability to calibrate rates to risk--pure community rating results in market disruption and works against cost containment in a variety of ways; and
- establish a form of reinsurance or risk-sharing to compensate for inequitable distribution of risk.

5. *Creates Sustained Cost Containment By Systemic Change in Financing and Delivery Systems*

Changing the health care delivery system is fundamental. The actual delivery of care must be substantially better organized than it is today to meet the needs of patients, purchasers, and providers. Therefore, managed care should be the primary vehicle for achieving sustained systemwide cost savings, and must be allowed to evolve and develop to its next generation. Managed care systems will serve the health care needs of communities by offering essential packages of care; they may also offer supplemental coverage.

Different forms of managed care coverage will compete on a level playing field. These competing forms of coverage include plans employing managed care techniques such as utilization review as well as managed care structures such as HMOs, PPOs, other network-based health plans, and evolving models. However, a defining element of all managed care systems will be their ability to collect and publish data which allow purchasers to compare outcome and price information across managed care systems.

Managed care systems will be permitted to pay providers in a variety of ways that encourage cost-effectiveness and quality care, including physician risk-sharing incentives, so that providers are rewarded for the cost-effective use of medical resources. New payment systems should encourage greater provider autonomy in decision-making and reduce the "hassle factor" that now results from micromanaging by payors.

Managed care systems will be user-friendly, efficient, and paperless. Administrative costs, and waste and fraud, will be significantly reduced. Improved alliances between providers and insurers will promote enhanced financial and managerial control of managed care systems, timely and responsive customer service, quality assurance programs, and fraud prevention.

Both managed care systems and employers will provide incentives that promote healthy behavior including discounts, promotions, and education. These incentives will reduce health care costs related to unhealthy lifestyle choices and will promote personal responsibility for one's health.

Given government's enormous buying power and its ability to influence provider costs, there should be strong incentives, perhaps requirements phased in over time, that Medicaid and Medicare beneficiaries fully participate in managed care systems to eliminate cost-shifting and control costs and utilization.

As managed care continues to develop, it will result in significant cost containment. However, managed care alone may not sufficiently control systemic health care costs. Therefore, alternative approaches (such as expenditure targets and provider rate regulation) should be explored as an additional means of controlling health care costs.

6. *Controls Systemwide Costs Via New Government Role*

Government will establish an entity that oversees and relies on one or more self-regulatory bodies to develop, implement and enforce rules of conduct for all players in the health care system. The regulatory framework will include all interested parties in the health care system--providers, insurers, employers, government, and the public. One, or possibly several, self-regulatory bodies will perform the following functions:

- establish consistent rules of market behavior for all health plans--those provided by insurers, self-insured employers, HMOs, government, or any other entity (see point 4);
- define essential package(s) of coverage that is made available to all, regardless of their income, age or employment status (see point 3);
- establish rules for providers to follow which ensure that they set consistent payment levels for all public and private payors for the same service. These rules should:
    - recognize that different payors may use different payment methods; and
    - assure that payments reflect real economic costs and value to providers and payors (such as convenience, service, adherence to quality standards, cost-effective practice patterns, or meeting additional contractual obligations).

      (In no case, however, should the rules allow providers to grant discounts to one payor simply by increasing the cost to another payor. The most important outcome of these new rules is to eliminate government's chronic failure to pay the true costs of care for poor and elderly Americans. In other words, Medicaid and Medicare should no longer receive special deals with providers at the expense of the rest of the population.)
- develop standardized guidelines for electronic data processing and a nationally uniform claim form to achieve an efficient and paperless system;
- evaluate technologies (i.e., drugs, procedures, and equipment) for their cost-effectiveness; sanction clinical guidelines (developed by appropriate professions) that can be used as legal defense against malpractice claims; determine valid experimental treatments eligible for reimbursement through participation in clinical trials;
- establish standards for the reporting of outcome and cost information published by managed care systems;

- establish a mechanism for pooling certain cost and utilization data on a regional, state and/or national basis to assist all payors in controlling costs and utilization, to help managed care systems produce outcome and cost data, and to help the government-authorized entity to develop guidelines that ensure that providers set consistent payment levels;
- enact legislative reforms of the malpractice adjudication system;
- enact legislation that allows insurers to exchange information for the purpose of identifying fraudulent providers; and
- consider actions needed to change the mix and supply of physicians and to increase the supply of physicians in inner cities and rural areas.

7. *Establishes Equitable Rules for All*

Government will require all public and private payors to play by the same rules. To achieve this level playing field, the regulatory framework must:

- avoid duplicative or overlapping regulation among the states or between the state and federal levels;
- remove all state regulatory control over anti-managed care laws, mandated benefits laws, and provider contracting laws;
- prohibit states from mandating additions to the essential benefit package; and
- amend ERISA to allow this regulatory structure to successfully implement the above responsibilities.

8. *Promotes Equitable Tax Policy*

Government must implement tax policies that eliminate perverse incentives for health care spending.[1] An unlimited tax preference for employer-sponsored health benefits does not promote cost-consciousness among employees. Instead, tax preferences for the essential package of coverage should be:

---

[1]As noted earlier, this vision addresses reform of the acute care medical system; it does not address long-term care financing reform. HIAA continues to support several recommendations in the latter area, including favorable tax treatment of long-term care insurance, on the grounds that the increased availability of affordable private insurance will have a significant impact on reducing future public (Medicaid) spending on long-term care.

- capped at a level equal to the essential benefit package;
- extended to the self-employed and to those who purchase the coverage outside of an employment setting;
- inapplicable to any premiums for health benefits in excess of the essential package; and
- inapplicable to cost-sharing requirements, such as deductibles and copayments, for the essential package.

Employers would continue to be allowed to deduct 100 percent of their contributions to employees' health coverage, even if their contributions are for coverage in excess of the essential package. (But employees are taxed on the excess.) In addition, the inequitable taxation of various payors must also be addressed to help level the playing field in the new system.

The revenues from these tax changes should be used only to help pay for health care reform. HIAA could not support these tax changes if cost-shifting is not adequately addressed or if the revenues generated from these changes are not specifically applied to health care reform.

SYSTEMIC FACTORS DRIVING COSTS ARE SLOWED

We have proposed many ways to create a sustained reduction in the growth of health care spending. Everyone will have continuous coverage so people will not wait until they are ill before seeking care. Managed care systems will discourage excess doctor visits, unnecessary hospital and specialist care, and technology use that is not cost-effective. Physicians will be empowered to practice effective, not defensive, medicine. Managed care systems will offer essential packages of care that will compete on price and value.

Providers will not be able to shift costs among payors, so true market competition will compel providers to become more efficient. A government-authorized entity will evaluate, and slow the use of, expensive technologies that are not cost-effective. Administrative simplicity, a paperless system, and standardized claim forms will save money and help control fraud and waste. Coverage of preventive care and incentives for healthy lifestyles will pay off over the long-run. Tax advantages will be limited to the value of the essential package of care, thereby motivating everyone to seek the best value.

Successful reform will yield measurable results and trends that will compare favorably to those of other nations on costs and on a variety of quality measures (such as mortality, percent who smoke, and height/weight standards).

HIAA will continue to refine its vision of health care reform. However, we are committed to achieving the objectives outlined.

Fixing the health care system will lift a sizable burden from our collective shoulders, yielding resources and liberating energies for other critical issues on the nation's social agenda.

SEPARATE ISSUE PAPERS

Additional issue papers are being developed on selected subjects. In some instances, these are descriptive papers discussing the pros and cons of the issue. In other cases, these are supplemental papers providing more detail than what is proposed herein. Topic areas include:

1. Price controls
2. Global budgets or expenditure targets
3. Extent of tax-favored treatment for health insurance
4. Precise nature of federal and state responsibilities
5. Cost estimates and revenue sources for reform
6. Implementation and enforcement of employer and individual mandates (including how much an employer contributes, which employees qualify under the employer mandate, and how a subsidy program could be structured)
7. Centrality of employers in providing coverage (including a discussion of the concept of group purchasing arrangements)
8. Insurance in the new market
9. Determining the essential package of coverage (including a discussion of supplemental coverages)
10. Medicare and Medicaid
11. Technology assessment
12. Tort reform
13. Individual responsibility, wellness and prevention
14. Measuring and assessing results with other nations
15. Medical care coverage under Workers' compensation and auto insurance

AMERICAN HOSPITAL ASSOCIATION PLAN

American Hospital Association. National Health Care Reform: Refining and Advancing the Vision. Chicago: AHA; 1992:1-16.

National Health Care Reform:
Refining and Advancing the Vision

This document was approved by the AHA Board of Trustees in May 1992. It is the Association's most current policy on health care reform. The AHA will continue to develop and improve its vision for change.

Executive Summary

Hospitals and their leaders have a professional responsibility to their patients and their communities to provide leadership in solving the problems of our health care system and making this nation the healthiest in the world. Toward that end, our nation must come together on strategies to promote health and well-being and to assure judicious use of a health care system reshaped to put patients first.

The challenge of health care reform is to simultaneously expand access to health care and contain costs while at the same time promoting improvement in the quality of care. The AHA's vision for reform, described below, provides for universal access, economic self-discipline for the delivery system, and quality care.

Universal access to health care coverage would be provided through:

- ❑ A pluralistic system of financing, combining private coverage and a new single public program consolidating and expanding Medicare and Medicaid.
- ❑ An emphasis on private coverage through the workplace, where employers ultimately would be required to provide and help pay for health coverage for their employees and dependents, with employees ultimately required to accept and pay their share of the cost of coverage. A significant phase-in period, with tax breaks for employers and low-wage earners and other types of assistance, would protect against economic dislocations.
- ❑ A basic benefit package in the public program that would serve as the floor for coverage offered in the private sector. Benefits should cover the full continuum of care, from preventive through long-term care. Issues of affordability should be addressed first by reducing unnecessary or marginal care and by adjusting cost sharing, before consideration of limitations on the scope of services. Following an opportunity for public comment, an independent commission would select the most beneficial combination of coverage and cost sharing, given the funds made available for the public program by the Congress.
- ❑ A plan to ensure the availability of physicians and other health professionals needed to provide adequate access to health care services for everyone.
- ❑ Insurance reforms that prohibit practices such as the use of pre-existing condition clauses, which result in avoiding rather than managing risk, diminishing the value of private health insurance.

Economic self-discipline in the health care system would be provided through:

- ❑ Fundamentally restructuring health care delivery through the establishment of community care networks that would provide patients with integrated care organized at the community level.
- ❑ Restructuring financial incentives using risk-adjusted capitated payments to networks to encourage providers within the network to promote the health of patients through primary and preventive care, collaborate with other providers to avoid unnecessary duplication of services, and conserve health care resources.
- ❑ Other complementary efforts, such as development and dissemination of medical practice parameters, medical liability system reform, reform of antitrust and other laws that impede efficient use of resources, and strategies for reducing administrative costs in the system.

The quality of care would be improved through:

- ❑ Reorienting the system to focus on improving the health status of communities and on coordinating and better managing patient care.
- ❑ Focusing attention on continuous quality improvement, which will further facilitate the integration of care and referral of patients within networks.
- ❑ A sustained level of governmental and private support for innovation and the evaluation of new clinical approaches.

The Need for Change

The U.S. health care system is unique, both in its strengths and weaknesses. In the aggregate, the United States has a wealth of health care facilities and highly trained personnel. We have long been recognized as a leader in the high quality of care provided. Our health care system has encouraged clinical innovation and is known for state-of-the-art treatments and technologies.

Despite these strengths, many problems remain. Chief among these is inadequate access to health care coverage in this country. There are currently 36 million uninsured individuals in the U.S., 10 million of whom are children. Half of the uninsured live in families with incomes below the poverty threshold. Medicaid, a program originally designed to provide health insurance for the poor, now provides care for only about 40 percent of the poverty population. Because of strained federal and state finances, even those who qualify for Medicaid face limitations on the services they receive. Many state Medicaid programs, for example, do not pay for screening and preventive services. Even for the privately insured, coverage limitations are more commonplace today as many employers and insurers resort to benefit cutbacks to limit their rising costs.

A compounding problem is the continuing rapid growth in health care spending. National health expenditures in 1992 are expected to exceed $800 billion, rising at an annual rate of over 10 percent. We currently devote more than 13 percent of our Gross National Product to health care spending, more than any other nation in the world. Despite this level of spending, the U.S. still suffers significant deficits in health status. For instance, among the western industrialized democratic nations, the U.S. ranks first in spending per capita, but 21st in infant mortality.

Faced with growth in health care costs, federal and state lawmakers have frequently opted to reduce payments to hospitals and physicians over the last 10 years. In the aggregate, the Medicare program now pays hospitals for only 90 percent of the cost of treating Medicare patients. State Medicaid programs frequently pay even less. While payment varies from state to state, in the aggregate Medicaid now pays hospitals for only 80 percent of the cost of treating Medicaid patients. In addition to these payment shortfalls, hospitals in 1990 provided over $9 billion in unsponsored care to the medically indigent for which no payment was received.

To cope with payment shortfalls and unsponsored care, health care providers have often shifted these unfunded costs to privately insured patients by raising their prices. For these and other reasons, private insurance premiums have increased even faster than hospital costs. These rising insurance costs which affect so many Americans, including middle-class Americans, have brought the issue of health care to the political forefront.

As costs rise, policy makers are increasingly dissatisfied with the health care system. While we have considerable capacity for providing care, our capacity is excessive in some areas and inadequate in others. The proliferation of freestanding health care facilities has added to the problem of excess capacity and encouraged further fragmentation of care.

Most importantly, rising costs, fragmentation of care, and coverage limitations and complexities have led to patient dissatisfaction with the health care system. In the current system, individuals generally receive health care from a changing array of providers, and only after they become ill. Patients are often left to patch together services in a variety of settings from unconnected providers. Adding to patients' frustrations are the paperwork and billing associated with an episode of care. After a hospital stay, for example, patients may receive one bill from the hospital, several more from attending and consulting physicians, and a notification of payment from an insurance company. All of this has begun to raise questions for all Americans as to the value they receive for the health care dollars spent.

AHA's Vision for Health Reform

Hospitals and their leaders have a professional responsibility to their patients and their communities to provide leadership in solving the problems of our health care system and making this nation the healthiest in the world. Toward that end, our focus is on affordable access to needed health care, including preventive services. This nation must come together on strategies to promote health and well-being and to assure judicious use of a health care system reshaped to put patients first. Leadership is required to forge partnerships among hospitals, physicians, other health professional groups, business, government, labor, insurers, the educational system and, above all, the American public.

AHA supports 10 goals for improving our health care system that everyone — citizens, providers, insurers, purchasers, and governments — must work toward. Our health care system should provide:

1. **Basic health services coverage for all.** All individuals, at a minimum, must have access to a benefit package of basic health care services.
2. **High-quality care.** Medical conditions must be effectively managed and coordinated and continuous improvement in the quality of care must be promoted.
3. **Community-focused, patient-centered care.** Care delivery and financing must be managed at the local level to recognize appropriate community variations in health care needs, available resources, and medical practice patterns consistent with national standards.
4. **Timely access.** Individuals must be encouraged to obtain care when and where it is most likely to change the course of a disease or prevent avoidable illness, loss or impairment of function, or death.
5. **Affordable care.** Patients must be able to obtain needed care for what they are willing and able to pay.
6. **Efficiently delivered care.** Financial and other incentives for participants in the health care system must be aligned to eliminate conflicting interests, discourage unnecessary duplication of services, and promote continuous improvement in the efficient use of resources to restore or preserve health.
7. **Adequately and fairly financed care.** To mitigate cost-shifting, any public or private financing program must itself bear the full cost of the services provided to its enrollees or beneficiaries.
8. **User-friendly care.** All participants in the health care system must be able to obtain, deliver, and pay for care with minimum confusion and paperwork.
9. **Adequate and appropriate supply of health care professionals.** We must ensure the availability of the number and types of physicians and health care professionals needed to provide access to health care services for everyone.
10. **Innovation.** We must encourage the continued development of new and more effective methods of treating and preventing illness and delivering services.

There are currently over 100 proposals being considered for reforming the U.S. health care system. But most do not address all of the goals we consider critical to improving the health care system. The current health reform debate centers on two priority, but competing, needs: expanding access and containing costs. The challenge of health care reform is to find an acceptable balance between expanded access and cost containment while at the same time promoting continued improvement in the quality of health care we provide. We believe that the AHA's vision for reform, described below, strikes an appropriate balance, providing universal access to coverage, cost containment, and quality care.

Universal Access

Universal access is the first priority. The AHA's proposal provides universal access to coverage for basic care through a pluralistic system of financing — a combination of private coverage and a new single public program consolidating and expanding Medicare and Medicaid.

Private Coverage

As in our current health care system, employer-sponsored private coverage would be the principal source of health care coverage for individuals under the AHA vision. This is the most practical road to universal access. It builds on the strength of current employer, employee, and insurer relations. Employer-based groups currently cover 88 percent of the nonelderly, privately insured population and more than 85 percent of the uninsured are connected to the workforce — either as workers or living in a family headed by a worker. Required employment-based coverage encourages employers to treat health care coverage like Social Security or workers' compensation — as a cost of doing business. It also provides the best means of maintaining a local relationship between providers, consumers, and payers.

AHA's approach would strengthen employer-sponsored coverage. Required employment-based coverage would be phased in and preceded by insurance reforms, tax breaks, and hardship funds for small and new employers to allow time to put in place more affordable coverage. Underwriting practices, such as pre-existing conditions clauses, designed to avoid rather than manage risk, would be precluded. Reinsurance mechanisms and insurance pools would be developed where necessary to spread risk so that more affordable insurance is available to small businesses and to self-employed and medically uninsurable individuals.

Ultimately, employers would be required to sponsor group health coverage and pay at least 50 percent of the cost of doing so for full-time permanent employees and their dependents and a prorated amount for part-time permanent workers and their families. Employers would retain the ability to self-fund coverage, but they would assume responsibilities and obligations for health care coverage that are equal to those of insured businesses, such as participating in state risk pools.

The employment-based coverage provided would have to meet minimum specifications of a federally-defined basic benefit package, described below, thereby pre-empting state mandated benefit laws. Employers would be free to offer more than basic health benefits if they and their employees so desire. Employees would be required to accept employer-sponsored coverage (unless they were otherwise covered) and pay their share of the cost of coverage. Low-income employees would be assisted by tax incentives (e.g., tax credits) to help cover their share of premiums.

In the area of taxes, Congress would grant the same tax advantages to self-employed individuals and unincorporated businesses for the purchase of health benefits (100 percent, rather than 25 percent, deductibility of premiums as a business expense) that large employers and their employees currently enjoy.

Incentives such as these can be used to maintain a pluralistic financing system with heavy reliance on employer-sponsored private coverage. The key is to design incentives that make private coverage economically feasible and desirable for employers and employees.

A New Public Program

On the public side, a new program would consolidate and expand upon Medicaid and Medicare, providing basic health benefits to these individuals as well as to all others unable to obtain private coverage. Government's first priority in subsidizing coverage under the public program should be targeted at those least able to afford coverage.

Enrollees in the public program with income less than 150 percent of the federal poverty level would receive fully subsidized basic benefits, with the possible exception of nominal cost sharing. Those with income greater than 150 percent of the federal poverty level would make contributions to premiums scaled to their ability to pay, in addition to copayments and deductibles. The public program would pay for all Medicaid recipients in full and would pay all or part of the premiums and cost-sharing for most Medicare beneficiaries.

The public program would be financed by a combination of broadly based federal tax revenues and premium contributions from those covered who can afford them. These monies would be dedicated to an off-budget trust fund that would pay for covered health care costs for public program enrollees. With a single public program, states' financial responsibility for Medicaid could gradually be phased out, but they could continue to subsidize those unable to pay the long-term care deductible proposed as part of basic benefits coverage. Federal and state financial responsibilities for other domestic programs could be realigned to maintain current levels of state health funding support.

BASIC BENEFIT COVERAGE

Private Coverage	Public Coverage
Employer-based coverage of employees and dependents Other privately covered Individuals	Medicare Medicaid Individuals unable to obtain private coverage

Basic Benefits

AHA believes that coverage of the full continuum of care is a necessary first step in refocusing on efficient clinical decision making. AHA calls for a broad basic benefit package covering the full continuum of care from preventive care through long-term care. Historically, public and private benefit packages have addressed the affordability issue by excluding or severely limiting coverage of certain types of services. This approach has had several practical but unfortunate effects: discrimination against certain types of illnesses (such as Alzheimer's disease) and creation of incentives for health care practitioners and providers to deliver whatever services are covered, rather than the most efficient service to meet a patient's need.

In order to provide incentives for the responsible use of health care services by consumers, some cost sharing would be required. To create the right incentives, cost sharing would not be applied to preventive services, but would be focused on those points where consumer judgment on whether, when, and where to seek services plays a significant role in appropriate utilization. For example, if enrolled in a network where a primary caregiver oversees access to specialty care, cost sharing might focus on primary care visits, emergency room visits, and outpatient prescriptions. If not enrolled in such an arrangement, cost sharing might apply to all but preventive services. This approach, in addition to being sensitive to the consumer's decision making role, has the added advantage of providing the incentive of reduced exposure to out-of-pocket costs for those consumers who enroll in networks where utilization could be better managed.

To maintain incentives for families to continue their role as caregivers, long-term care (other than post-acute recuperative care) would carry a $10,000 deductible. These deductibles and copayments would be waived for low-income individuals to assure that they do not serve as barriers to access.

Determining the basic set of benefits is perhaps the most difficult and critical element of this proposal — difficult because it means reconciling benefits with available funding; critical because it determines the core of health care coverage. An independent commission, established outside the federal political and budgetary process, would be responsible for defining the basic benefits package. On a biannual basis, Congress would determine the aggregate funding level for the new public program. The independent commission would then determine the specific benefits that could be provided by the public program within that budget. This set of benefits also would serve as the benefit floor for coverage offered in the private sector, thereby pre-empting state mandated benefit laws. Coverage under the benefit package would be defined by health care needs and services, not specific provider settings, leaving latitude to assure that care is delivered in the most appropriate, cost-effective setting.

The primary objective of establishing an independent commission is to stimulate a public debate on the proper balance between the health care benefits to be promised and the funds available. The independent commission would first provide Congress the information and advice it needs to set a budget target for the public program. This might include information on benefit levels and cost sharing, the adequacy of public program funding, and the adequacy of provider payments under the public program. Given the funds made available for the public program by Congress, the independent commission would select the most beneficial combination of coverage following an opportunity for public comment. If the funding level is inadequate to cover some services that the public wants, Congress and the President would be pressured by voters to increase health care funding levels.

Several approaches are available for balancing health care benefits with available funding. The first step would be to identify and eliminate inappropriate and unnecessary care from the health care system. This can be facilitated by promoting effectiveness and outcomes research to identify where care currently provided to patients yields marginal benefit to their health or quality of life. Equally essential is the development and use of medical practice parameters, which operationalize what we learn from such research by improving our understanding of what types of care are appropriate under specific clinical circumstances. Reforming our medical liability system can also be helpful by obviating the need to practice defensive medicine, as well as reducing the excessive costs currently associated with the tort system. Promoting the widespread use of living wills and other advance directives would make it easier for patients and their families or guardians to reject non-beneficial final care.

If savings from reducing inappropriate and unnecessary care are not enough to bring benefits and costs into balance, the independent commission, through a public process, would develop and apply criteria for determining which services and clinical conditions would be covered in the basic benefits package. Once the commission has included coverage for a particular clinical condition, it would be expected to cover all services necessary to treat the clinical condition including long-term or rehabilitation care. The intention is that no type of service would be excluded arbitrarily from coverage in all cases. Rather, criteria would be developed to include services for specific clinical conditions. Heath care practitioners and providers would not be required to provide services excluded from the basic benefit defined by the commission.

Another avenue available to the commission in reconciling the definition of basic benefits with available funding would be the adjustment of cost-sharing and premium levels. The implications of the commission's decisions would be significant. Coverage and cost-sharing variations can have two primary effects: shifting expenditures from premium costs to patient out-of-pocket costs or vice versa, and stimulating or curbing utilization of services which would affect total health care expenditure levels.

For example, if the commission chooses to augment capitated premium payments with high consumer cost sharing (e.g., a deductible of $500 for inpatient and outpatient care, a $10,000 deductible for institutional long-term care, and coinsurance of 20 percent except for preventive care) the average annual premium would be about $2,630, at least half of which ($1,315) would be paid by the employer. By comparison, the average premium in existing employer plans is about $3,440, of which the average employer pays about 75 percent ($2,580). An approach that incorporates high consumer cost sharing, however, would need to be coupled with some sort of limit on out-of-pocket expenses based on income to assure that no one would be impoverished as a result of these cost-sharing requirements.

Alternatively, the commission could select an intermediate approach, with capitated premium payments and fixed dollar copayments for just those services where the consumer has significant influence over utilization (e.g., routine care). Under this scenario, the average annual premium would be about $3,940. The higher annual premium amount reflects lower consumer out-of-pocket spending. Because this type of approach means that networks are more reliant on capitated payments and must bear the associated financial risk, networks might be required to carry stop-loss insurance coverage to guard against unpredictably large expenses.

The commission also could choose to finance benefits entirely through capitated premium payments, imposing no cost-sharing on consumers except for long-term care services. The average annual premium in this case would be highest — about $4,305 — reflecting no additional spending required on the part of consumers. However, an approach that requires no consumer cost-sharing is likely to result in increased utilization of services since consumers would not be asked to bear any additional cost of care.

Economic Discipline

In this environment of limited financial resources and competing public priorities, our nation must seriously address the issue of cost containment beyond the question of benefit coverage. Because our current health care system encourages further fragmentation of care as well as unnecessary use and duplication of services, the AHA believes that simply increasing access to the current system will deepen frustrations with health care costs and invite more intrusive regulation by government and insurers without corresponding benefit to patients.

Competing incentives for health care providers and consumers have led to a system that is costly and fragmented. Physicians are paid for each service rendered, giving them an incentive to provide more services. Hospitals, on the other hand, are often paid a fixed amount per patient for each admission, particularly for Medicare patients. Once a patient is admitted, hospitals are encouraged to conserve health care resources by providing medically necessary services, but no more. There is no incentive, however, to keep people out of the hospital in the first place. In the absence of such incentives, insurers use external utilization review to constrain access to hospital care. Consequently, more tests and more surgeries are being provided outside hospitals in physicians' offices or in freestanding facilities where financial incentives to conserve are generally absent and quality assurance mechanisms seldom are in place.

The result is that patients must navigate a fragmented health care system, going from provider to provider in order to seek the full spectrum of care they need. Because most consumers have insurance and do not pay directly for the cost of much of the health care they use, consumers have little incentive to conserve their use of health care resources, to weigh potential benefit compared to cost, or to shop for the most cost-effective providers.

Responsible and effective cost containment begins by restructuring the health care delivery and financing systems to realign incentives and encourage the efficient use of resources by everyone.

Restructuring Health Care Delivery

Health care delivery should be fundamentally restructured by establishing community care networks that would provide patients with integrated care organized at the community level. Networks would be responsible for providing all of the services covered for their enrolled population and would coordinate patient care over time and across various provider settings. Patients would turn to their network for everything covered — from preventive care to acute care to long-term care services.

Where possible, consumers would have a choice of networks as they became available in each community. Required annual open enrollment would ensure that no one was "locked in" to an unsatisfactory network. In smaller communities where only one network may be available, other safeguards would be needed to ensure that the network is held publicly accountable for patient satisfaction and the quality of care it provides to the community.

Community care networks are the keystone to universal access. They are designed to:

Focus on community health status. Networks would be responsible for maintaining and improving the health status of their enrollees, giving them an incentive to reach out into their communities and to work with public health, social service or other organizations that can help to measure and improve health status.

Focus on patients. Networks would minimize patient hassles by truly managing and coordinating care, by making available a broad spectrum of care, and by giving patients a consistent point of access to the health care system.

Focus on prevention and primary care. Networks would emphasize wellness in addition to the treatment of illness.

Focus on community-level solutions to community problems. Networks would match local health care resources and strategies to local community needs and circumstances.

Community care networks represent a self-disciplining system with coherent and consistent incentives that encourage providers to do what they do best — manage the health care of their patients.

Community care networks hold the promise for true management of patient care. Many of the current "managed care" arrangements are simply insurer programs that contract with a selected group of providers who agree to discounted prices. The providers participating in the plan often change each year as the insurers use their leverage to seek deeper discounts from providers. The insurer then controls access to those providers through a complex system of authorizations that must be obtained from the insurer before anyone can receive non-emergency care. While this approach emphasizes managing *costs*, it does not manage *care*.

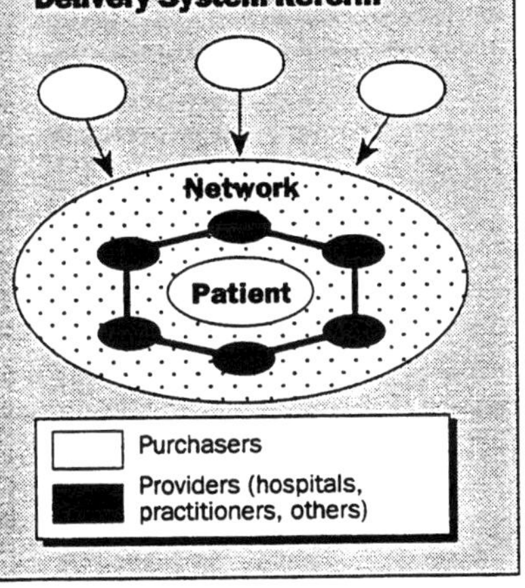

AHA Proposal for Delivery System Reform

True managed care requires assessing patient health risks and needs. It means planning and organizing care so that problems are averted or treated early and all needed services are efficiently provided without unnecessary duplication of capacity. Within community care networks, patient needs would be returned to the focus of the delivery system and the management of care responsibility would be returned to the caregivers.

To meet these goals, as well as to create a more user-friendly system, each network enrollee would choose a primary caregiver to assure a consistent, specified point of entry into the network. The primary caregiver would act as the care manager for that individual. It would be the primary caregiver's responsibility to ensure that an initial evaluation of health status is conducted, that appropriate primary care and preventive services are provided, and that services throughout the system are coordinated for the patient, particularly when specialty services are needed.

Restructuring Financial Incentives

The key to successful community care networks is creating strong incentives for Americans to choose them and aligning provider incentives through risk-adjusted capitated payments to the networks. Capitation — a set fee paid to the network per enrollee — provides the network with its budget for delivering care to the enrolled community. It allows the public program, employers, and employees to manage their outlays, but leaves the allocation of resources to local decision making. Most important, it provides the stimulus for reorienting our health care focus from sickness to wellness. This type of approach encourages providers to:

Promote the health of patients and prevent future, more costly illnesses. If the network's enrolled population is relatively stable, then the network has an incentive to provide its enrollees with low-cost preventive care now in order to avoid the use of more costly acute care in the future.

Collaborate with other providers to avoid unnecessary duplication of services. Once providers are linked within a network, the financial incentive will be to avoid duplicative facilities and services that were encouraged previously by the competitive system.

Conserve health care resources by providing only appropriate and necessary care. The collective challenge to providers within networks will be to provide needed health care services within the fixed capitation amount through better patient care management by practitioners and institutions.

The independent commission responsible for determining the basic benefit package would also be responsible for setting actuarially sound capitated rates under the public program to be paid to networks. This commission would balance the public need for cost containment with hospitals', practitioners', and other providers' need for fair payment.

The independent commission also would adjust those rates to reflect the underlying risk of the population covered and the geographic conditions under which services are delivered. By broadly adjusting the capitation payments to networks, the payments would better reflect the expected costs of serving each network's enrolled population. This gives networks the incentive to treat everyone in their community; young or old, sick or well.

Placing capitation rate-setting for the public program in the hands of an independent commission does not guarantee elimination of government cost-shifting to the private sector. The AHA believes it can go a long way, however, toward minimizing it. In the private sector, network payment rates would be negotiated between networks and employers. It would be left to individual states to decide whether to regulate those decisions in any way.

Because capitated payments require the network to take on some financial risk, networks might be required to carry stop-loss insurance coverage to protect against unpredictably large expenses.

Network Characteristics

Networks are designed to foster new relationships among physicians, other health professionals, hospitals, community health centers, and nursing homes as well as private insurers. As the major sources of care in most communities, hospitals and physicians would need to be key partners in the formation of networks.

Hospitals often provide services beyond inpatient acute care, and are the locus of most specialized technology. Moreover, as generally the largest health delivery organizations in their communities, hospitals can provide many of the management and service coordination skills and systems necessary to integrate and manage the delivery of high-quality services.

Physicians and other health professionals are essential to successful formation and operation of networks. Patients build strong relationships with their physicians. For many people, their primary care physician is the first point of entry into the health care system. Networks must actively involve local physicians in order to coordinate and manage patient care.

Networks also offer a range of opportunities for private insurers. Insurers may choose to partner in a network, with providers and the insurer underwriting the risk of the enrolled population. Alternatively, insurers may participate in networks by providing reinsurance to networks, marketing and promoting networks to prospective enrollees, assisting networks in evaluating their cost and quality performance to support marketing, helping with regulatory compliance and insurability decisions, processing provider payments within the network, etc.

Hospitals, physicians, insurers, and other participants may choose from a variety of roles in the network. They may assume a leadership role as a network owner, a partnership role, or more traditional roles. Networks may form between selected providers and major employers, local government, or insurers. Even where hospitals and physicians are not network owners or partners, some may wish to negotiate a payment arrangement to share in the overall operating results of their network. Ownership and governance of networks could take a not-for-profit, investor-owned, or public form, depending on local values, interests, and practical realities.

Larger communities may be served by several networks while smaller communities might be served by only one. The number of networks would be determined in part by the number of parties willing to organize into partnerships in an area. The number of networks in an area also would be affected by each network's need to pool health costs and risks over a sizeable enrolled population.

Broad government parameters would guide network formation. Some of these guidelines would provide assurances to the public as to the financial stability of networks. Other guidelines might address networking with hospitals that have special missions such as teaching, research, or care to the indigent, to encourage the participation of these institutions. Similar guidelines might address the inclusion of physicians offering specialized services. No requirement would be made to include all area providers in a network.

Above all, the network concept is flexible and must remain so. Because networks are designed to reflect the individual needs and preferences of each community, no two networks will look exactly alike. Network arrangements will vary by geographic location in order to recognize appropriate community differences, preserve latitude for local decision making, and provide for appropriate involvement of state and local governments. A uniform approach to the organization and operation of networks would defeat the goal of community-tailored health care.

Flexibility also means open arrangements for the payment of providers within the network. While most networks would operate on a budget determined by the fixed annual payments per enrollee, the network could choose to pay its providers in a variety of ways. Hospitals might by paid based on costs, prospective rates, per admission or other unit of service, a capitated rate, or a global budget. Similarly, physicians might be paid based on costs, a fee schedule, a salary, or a capitated rate. Hospitals, physicians, and others might share in the operating results of their network.

In looking to the future, collaboration among providers within networks, with constructive competition across networks where two or more are formed, seems to hold the best promise for expanding access to health care while controlling costs. But to reassure the public of the value that can be achieved under this approach, public accountability is essential. Networks would be structured to give providers greater freedom to make decisions without the micro-management by government payers and insurers. In exchange, networks of providers must be willing to be accountable to government, employers, and the public for their financial and quality performance.

Public accountability might be demonstrated in various ways. Networks might provide regular reports to their communities on health status improvement, patient satisfaction, and provider satisfaction with network relationships. Public accountability might be achieved by reporting on selected indicators related to network costs, quality, and overall efficiency. This information could be compared across networks if adjusted to reflect population risk and use factors such as age, sex, or socioeconomic status. In communities served by only one network, a greater measure of public oversight might be needed. Public accountability in this case might be demonstrated through more direct public oversight of network operations and capitated rates or through public representation on the network's governing body. The goal is for networks to strengthen, not diminish, accountability to patients and the public.

Community care networks hold the promise for improving the health of our nation in a cost-efficient way. But how much society can save on its health care bill depends in large part on what society is willing to do. Saving money will depend on the extent to which community care networks are established throughout the country and used by consumers as their health care source. The formation of networks and consumer selection of networks would be encouraged by tax and other incentives, moving at a pace determined not only by the strength of the incentives but also by how fast the advantages of networks are realized.

If strong incentives are provided to encourage the formation and use of networks, 80 to 85 percent of the population is expected to enroll in networks. If society requires participation in networks and everyone enrolls, system efficiencies and administrative savings would be about 20 percent greater. If, however, no changes are made in incentives to form or use networks, only 20 to 25 percent of the population would be expected to enroll. In this case only about one-quarter of potential system efficiencies and administrative savings would be achieved.

Human Resources

The United States must adopt a more coherent and comprehensive approach to ensuring the availability of physicians and other health professionals needed to provide adequate access to health care services for everyone, particularly access to primary care as universal access to health care coverage becomes a reality. The human resource policy goals are adequate supply, efficient use of health care professionals, and appropriate geographic distribution of needed human resources. Steps to achieve these goals must be based on sound assessments of human resource needs and should focus on both the near and long term.

To accomplish this, a second public/private commission would be established to provide a regular and comprehensive assessment of future human resource needs. Advice from this commission could be used to develop both national and state strategies. The commission also would provide advice on national health care training policies and federal funding priorities for educational program and student support. The direction and organization of graduate medical education should be a collaborative effort by hospitals, medical schools, affiliated programs in alternative settings, appropriate national standard setting agencies, and the commission.

Community care networks, through their providers, should be responsible for conducting or supporting educational programs in the health professions and allied fields to ensure a continuing supply of trained professionals for their community. Further study is needed, however, on the appropriate methods for paying providers for the cost of educating physicians and other health professionals within the framework of community care networks paid on a capitation basis.

Initiatives would be designed to stabilize training programs, promote new programs where needed, reorient training programs to future needs, and attract qualified students to the health professions. For example, efficient use of health care professionals would be promoted by enhancing career mobility within professions and eliminating barriers that unnecessarily limit flexibility and discretion in the use of personnel. Appropriate geographic distribution of health care professionals would be achieved by attracting and retaining personnel in poor, remote, or underserved areas so that everyone has reasonable access to needed services.

Research

Health system reform must include a sustained level of governmental and private support for innovation and the evaluation of new approaches. Biomedical research enhances our capacity to diagnose and treat illness; health services research is essential for more complete information on such critical issues as assessing the efficacy of diagnostic and therapeutic regimens and establishing the relationship between treatments and outcomes. Our future ability to improve the value of health care services will depend in significant part on rigorous evaluation of today's and tomorrow's delivery and payment system innovations.

From Vision to Reality

AHA's vision for reform could be implemented incrementally in order to minimize disruption in current coverage patterns and facilitate the broadening of benefits. For example, access could be expanded in stages. Starting with mothers and children, coverage of the poor and near poor who are not currently covered by Medicaid should be provided by the public program over a pre-established period of time. Next, individuals with incomes exceeding 150 percent of the poverty level could be phased in, making premium contributions according to ability to pay.

Similarly, community care networks could be developed in stages, growing in concert with community values and needs. Listed below are some of the changes needed to make the health reform vision a reality.

Changing the Health Care Environment

- ❏ In hospital strategic planning and operations, shift emphasis from provider competition to collaboration and integration. Focus on both hospital/physician relationships and hospital-to-hospital relationships
- ❏ Seek antitrust reform to allow for greater provider collaboration
- ❏ Seek tort reform to reduce the cost of the malpractice system and its effect of stimulating defensive medicine
- ❏ Seek insurance reform to make health insurance more available and affordable for employers and individuals
- ❏ Equalize tax incentives for all employers to provide health insurance for employees and their dependents
- ❏ Seek new programs or waiver authority that offer options for reorienting care delivery in government programs
- ❏ Improve funding for Medicare and Medicaid

Developing Resources and Skills

- ❏ Develop provider skills in accepting and managing financial risk
- ❏ Expand emphasis in medical education programs on primary care careers
- ❏ Invest in medical practice parameters, clinical guidelines, and outcome measures with rapid implementation
- ❏ Develop community health status and needs assessment tools
- ❏ Encourage community reports on population health status
- ❏ Establish uniform data requirements and implement electronic methods to collect, store, and share community and patient data across providers

Encouraging the Formation and Use of Networks

- ❏ Work with physicians and other providers in transitional network arrangements such as IPAs and PPOs
- ❏ Develop networks consistent with existing waiver authority under Medicaid and Medicare HMO/CMP options, and employer opportunities at the local level
- ❏ Require employment-based coverage for basic benefits package
- ❏ Strengthen financial incentives for public program beneficiaries to use networks, including required network enrollment where there are at least two networks from which to choose
- ❏ Offer tax or other incentives aimed at employers, employees, insurers, and providers to offer and use networks

JACKSON HOLE GROUP PLAN

Ellwood PM, Enthoven AC, Etheredge L. (1992). The Jackson Hole Initiatives for a Twenty-First Century American Health Care System. *Health Economics.* 1:149-168.

Enthoven A. (1992). Commentary: Measuring the Candidates on Health Care. *N Eng J Med.* 327:807-809.

Toner R. (February 28, 1993). Hillary Clinton's Potent Brain Trust On Health Reform. The New York Times. F1, F8.

HEALTH ECONOMICS, VOL. 1: 149–168 (1992)

THE JACKSON HOLE INITIATIVES FOR A TWENTY-FIRST CENTURY AMERICAN HEALTH CARE SYSTEM

PAUL M. ELLWOOD, ALAIN C. ENTHOVEN AND LYNN ETHEREDGE

INTRODUCTION

The 'Jackson Hole Group' is an informal collection of health industry leaders, public officials, and health services researchers that started meeting in the mid-1970s in Paul Ellwood's living room in Jackson Hole, Wyoming. Ellwood, a paediatric neurologist, is CEO of InterStudy, a non-profit health policy research institute. Usually there have been about 15 to 20 participants. The composition of the group has varied as focus shifted from one to another aspect of the health care system. Alain Enthoven, an economist and Stanford professor, participated from the outset. Lynn Etheredge, former official in the Office of Management and Budget and now an independent health policy analyst, joined in the late 1980s. A list of attendees who have been active in recent discussions is in the appendix to this article.

In recent years, the Jackson Hole discussions have focused on understanding the shortcomings of existing private sector institutions and public policies that make up the nation's health care system. Each attendee presents an analysis of the subject of the meeting from his or her own perspective, not necessarily reflecting the official positions of his or her organization. The focus was on mutual education and understanding, not necessarily on reaching agreement. It has been very instructive for participants to hear how the problems in health care appeared from such diverse vantage points: insurers, HMOs, medical groups and associations, hospitals, governors, members of Congress and other public officials, employers, equipment and pharmaceutical manufacturers, and economists.

Address for correspondence: Alain Enthoven, Graduate School of Business, Stanford University, Stanford, California 94305, USA.

1057–9230/92/030149–20$15.00

Based on these sessions, the present authors came to believe that there was emerging a common ground that could become a consensus on the outlines of health system reform. We concluded this ought to be recorded in writing and privately circulated because it could serve as the basis for a broadly supported compromise. Thus, this 'Jackson Hole Initiatives' paper came to be written in 1991. The key elements have stood up well through steadily-expanding discussions in both the private and public sectors.

Of course many of the participants are heads of large organizations that have their own official positions on health system reform. So they cannot speak unilaterally for their organizations. And not all agree with every point.

But the initiatives do reflect broad consensus on the outlines of what has come to be labelled the 'managed competition' approach to health care reform. This strategy requires far-reaching changes in the health system's information, institutions, incentives and regulation, as well as basic health insurance coverage for all citizens. It is a blueprint for both private and public sector actions.

1. The reformed system must be based on organizations that integrate the financial, clinical, managerial and preventive aspects of health care, that are publicly accountable for their cost, health outcomes produced, and patient satisfaction. We refer to them as 'Accountable Health Partnerships'. Such organizations would replace the traditional fee-for-service fragmented practice, remote third-party intermediary model.
2. These organizations must be made to compete on value for money for the custom of well-informed price-conscious consumers in a

restructured market designed and managed to counteract important sources of market failure. A market-oriented regulatory framework is needed to assure the supply of information necessary for uniform health outcome accountability, and to oversee the functioning of the competitive markets.

3. The demand side of this market, now fragmented and ill-informed, must also be empowered and restructured with appropriate incentives. Small employment groups must be pooled into purchasing cooperatives that are large enough to spread risk, achieve economies of scale, offer choice of plan at the individual subscriber level, and manage competition effectively. Tax code changes must limit public subsidies to the costs of economical health plans.
4. An authoritative public body and process must make collective determinations of which health services should be included in the uniform basic health benefit coverage. Such determinations should be based on outcomes research and judgments about value for money, not political influence.
5. There should be universal coverage of these uniform basic health benefits through Accountable Health Partnerships.

Recent months have seen broadening consideration of these Jackson Hole concepts. A New York Times editorial (April 25, 1992) proposed 'Jackson Hole Compatible' as the standard by which all health system reform proposals should be judged. A more recent editorial (June 22, 1992) noted 'Many Democrats have taken a hard second look at the approach called managed competition and like what they see. Managed competition, which has always seemed the best idea for insurance reform on the merits, may now become the best approach for political reasons as well.' Managed competition in its Jackson Hole variety also has appeal for market-oriented Republicans.

As of the summer of 1992, it has clearly achieved status as one of the main approaches in the contest for American health system reform. The Jackson Hole concepts are compatible with a wide range of possible financing schemes from universal taxpayer financing to employment-based financing of coverage under the lowest-priced plan in each area. (Consumers electing coverage in a plan costing more than the least costly must always be required to pay the difference with their own money.)

The American health care system with more than $800 billion of revenues now ranks among large nation-states in scale, complexity, political and economic dynamics. To most economists, the potential advantages of market-oriented approaches—in promoting efficiency, rewarding the best performers, and serving the consumer—will be readily apparent, as will the problems of centralized command-and-control regulation and attempts to put the U.S. health care system on a national budget. There is great uncertainty and complexity ahead on either route. Thus, in circulating this paper now to a wider audience, we emphasize that it remains a 'working draft' for continuing discussions. It will change as debates evolve, other ideas are suggested, and as events and reflections on them unfold. We keep this document on the word processor.

I. OVERVIEW AND ACCOUNTABLE HEALTH PARTNERSHIPS

The environment of the American health insurance system is changing dramatically. From 1965 on, the responsibility of insurers was clear: for the private sector, to provide people with protection against financial catastrophe and to assure them and their families of access to the health care system; and for government, to administer health care programmes for the elderly, the poor, and the disabled.

More recently, HMOs, PPOs, and other forms of managed care were conceived to gain greater control over both the cost and quality of health care by changing the structure and incentives of the health system. Too often, however, 'managed care' has increased administrative complexity and arms-length conflict without equivalent improvements in cost and quality. Preauthorizations, utilization reviews, and financial incentives intended to motivate or channel physicians' energies have too frequently generated distrust and wasted effort as insurers, payers, and providers seek to manipulate each other. The effectiveness of the current system has been further eroded by segmentation of markets, biased risk selection and inequitable underwriting practices in the private sector, and uneven or incomplete coverage of the elderly, poor, and disabled in the public sector.

The 21st century health system requires a different relationship between insurers and providers than the one that exists today. Its success depends on information that can facilitate better decision making regarding the selection of patients for medical interventions, and a closer, collaborative relationship between all of the components of the health system. Changing the structure and incentives in medicine has not been enough to correct the deficiencies inherent in the way medical decisions are made. Well-motivated physicians practising at the state of the art are unable to select interventions with sufficient precision to assure the quality of the care delivered while at the same time controlling costs. Physicians do not have access to an information base from which such responsible, informed choices can be made. The new health care system must create a mechanism by which medical practices can be continuously updated based on robust epidemiological insights, along with more traditional mechanisms such as clinical trials and expert professional judgment.

Now, hyperinflation in U.S. health services without commensurate increases in value is leading critics to demand increasing public intervention, global spending limits, area-by-area and service-by-service budgets, and elimination of a multiple-payer, private insurance industry. The private insurance industry and the private practice of medicine face a formidable challenge. In addition to providing financial protection, both private carriers and providers must justify their independence from extensive government controls or from being supplanted by a government programme by proving they can produce better health, satisfied patients and payers, and slow the rapid rise of health care costs.

At stake is whether the 21st century American health system will be built around competitive markets. The ability of consumers, insurers, employers, and health care providers to shape a competitive medical care system through their informed choices is at issue. Without effective markets, the government will be forced to regulate and take over health care financing and to ration medical care spending and services.

For the American health insurance industry, minor reforms, let alone business as usual, are not sufficient to assure a future role in the new health care system. Providers and insurers alike require:

- vast improvements in clinical information systems to improve medical decision making;
- accountable insurer and provider organizations and relationships that are effective, yet unobtrusive in day-to-day decision making; and
- a competitive market structure that rewards insurers and providers for balancing medical care costs, quality, and patient satisfaction—that is, for improving the *value* of medical care—and prohibits competition based on biased risk selection and underwriting practices.

A sound private sector health system is achievable, but its foundation must be a 21st century health insurance system. The goal for American health care providers, insurers, and managed care companies (including HMOs) must be to move from managing care based on patient-by-patient and claim-by-claim reviews to Accountable Health Partnerships. These health partnerships must be publicly accountable for their cost (in dollars) and effectiveness (in terms of their impact on clinical status, function, and well-being) of medical services, as well as for patient satisfaction with that care. This new health system will be based on informed choices, diversity, flexibility, and the professional and cultural values of a private system working in concert with governmental efforts to assure public accountability, universal coverage, and cost containment. Accountable Health Partnerships that fully integrate the financial, managerial, clinical, and preventive aspects of health care are the vital elements of this 21st century system.

These necessary reforms will require investments in people, ideas, and innovation. For providers, this means structuring personnel and resources into groups that are capable of delivering the full array of Uniform Effective Health Benefits. The numbers and types of providers as well as the quantity of resources in each of these groups should match the needs of the particular population that the group is intended to serve. Further, each provider group must be held publicly accountable for the impact (in terms of cost, effectiveness, and patient values) of the care they deliver.

Some health insurance firms have the immediate potential—the leadership, customer base, capital, and management skills—to improve the way medicine is practiced by taking an active interest in the effects of that medicine on their policy holders' health. This 'active interest' in medical care implies nothing less than integrating, coordinating, collaborating in, and actively contributing to the process of enabling providers and patients to make better health care decisions while at the same time providing the financial means for making a set of Uniform Effective Health Benefits accessible to everyone who needs it.

Health insurers are not uncontested heirs to these responsibilities. The opportunity to shift their resources and emphasis from risk-spreading and bill-paying to clinical and quality of life-enhancing functions is now at hand. At issue is whether this transition can be achieved quickly enough, and, whether it will be sufficient to forestall massive public intervention into the U.S. health care system.

The Jackson Hole Group (JHG) initiatives for establishment of The 21st Century American Health System are based on the assumption that provider groups, health insurers, and managed care companies will agree, to assume responsibility for the kind of internal restructuring that is crucial to what will become the new competitive bottom line in health care: public accountability for health care's impact on patient satisfaction, function, and well-being, all at a reasonable cost. The proposals assume that providers and insurers will take the initiative to compete effectively and, at the same time, foster collaboration among themselves, purchasers, patients, and the government. The JHG initiatives require providers and insurers to:

- voluntarily undertake the design and promotion of a common approach to building the organizations that will form the foundation of the next generation system of health care;
- enlist the help of business, labour, and consumer groups in a united effort; and
- secure the legislation necessary to make the system operational.

This paper describes major elements of the JHG initiatives and their implications for providers, insurers, and purchasers. It also identifies steps to be taken in formulating private sector initiatives, as well as state and federal legislation.

MAJOR POINTS OF THE JACKSON HOLE GROUP INITIATIVES

- Federal legislation will ensure that all persons have access to Uniform Effective Health Benefits provided by Accountable Health Partnerships financed through a combination of mandated employer contributions, government assistance, and their own financial resources. (Universal Access—JHG Document II).
- Within each state, at least one Health Insurance Purchasing Cooperative will be established to act as collective purchasing agents for small employers to take advantage of economies of scale and ability to spread and manage risk (see Health Insurance Purchasing Cooperative—JHG Document II).
- A trio of health care standards-setting boards will be established, sponsored by consumers, insurers, health care providers, and industry groups. The charter of these boards is to assure uniform definitions and standards of performance, to improve clinical effectiveness information, and to put in place the necessary ground rules that will allow market forces to work most efficiently (see JHG Document IV). These standards boards are:
  - The Outcomes Management Standards Board (OMSB), responsible for establishing 'generally accepted health services accounting practices' including standards for the content and format of data to be used in accounting publicly and internally for the results of medical care. The OMSB will establish the framework within which Accountable Health Partnerships will be evaluated;
  - The Health Standards Board (HealSB), involving providers, insurers, consumers, medical scientists, and others will undertake technology assessment and benefit plan design. Accumulating clinical epi-

demiological data will be used to identify those technologies and treatments that are sufficiently effective, in relation to their costs and risks, to justify inclusion in 'Uniform Effective Health Benefits.' (see Uniform Effective Health Benefits—JHG Document III) Only this benefit package will receive favourable tax treatment.

— The Health Insurance Standards Board (HISB), which will establish underwriting practices with emphasis at the outset on the small group insurance market, ensuring that competition can take place on the basis of health services cost, quality, and patient satisfaction rather than on risk selection and market segmentation.

Private sector leadership will ensure that purchaser, patient, and industry experience and consensus building is used to shape future health policies. To ensure a competitive market orientation, an independent, quasi non-governmental agency, called the National Health Board (NHB) (see National Health Board—JHG Document IV), will be established, modelled on the Securities and Exchange Commission (SEC).

The private sector standards boards (OMSB, HealSB, and HISB) will provide recommendations to the NHB for review and application, just as the Financial Accounting Standards Board (FASB) works with the SEC. The NHB, for its part, will facilitate the transition to the 21st Century American Health System, publishing and revising a list of Uniform Effective Health Benefits; registering and overseeing Accountable Health Partnerships and Health Insurance Purchasing Cooperatives; setting the rate of transition from the present system to the new one; ensuring that standards and methods are appropriate and effective; proposing new standards/methods where necessary; and in general guiding the system as it evolves.

The insurance industry, provider groups, and purchasers will initiate or expand a series of programmes aimed at establishing working prototypes of these standards-setting advisory boards and systems. They will immediately apply the resulting standards to themselves.

The state and federal governments will:

- Revise the federal tax code so that only Accountable Health Partnerships providing Uniform Effective Health Benefits according to the standards set by the NHB will qualify for employer and individual 'tax-advantaged' premiums. These requirements will be phased, administered through agreements with state insurance regulators where acceptable, or directly by the NHB. To encourage competition, qualifying Accountable Health Partnerships will also receive ERISA-like exemptions from incompatible state laws.
- Set limits on the amount of the employer and individual premium contribution that will be excludable from taxable income, tied to the competitive rates (to be established through a Health Insurance Purchasing Cooperative conducted bidding process in each state) of Accountable Health Partnerships providing Uniform Effective Health Benefits to a pooled small group insurance market (see JHG Document II).

MAJOR CHARACTERISTICS OF ACCOUNTABLE HEALTH PARTNERSHIPS

- The critical, defining characteristics of Accountable Health Partnerships will be their participation in a system of public accountability reporting for the health of enrolled populations and their ability to compete successfully on the basis of costs.
- Accountable Health Partnerships will be judged on their ability (a) to organize and deliver the full array of Uniform Effective Health Benefits that produce a high level of patient-oriented results (i.e., favourable impacts on satisfaction, clinical status, function and well-being), and (b) to keep cost increases at a level that closely parallels the Consumer Price Index.
- Accountable Health Partnerships will be registered by the NHB based on the submission of publicly available reports of their health outcomes prepared in accordance with standardized 'generally accepted health accounting practices' much as the SEC registers securities based on the presence of an accounting system that fulfills generally accepted accounting practices. The design and installation of these health accountability systems will be a joint project of all Accountable Health Partnerships, coordinated by OMSB and other advisory groups discussed

earlier. To the extent that the means for achieving full, outcomes-based accountability in health care are, as yet, in developmental stages, it will be necessary to rely during the early years of registration on some of the more traditional, but historically less effective means of health care quality assurance, such as credentialing of professionals and the presence of internal quality assurance systems.

- Registered Accountable Health Partnerships can be single, vertically integrated organizations consisting of providers who are, at a minimum, capable of delivering health care services that meet the required set of Uniform Effective Health Benefits, and insurers who are, at a minimum, able to meet the underwriting standards for the industry. Registered Accountable Health Partnerships may also be made up of two affiliated, but independently registered organizations—a provider who is publicly accountable for outcomes, and a carrier who can meet industry underwriting standards—working collaboratively to achieve the same goals as an Accountable Health Partnership.
- The formation of an Accountable Health Partnership requires the creation of a new relationship between insurer and provider that integrates corporate policies for compensation, price, and continuous quality improvement. Regardless of the specific organizational model used to achieve this integration, Accountable Health Partnerships will be characterized by:
  - a corporate commitment to improve their health care organization's cost effectiveness, quality, patient service, and impact on patient health as a primary business strategy;
  - offering a 'Uniform Effective Health Benefits' plan covering those services ultimately determined by the NHB to be appropriate and effective;
  - responsibility for the professional expertise, staff, infrastructure, resources, data systems, and corporate culture necessary to optimally conduct, integrate, and manage medical health outcomes and consumer satisfaction;
  - participation in an outcomes management reporting system, and the provision of standardized reports that will allow employers, patients, other interested parties to reliably compare the performance of various Accountable Health Partnerships;
  - registration with the NHB covering insurance practices, scope of coverage, and accountability for the quality of care; and
  - expansion of the proportion of insured who participate in Accountable Health Partnerships consistent with legislatively-specified targets for the proportion of business that must be enrolled in order to qualify for employer premium tax exclusions.

DISCUSSION: NEXT STEPS

Insurance carriers must join forces with HMOs, health care providers, employers, labour and consumer groups in a bipartisan political effort with the government to reshape the health care system. These proposed policies have been informally introduced and well received by policy makers at the state and national levels. Several initiatives in various states and the federal legislature incorporate elements of this approach. But refinement and implementation of these models require coordinated provider and insurance company action, collaboration with purchasers and policy makers, new legislation, continuing refinement of health service accounting and reporting standards, and transition planning for implementation of the new standards and accounting techniques.

Insurer initiatives have already built a strong foundation for the three new private sector standards-setting organizations through prototype demonstrations of outcomes reporting in the Managed Health Care Association projects (OMSB), information exchanges among insurers for medical technology assessments (HealSB), and the National Association of Insurance Commissioners development of business practice standards and model laws for small group market reforms (HISB). These initial exploratory activities will be expanded and enhanced to rapidly move from research and development to decisive industry-wide application.

II. MARKET REFORM AND UNIVERSAL COVERAGE

THE CASE FOR MARKET REFORM

Market failure

The market for health insurance and covered health care services in the United States has clearly failed to contain expenditure growth to acceptable levels or to produce an equitable distribution of coverage and services. National health expenditures have grown much faster than incomes. Roughly 35 million Americans have no coverage, public or private. Market forces are not motivating the realization of even obvious potential gains in efficiency. The practices of underwriting and experience rating for small groups are driving up premiums to unreasonable levels for individuals and small groups with poor experience.

The main sources of market failure are:

1. *Cost-unconscious demand.* While cost-effective systems of managed care exist, they are largely denied the opportunity to market their superior cost-effectiveness by employers who systematically contribute more on behalf of employees who choose the less efficient fee-for-service arrangements. These employer practices grow out of past commitments made when efficient managed care was not available; they are sustained by collective bargaining and the open-ended exclusion of employer contributions from employee taxable incomes.
2. *Biased risk selection as an important source of profit.* Individual health care costs vary widely. In the absence of corrective action by purchasers it can be more profitable for insurers to select good risks for coverage while avoiding poor health risks than it is to organize and manage care efficiently.
3. *Market segmentation minimizes price competition.* Because of the huge number of complex services covered in health insurance contracts, carriers and managed care organizations can segment markets and minimize the number of persons who would actually change health plan because of price. Thus, price competition in premiums is attenuated or destroyed.
4. *Lack of information.* Because of the very high cost or actual unavailability of standardized comparative information about quality (health outcomes) on which purchasers could base rational decisions, people are reluctant to make decisions to change health plans because of price.
5. *Small groups unable to offer individual choice.* Roughly half of employed Americans get their coverage through groups of 100 or less. Most such groups are not big enough to offer multiple choice of plan at the individual level. It takes near unanimous consent to get a small group to switch from a wide access fee-for-service plan to a cost-effective managed care plan. Thus, price competition is blocked in this important market.
6. *Perverse public subsidies.* Public subsidies to individuals for health insurance purchases are distributed inequitably. Upper income persons choosing relatively costly coverages get substantial subsidies and incentives to purchase more coverage through the tax system; low income persons—whose decisions are likely to be much more sensitive to out-of-pocket costs—get much lower subsidies or none at all.

Other factors contributing to unacceptable market performance include inadequate information on clinical effectiveness, and a lack of an adequate number of managed care organizations actually capable of improving quality and efficiency. Proposals to address these problems are more fully developed in the papers on Uniform Effective Health Benefits and the 21st Century Health Insurance System. (Documents I and III.)

Managed competition and tax reform

The Jackson Hole Initiative promotes managed competition by structuring the process of consumer choice to reward, with more subscribers, those health plans that provide high quality care and control cost. It seeks to overcome the above mentioned (and other) sources of market failure and inequity. Major components of the managed competitive structure include:

1. A sponsor (large employer or other agency purchasing coverage and managing competition for a defined population) must select high quality cost-effective Accountable Health Partnerships (AHPs) to participate, and must contract with them regarding terms of participation.
2. The consumer who chooses a health plan whose premium exceeds that of the least costly plan must pay the full premium difference out of net-after-tax income. The point of this is to create for every health plan the normal market reward for offering a lower price, i.e., more customers.
3. The sponsor must risk adjust its contributions (or premiums) for health risks enrolled in the different plans, contributing more on behalf of subscribers in plans that enroll people with higher predicted health expenses to compensate the health plans for enrolling higher risks and to remove or eliminate the competitive advantage for selecting good risks. The sponsor should maintain active surveillance over the processes of selection and enrollment to counter biased risk selection or compensate for it.
4. The sponsor should contract with the AHPs for standardized Uniform Effective Health Benefits; it should not let individual carriers offer their own coverages that might select risks and segment markets.
5. The sponsor should actively seek to inform consumers about quality of care and service in the competing plans, relying on a nationally standardized system of generally accepted health care accountability.
6. Federal and state income and payroll tax laws should be reformed to limit tax-free employer contributions to the price of the least costly Accountable Health Partnership available to the taxpayer; the savings (which can be substantial) should be used to subsidize coverage for people not now covered.

Very large employers already contributing most of the premium and performing a management role can carry out sponsor functions. But for the many thousands of small employers and individuals who do not have the resources to purchase effectively and economically, new sponsorship organizations are needed. These new sponsor organizations are also needed because of special sources of market failure in the small group market.

Market failure in the small group market

A key to success for a health insurer in a free market situation is to price coverage for each group at an amount that just covers claims cost, administrative expense, and normal competitive profit. Claims costs vary widely among individuals and small groups. Premiums vary widely among small groups, with premiums for some groups of ten or more times those for others. In extreme cases, insurance may simply be unavailable to high cost individuals and groups.

Wide variations in premiums among groups have several negative consequences. First, this creates inequity. Second, many small groups find that insurance is not available when they really need it—when members of the group become seriously ill. Third, high premiums can simply price coverage out of the market and lead to increased numbers of sick people being uninsured. Employers may decide they simply cannot afford the premiums. Employees may decide that they are better off seeking free care from private or public providers.

Such wide variations (or unavailability) have particularly negative consequences with respect to two proposed public policy initiatives. First, opposition to an employer mandate to provide coverage is likely to be particularly—and understandably—intense from employers who face high premiums. Second, any attempt to limit tax-free employer contributions based on community average costs is likely to be perceived as particularly unfair to those groups facing premiums much above average.

Thus, attempts to enact these policies must be preceded by attempts to reduce variation in small group premiums.

Small employment groups—of 100 or fewer employees—are simply too small for the spreading of risk in an era in which $100,000-plus cases are no longer unusual. Moreover, such groups are far too small for acquiring and supporting the data and expertise needed to function effectively in this very complex market where information is so costly. Furthermore, administrative expenses (as a percent of premium) are much higher for small than large groups: e.g.,

35 percent for groups of 5 to 9 employees and 18 percent for groups of 50 to 99 employees, compared to 5.5 percent for groups of over 10,000. Recent federal legislation—which extends Medicaid coverage to family members of low-wage workers, plus adding a new health insurance earned income tax credit—will sharply increase the complexities and coordination of coverage problems already confronting many small employers. Thus, the purchasing power of small groups must be aggregated and pooled, both for risk spreading and for economies of scale in management.

HEALTH INSURANCE PURCHASING COOPERATIVES

The Jackson Hole Initiative proposes establishment of a new national system of sponsor organizations—Health Insurance Purchasing Cooperatives (HIPCs)—to function as a collective purchasing agent on behalf of small employers and individuals. These HIPCs are designed to correct the problems of market failure in the small group market, and to sharply cut employers' administrative burdens to a minimum (primarily sending premium payments to the HIPC). They offer an administrative mechanism to handle coordination of employer contributions with Medicaid coverage, tax credits and other public subsidies without resorting to 'play or pay' approaches that transfer tens of millions of small employers, their employees, and family members into the Medicaid programme. They can also administer COBRA continuity for small employers. They provide a solid basis for determining the competitive costs of offering uniform benefit plans that can be used for establishing a tax exclusion limitation for each market area.

The need for incentives, institutions, and active management

Creating a purchasing pool means that persons and groups with low health care costs share in the costs of people and groups with high costs. If given a choice, people expecting low costs are not likely to do so voluntarily. There need to be compelling incentives or legal requirements for all small employers to participate. One form of compulsion that has been suggested is to require all insurers to practice community rating (or observe rating bands narrower than the variation in unconstrained premiums) and 'guaranteed issue' (i.e., guarantee to sell the community rated coverage to any group that seeks it). The problem with such compulsion is that it requires carriers to do business they do not want to do because they know they will lose money at it. This approach gives them powerful incentives to find ways of avoiding enrollment of high cost groups. And the most successful carriers will be those who are most skillful at evading the intent of the rule. Low cost groups will inevitably seek coverage at premiums fitting their low costs or remain uninsured.

The alternative to compulsion is to offer incentives for small employers to join a pool. The Jackson Hole Initiative offers several inducements for low-cost groups to participate in the pool and to prevent insurers from splitting off low-cost groups.

1. The economies of scale inherent in a large pool will reduce employers' and carriers' administrative costs substantially, making pool membership attractive.
2. Enactment of legislation to allow pools an 'ERISA-like' exemption from state provider mandates and require them to offer Uniform Effective Health Benefits.
3. Possible use of age-rating to attenuate cross-subsidies within pools so that younger groups can still get premiums somewhat lower than older groups.
4. Small group participation in a pool should be a condition for exclusion of employer contributions from employee taxable income.

Health insurance is a very complex and dynamic business in which many varieties exist and many innovations occur. The administration of rules governing rating, guaranteed issue and the like, not to mention managing competition, requires institutions, active intelligent management, and expertise. Passive inflexible state regulation cannot manage this market. Active management through voluntary contractual relationships is needed.

The HIPC described

An HIPC would be a collective purchasing agent for small employers. It would be a voluntary, nonprofit membership corporation whose board would be made up of people elected by participating employers.

In a manner reminiscent of the HMO Act, the National Health Board would recognize qualified Health Insurance Purchasing Cooperatives which, in return, would offer coverage through competing Accountable Health Partnerships. The federal government would make grants to subsidize start-up expenses, override opposing state laws if any, and grant appropriate anti-trust exemptions.

Small business associations, chambers of commerce, the National Federation of Independent Businesses, etc., would be invited to form HIPCs. They would compete for designation just as various private entities compete to be designated Peer Review Organizations. However, the boards of directors of HIPCs would be elected by a vote of all the participating employers and self-employed.

State governments would select and designate HIPCs (as governors once designated Health Systems Agencies), based on geographic units. Formal approval and registration of HIPCs would be the responsibility of the National Health Board. The HIPC would contract with AHPs to offer enrollment to all employees of participating employers in periodic open enrollments (similar to practices in large employment groups). Participating AHPs would cover Uniform Effective Health Benefits as defined by federal law. (Each HIPC needs to standardize coverages for its participating plans for reasons of managed competition. The use of a federal Uniform Effective Health Benefits standard is related to the limit on tax-free contributions—see below).

The HIPC would also contract with participating employers. It would accept all appropriate employment groups located within its area. It would not be allowed to exclude groups or individuals based on health status. It would assure continuity of coverage and not allow exclusions for pre-existing conditions. The HIPC would manage competition, applying business judgment in determining the numbers and identities of competitors. At the outset, the availability of managed care varies so widely from one geographic area to another that HIPCs would be allowed wide latitude in their initial choice of plans until registered AHPs are generally available.

The HIPC would serve as the health benefits office for participating employers—saving employers time and expense and allowing them the benefit of superior expertise. The HIPC would seek to measure and monitor quality and compliance with programme goals. It would manage relationships between consumers and carriers (grievances, etc.). It would prepare informative materials for consumers. It would manage 'COBRA continuity' on behalf of employers, as well as receiving Medicaid 'buy-in' payments so that employers of low-wage persons can retain private insurance coverage, and dealing with questions about using the new health insurance EITC benefits.

To achieve economies of scale, each HIPC should purchase coverage for at least several hundred thousand people. The favourable experience of the California Public Employees' Retirement System (PERS) which acts as a HIPC for over 800 local government agencies in California—some with as few as two employees—and which covers 800,000 people, suggests that one million covered lives might be a good target. However, it would be desirable to keep HIPCs small enough that they would be able to carry out their functions acting on business merits, not becoming political entities whose every move would incite a march on the legislature. Moreover, it would be desirable to keep HIPCs close to the employers they serve.

Participating health plans

The requirement that participating health plans should be registered Accountable Health Partnerships will be phased in.

Accountable Health Partnerships would agree to accept all enrollees without medical review, waiting periods, or exclusion of coverage for pre-existing conditions, and cover them for the year of enrollment for a price set in advance (just as they do now in large employment groups). They would be allowed to set temporary geographic capacity limits as part of a plan negotiated with the HIPC.

Participating health plans would set a 'community rate' (no experience rate or health status adjustment). This might be demographically adjusted to each employment group, a policy decision that would have to be made.

Participating employers would agree to:

1. Coverage of all full-time employees and their dependents without waiting periods or exclusions.
2. Conduct an annual open enrollment, using materials supplied by the HIPC, in which

each employee is able to select from the full menu of choices offered by the HIPC.

3. Continuity of participation (i.e., rules to prevent opportunistic switching in and out).
4. Payment of fixed, defined contributions toward employee coverage not to exceed the price of the lowest-priced plan offered by the HIPC.
5. Payroll deductions and secure payment arrangements for employer and employee contributions.
6. Timely notification to the HIPC of changes in enrollment.

IMPLEMENTATION STEPS TO MARKET REFORM

1. Establish the National Health Board and its advisory groups (see JHG Document IV).
2. Enact a federal law inviting governors to designate HIPCs in their states that together cover the whole state. (This would allow for the possibility of inter-state HIPCs to cover metropolitan areas crossing state lines.) The law would:

   - set standards for HIPCs;
   - override restrictive state laws;
   - provide anti-trust exemption.

   As of a specified date, at least one year after enactment, the exclusion of employer contributions to employee health benefits from employee taxable incomes would become conditional on purchases of coverage through a qualified HIPC for all employment groups of less than 25 employees. The public policy rationale for the tax exclusion is to make private health insurance widespread, a goal now thwarted by market failure in the small employment group market.
3. In the second year after enactment, raise the threshold to employment groups up to 50 employees.
4. In the third year, raise the threshold to groups of 100 employees. Further subsequent steps could then be considered.
5. In the final step, all tax-free employer contributions for employment groups of all sizes would be limited to the price of the lowest-priced plan covering Uniform Effective Health Benefits offered by the HIPC covering the employee's place of employment. In effect, Congress would declare that the excludable amount in each area would be the minimum necessary to purchase Uniform Effective Health Insurance Benefits, as evidenced by the price of coverage sold by the HIPC.

This policy deals with three major objections to a flat-dollar 'tax cap': First, because of wide variations in premiums, a flat-dollar tax cap would be unfair to high-cost groups. Under this concept, small groups would be guaranteed the ability to buy at the tax cap price. Second, a flat-dollar tax cap does not allow for geographic variations; this approach would.

Third, there is concern that a fixed-dollar tax cap would not rise with health care cost, thus declining in real value. This approach would tie the cap to a real price. The HIPC proposal will allow for setting a tax cap that accurately reflects the cost at which individuals can purchase Uniform Effective Health Benefits, efficiently provided, in each health care market.

Some might be concerned about setting a precedent for indexing a part of the tax code to geographic costs. However, this is not geographic indexing. Rather, it is an extension of an idea already present in the Tax Code—deductible amounts are 'ordinary and necessary amounts' to achieve certain purposes.

This approach thus provides a basis for government intervention into health care markets that responsibly limits public tax subsidies to amounts needed to cover the cost of Uniform Effective Health Benefits efficiently provided. This is in fundamental contrast to national budgeting schemes that ration spending and seek to control every expense in a $800 billion industry. The JHG approach allows individuals the continuing freedom to spend their own after-tax incomes for medical benefits.

As is normal in tax or Medicare regulations, many specific situations would have to be defined and rules established. For example, would firms that started under 100 employees and subsequently grew beyond that be required or allowed to stay in the HIPC? The answer is probably 'yes' until they reached some specified larger size. Would firms larger than 100 employees be allowed to join the HIPC? The problem posed is that such choice on the part of the firm could lead to adverse selection against the HIPC. So the answer would probably be that HIPCs could accept the entry of larger employment groups on terms negotiated to protect them from adverse risk selection.

BEYOND MARKET REFORM TO UNIVERSAL HEALTH INSURANCE

The JHG is committed to the goal of universal health insurance in a decentralized market guided by responsible and informed individual choices. These market reforms will greatly reduce the cost and difficulty of taking further steps toward universal coverage. Universal coverage is important for a number of reasons.

First, nobody defends the proposition that people without coverage or money to pay should go without necessary medical care, or should be allowed to suffer, be disabled or die for lack of reasonable care that could prevent it. For this reason our society has developed a very complex patchwork of institutions to care for and finance the care of the uninsured. These institutions are extremely wasteful and often unfair, permitting preventable medical bankruptcies and disabilities. They lead to delayed care which can often mean serious and costly illness that could have been prevented by early treatment. They lead to care in very costly settings—hospital emergency departments—when the care could have been delivered at much lower cost in the primary care physician's office. They permit epidemics of communicable diseases (e.g., measles) that could have easily been prevented. They generate requirements for very costly eligibility determinations—millions of dollars spent on lawyers. They lead to cost shifting from those who do not pay and those who provide free care to those who do pay for health insurance. They lead to the closing of hospital emergency departments because they are the major source of patients who cannot pay. This, in turn, deprives whole communities of an important resource.

By putting market pressure on providers to cut costs, market reforms promoting competition, not accompanied by universal coverage, could make access problems for the uninsured worse. It would be more humane, economical, and rational simply to adopt a policy providing coverage to virtually everybody through an Accountable Health Partnership that provides primary care and preventive services as a part of comprehensive benefit package. (The remaining few uncovered, such as the homeless would, as now, be cared for by public providers.)

A necessary condition for universal coverage is that everybody who can contribute to financing the system must do so, in some reasonable relationship to ability to pay. A system of universal coverage will not work if everybody is covered, but only those who voluntarily choose to do so pay for it. Such a system would be destroyed by 'free riders'!

Taxes are unpopular. 'Employer mandates' are a form of employment tax, but many are now being taxed in an irrational system of hidden levies often most burdensome to those who behave responsibly. Some employers pay three times: for their employee, for their employee's spouse who works for an employer who does not provide coverage, and through taxes and 'bad debt' or 'free care' surcharges to cover those with no insurance. Generally, the insured pay for much of the care of the uninsured. The real choice is between explicit, relatively efficient and equitable taxes versus inequitable and inefficient hidden taxes.

For many years in this country we have had an employment-based system of health care coverage. Seeking politically feasible incremental change, the JHG proposes to build on that system and correct its deficiencies rather than to replace it radically.

To summarize, the Jackson Hole Initiative calls for:

1. Limitation of tax-free employer contributions to employee health benefits to the price of Uniform Effective Health Benefits in the employee's area of residence as evidenced by the premium charged by the lowest-priced plan contracting with the HIPC in the employee's area of residence. Because many households have multiple employers, the limit should be applied at the taxpayer level (e.g., one tax-free family coverage per family). If employer contributions fall short of the limit, allow the taxpayer to exclude his or her contributions up to the limit applied to the combined total.
2. Mandating all employers to 'cover' all full-time employees, i.e., offer coverage, make a defined contribution equal to an amount in the range of 50 to 100 percent of the price of the lowest-priced Accountable Health Partnership covering Uniform Effective Health Benefits in the applicable HIPC area, and make payroll deductions and payments to the HIPC or the AHPs. The reason for the 50

percent requirement is to make employee purchase of coverage sufficiently attractive to healthy employees that they will be motivated to buy coverage. The reason for the 100 percent limit is that employees should be required to use their own money for the extra cost of coverage if they choose a plan whose price exceeds the lowest-priced plan.

3. The payroll tax on all non-covered employment (e.g., part-timers) combined with opportunity for part-timers to make subsidized purchases of coverage through a HIPC. A similar tax will be placed on the Adjusted Gross Income of nonemployed people with incomes (e.g., early pre-Medicare retirees), with proceeds used to subsidize their purchases of coverage through a HIPC. This tax constitutes an individual mandate, with the tax level on the subsidy set to equal the price of the low-priced plan.
4. The federal government would collect the payroll tax (equalized among states). This money, plus the revenue savings achieved from the limit on tax-free employer contributions (roughly $12 billion in 1988 dollars) would be sent to the states based on the number of people covered under state sponsorship. States would combine these revenues with the sources of funds they presently use to subsidize care for the uninsured (e.g., the 'Bad Debt Free Care' Pool in Massachusetts, state subsidies to counties in California, etc.), and revenue savings they realize from the limit on tax free employer contributions. States would contract with HIPCs to enroll all people not covered through employment, Medicare, Medicaid, CHAMPUS or CHAMPUSVA. The states would pay the premium of the low-priced plan, and let the insured make additional contributions if they want to subscribe to a higher-priced plan.
5. Public programmes would have the opportunity to contract with HIPCs for coverage of their beneficiaries. For example, Medicaid programmes could contract with HIPCs and AHPs for coverage for acute somatic medical care for their beneficiaries. Medicaid programmes would continue to pay for nursing homes for aged, disabled, mentally retarded, etc., unless or until some alternative system is developed.

The Medicare programme must evolve from its present fee-for-service orientation to purchasing coverage through HIPCs and AHPs. Initially this should be done by creating per capita cost equivalents (the 'Adjusted Average Per Capita Cost') in each HIPC area, and making capitation payments on behalf of those beneficiaries who wish to choose coverage through AHPs. Eventually, all care should be purchased in this way.

III. UNIFORM EFFECTIVE HEALTH BENEFITS

THE CASES FOR UNIFORM EFFECTIVE HEALTH BENEFITS

For many reasons, it is important that basic health benefit coverage be both uniform and restricted to demonstrably effective and appropriate services. First, any proposal to provide universal access to health services for all U.S. citizens must include a specific definition of which services will be covered. Second, a well-conceived uniform set of basic health benefits can be used to more equitably distribute health care taxes and tax exclusions. A common definition of effective services will also help in capping tax exclusions reducing tax losses and containing health care costs. Third, uniformity of basic coverage puts private and government insurers on the same plane. People can move from private to public carriers, and vice versa, without gaining or losing health benefits coverage. Fourth, publicly defined uniform coverage can be used to eliminate state mandates and circumvent court-ordered coverage for individual cases. Finally, with a common definition of service offerings, the relative quality and efficiency of an Accountable Health Partnership can be more readily compared.

DEFINITION OF SERVICES

A definition of Uniform Effective Health Benefits should be responsive to public values about the appropriateness of various treatments, incorporate scientifically-based information on treatment effectiveness, and be sensitive to considerations of cost in terms of the net benefits of services.

- Appropriateness of services should be based on widely-held beliefs about the value of a service to society (e.g., public health impact, social costs, community compassion) the value of a service to the individual at risk of needing that service (e.g., personal ability to function, length of life, equity), and the extent to which a service is considered an essential component of a basic level of health below which no person should fall. Public values can be periodically assessed through surveys, focus groups, public hearings, and other community meeting formats.
- Effectiveness of services can be assessed initially through clinical trials, expert opinion, review of the literature, and short-term studies. Ultimately, accumulating epidemiological data based on naturally occurring variations in health practices will also be used to identify the most effective medical technologies and techniques for treating various conditions, as well as appropriate frequencies of intervention. Emerging techniques and technologies will be evaluated in the same way. HealSB will have responsibility for annually reviewing and revising the set of Uniform Effective Health benefits based on the latest available evidence, forwarding recommendations to the NHB which will have final responsibility for reviewing and incorporating those changes into policy.
- Cost of services and levels of tax exclusion will be assessed through a state-by-state competitive bidding process conducted by the Health Insurance Purchasing Cooperatives.

REVISION OF FEDERAL AND STATE HEALTH POLICIES

A principal incentive leading states, employers, and insurers to cooperate in establishing and offering a standardized benefit package will be the tax treatment of employer and individuals' contributions. Implementation of tax code revisions will be phased so as to allow time for the reorganization of health organizations. Major provisions include:

- Exclusion of employer and individuals' premium contributions from income and payroll taxes will be conditional on the purchase of coverage from an Accountable Health Partnership offering Uniform Effective Health Benefits.
- All tax-free employer contributions will be limited to the amount of the lowest-priced plan covering Uniform Effective Health Benefits within the employee's state of residence.
- All employers will ultimately be required to contribute to the cost of Uniform Effective Health Benefits for their employees.
- Uniform Effective Health Benefits will, if possible, be set to cost less than the amounts expected to be excluded from taxation. Tax exclusions will be capped, leading to a reduction in tax losses and freeing funds for coverage of those currently underinsured or uninsured.
- Standards for accountability or coverage that federal or state government imposes on the private sector must also be met by government entities.
- Federal law will be changed to circumvent ERISA and state mandates that tend to limit the capacity to establish a Uniform Effective Health Benefits standards.

RESPONSIBILITIES OF ACCOUNTABLE HEALTH PARTNERSHIPS

Accountable Health Partnerships will be required to provide and finance the full array of Uniform Effective Health Benefits.

- Accountable Health Partnerships will be held publicly accountable for the impact of Uniform Effective Health Benefits on the function and well-being of their beneficiaries.
- Accountable Health Partnerships will be expected to progressively increase the proportion of their clients who receive Uniform Effective Health Benefits.

DISCUSSION: NEXT STEPS

Within 12 months, a prototype HealSB will be established to begin:

- explicit definition of the first set of Uniform Effective Health Benefits;
- the description and establishment of a working prototype for monitoring and revising the benefits definition;
- the identification of changes in law and public policy required to implement a set of Uniform Effective Health Benefits.

Application of Uniform Effective Health Benefits to existing health insurance policyholders should begin within 18 months of the acceptance of the JHG initiative by private carriers.

IV. THE PUBLIC-PRIVATE HEALTH PARTNERSHIP AND THE NATIONAL HEALTH BOARD

The comprehensive plan for a 21st Century American Health System that is embodied in the Jackson Hole Group (JHG) initiatives will require both government and private sector actions. The new government roles will include implementing a public-private design for universal health insurance coverage, insurance market reforms, tax code revisions, and a national health outcomes accountability system.

These new government roles are necessary for the private health sector to perform its major role—to compete effectively on the basis of health care costs, high quality, and value to the patient. To foster this vigorously competitive and accountable private health care system, the JHG initiatives reflect three priority objectives:

- Assure effective national implementation of reforms consistent with a pro-competitive philosophy;
- Restrict new government authority to what is needed to implement these reforms;
- Provide for major private sector responsibility in standards-setting and advice.

There are a number of successful precedents for uniquely American blends of government and private sector responsibility and accountability to accomplish national objectives of importance and complexity. These include institutions with vital roles in our free-market economy such as the Federal Reserve Board, as well as the Securities and Exchange Commission (SEC) and Financial Accounting Standards Board (FASB).

In the JHG discussions, a 'SEC model' has seemed best suited for implementing the health sector reform plan. The JHG proposals include the following (see Figure 1).

- A National Health Board (NHB)—an independent federal agency, charged with overall implementation and oversight.
- Three private sector organizations that will have key advisory and standards-setting roles—a Health Standards Board (HealSB) for medical efficacy and benefit assessments; a Health Insurance Standards Board (HISB) for health insurance organization and market issues; and an Outcomes Management Standards Board (OMSB) for the new health outcomes reporting system. These new organizations would be jointly sponsored by major private sector groups, e.g., employers, consumers, health care providers, and insurers. The charter of these boards will be to assure uniform definitions and performance measurement standards, to improve clinical effectiveness information, and to put in place the necessary ground rules so that effective competition can take place on the basis of costs, high quality, and value to the patient.

This proposed structure is analogous to the relationship between the Securities and Exchange Commission, an independent federal agency, and the Financial Accounting Standards Board, a private sector organization broadly sponsored by user groups which establishes financial reporting standards for the nation's businesses and securities markets. As a matter of policy, the SEC normally accepts FASB-set standards. The new health sector standards boards would have similar standing with the National Health Board.

The three standards-setting boards will engage the private sector in the implementation effort. The national sponsor groups will select the boards' leadership. The new boards will operate through an open consultative decision process, have full-time professional staff—and a singular purpose of carrying out the proposed health care reforms. They will be built on standards-setting activities already underway in the health sector. As a result, the reform plan can be implemented quickly and will be able to take advantage of private sector expertise.

The key elements of this joint public-private implementation structure are discussed below.

NATIONAL HEALTH BOARD (NHB)

Structure

- An independent, i.e. 'quasi-non-governmental,' federal agency. Like the SEC, its members will be appointed by the President, with Senate confirmation.

Responsibilities

- Guide, oversee, and facilitate transition to a 21st Century Health System with universal health insurance coverage and effective competition based on costs, high quality, and value to patients.
- Recommend a set of Uniform Effective Health Benefits and tax exclusion amounts to the President and Congress (based on advice from HealSB and HISB).
- Establish registration requirements for Accountable Health Partnerships, including the Uniform Effective Health Benefits, small group marketing and underwriting rules, essential managed care requirements and a transition schedule to managed care, and patient outcomes reporting systems (based on HealSB, HISB, and OMSB standards). Only registered Accountable Health Partnerships can qualify for tax exclusion of employer contributions. Registered Accountable Health Partnerships are exempt from state benefit mandates and restrictive contracting laws.
- Establish registration requirements for Health Insurance Purchasing Cooperatives that will manage competition for the small group insurance market (based on HISB standards).
- Enter into agreements with state governments to administer some health insurance sector regulation, e.g., mandated benefits, registration, small group insurance reforms.

A national authority is required for implementing the reform proposals rapidly and as an integrated agency to bring health insurance to 32–37 million uninsured, to slow cost increases and to improve care quality. Overall responsibility could be assigned to the Department of Health and Human Services (DHHS), but this would give DHHS broad authority over both private and public sector spending—creating an omnibus regulator which it is a major objective of pro-competitive reforms to avoid. DHHS policy-making would also be subject to partisan political direction and lengthy administrative delays. Another possible implementation structure, an autonomous Federal Reserve Board model, would not have these drawbacks, but would have too little public accountability given the scale and public sensitivity of health care reforms.

Thus the best approach seems to be to establish the new National Health Board as an independent agency, like the SEC. The National Health Board will be responsible to guide, oversee, and facilitate implementation of all aspects of the 21st Century Health System policies and mandated to pursue a pro-competitive reform strategy. In carrying out its legal responsibilities, the NHB will rely extensively on private sector standards-setting boards and their broad consultative processes. The NHB will be free from day-to-day interference while still accountable to elected political officials. With Presidential nomination and Senate confirmation, nationally recognized leadership would be recruited to guide its efforts.

Three ways in which possible over-stepping or misuse of the federal government's new regulatory authorities can be 'checked and balanced' are reflected in the proposals: (1) a standards-setting process that designs in collaborative private sector roles through consensus development and technical expertise of new standards-setting organizations, (2) a 'registration' process, similar to the SEC registration of securities that meet FASB standards, that will limit the normal regulatory processes vis a vis the health sector to certifying compliance with these standards, and (3) a key state administrative role under agreements with the NHB.

HEALTH STANDARDS BOARD (HealSB)

Structure

- Sponsored by major insurance, employer, consumer, and health provider groups

Responsibilities

- Assess medical technologies, medical practice effectiveness, and consumer opinions on health
- Advise on a list of effective services that will constitute the 'Uniform Effective Health Benefits' set that will be used as a national standard, tax excludable health insurance package

HealSB will be a new private sector organization for coordinating national assessments of medical effectiveness and bringing these results into health policy and clinical practice. Based on clinical and epidemiological studies, its benefits standards will incorporate the most effective treatments for various conditions. HealSB advice will be used for defining Uniform Effective Health Benefits and for advancing managed care. Its standards-setting will rely on the patient outcomes reporting standards (OMSB) and required reporting from Accountable Health Partnerships. Its membership will be chosen by a private sector sponsoring committee that includes health provider groups and medical researchers, consumers, employers, and insurers.

The HealSB proposal builds on many private sector activities, including work by medical groups on clinical trials, practice guidelines, and clinical outcomes and insurer information exchanges for technology assessments.

HEALTH INSURANCE STANDARDS BOARD (HISB)

Structure

- Sponsored by major insurance, employer, and consumer groups

Responsibilities

- Advise on implementation of universal health insurance coverage and effectiveness of insurance market competition
- Set standards for Accountable Health Partnerships with respect to basic managed care requirements and insurer-provider relationships, underwriting and business practices, and a phase-in schedule for enrollment. (HealSB develops the Uniform Effective Health Benefits package; OMSB sets quality data reporting standards)
- Set standards for Health Insurance Purchasing Cooperatives, so that small group insurance competition takes place on the basis of cost, high quality, and patient value rather than risk selection. Report on Uniform Health Benefits premiums for setting tax cap limits
- Work with National Association of Insurance Commissioners (NAIC) to develop model state laws and regulations

Standards-setting for health insurance companies and the health insurance market will be assigned to the HISB. HISB oversight will help assure implementation of universal health insurance coverage and effective competition, as well as patient outcomes reporting. The HISB standards for Accountable Health Partnerships and Health Insurance Purchasing Cooperatives will provide a basis for NHB registration and use of the tax code to encourage rapid deployment of Accountable Health Partnerships. HISB will monitor health insurance premiums for the Uniform Effective Health Benefits, particularly premiums achieved by Health Insurance Purchasing Cooperatives, to help set tax cap limits that reflect what employers and individuals have to pay for benefits in each market area.

This proposal builds on the standards-setting activities, involving Blue Cross/Blue Shield Association, Health Insurance Association of America, and individual companies, in collaboration with the National Association of Insurance Commissioners. These activities have been notable in small group insurance market reforms.

OUTCOMES MANAGEMENT STANDARDS BOARD (OMSB)

Structure

- Sponsored by insurance, employer, consumer and health provider groups

NATIONAL HEALTH BOARD

- Independent federal agency. Appointed by President, with Senate confirmation
- Guides, oversees, and facilitates transition to a 21st Century Health System with universal health insurance coverage and effective competition based on costs, high quality and value to the patient
- Recommends Uniform Effective Health Benefits and tax exclusion amounts
- Establishes registration requirements for Accountable Health Partnerships that offer Uniform Effective Health Benefits, provide essential managed care elements, follow acceptable market practices, and meet quality accountability reporting requirements (based on HealSB, HISB and OMSB standards). Only registered Accountable Health Partnerships can qualify for tax exclusion of employer contributions
- Establishes registration requirements for Health Insurance Purchasing Cooperatives that manage competition for the small group insurance market
- Enters into agreements with state governments to administer insurance sector regulation, e.g., mandated benefits, registration, small employer market reforms

HEALTH STANDARDS BOARD (HealSB)

- Sponsored by insurance, employer, consumer, and health provider groups
- Assesses medical technologies and medical practice variations
- Advises on effective services to be used for 'Uniform Effective Health Benefits' definition

HEALTH INSURANCE STANDARDS BOARD (HISB)

- Sponsored by insurance, employer, and consumer groups
- Advises on health insurance coverage issues and insurance market competition
- Sets standards for Accountable Health Partnerships
- Sets standards for Health Insurance Purchasing Cooperatives. Reports on Uniform Health Benefits premiums for setting tax caps
- Works with NAIC to develop model state laws and regulations

OUTCOMES MANAGEMENT STANDARDS BOARD (OMSB)

- Sponsored by insurance, employer, consumer, and health provider groups
- Sets data collection and health outcomes reporting standards for Accountable Health Partnerships
- Oversees data centers and outcomes evaluation

Figure 1. The public—private health partnership: the Jackson Hole Group model

Responsibilities

- Establish national data system for patient outcomes and other quality measures
- Set data collection and reporting standards for Accountable Health Partnerships, including registered insurers and registered delivery organizations
- Oversee data centers and data evaluation

The OMSB will design and oversee a nationwide quality reporting system, based primarily on patient outcomes measures. The required reporting will provide a basis for quality accountability and competition by health insurers and health care providers. The data will also be critical for advancing the state-of-art of clinical practice and for determining the Uniform Effective Health Insurance Benefits.

OMSB will build on private sector R&D and field-testing of outcomes management reporting. Many of the nation's major insurers, in collaboration with large employers, are now field-testing such protocols through the Managed Health Care Association. The American Group Practice Association is carrying on parallel activities with large HMOs and multi-specialty clinics.

NEXT STEPS

There are three major steps in implementing these proposals.

- The current private sector standards-setting activities should be expanded to prepare for legislation. The outcomes management reporting system work can soon become a self-financed non-profit activity, sponsored by major users. To build the foundation for HealSB, organized cooperation should be expanded among groups involved in medical assessment studies, and a national private sector agenda established to identify and resolve key clinical practice issues, particularly those requiring resolution to deal with rapidly rising health care costs. To expand insurance industry standards-setting, major insurers should work for enactment of NAIC small group insurance market standards and participate in demonstrations of Health Insurance Purchasing Cooperatives. Finally, an Executive Secretariat can be established to provide for dissemination of information abut the JHG proposals, enlist a broad range of support, and coordinate the expanding range of these private-sector activities.
- Given the broad sponsorship and guidance role proposed for employer, consumer, provider, and insurer groups in the three new standards-setting organizations, their views should be solicited on the JHG design and their support enlisted in its refinement and implementation.
- Finally, legislative action, with active political participation by the many affected groups, will be needed to enact this joint public-private implementation structure.

JACKSON HOLE PARTICIPANTS

John R. Ball, M.D., J.D.
Executive Vice President
American College of Physicians

James Bentley, Sr. VP Policy
American Hospital Association

John B. Crosby, Sr. Vice President
Health Policy Development
Legislation and Advocacy
American Medical Association

The Honorable David Durenberger
United States Senate (RMN)

David M. Eddy, M.D., Ph.D
Jackson, WY

Paul M. Ellwood, M.D.
President and Chairman
InterStudy

Mary Jane England, M.D.
President
Washington Business Group on Health

Alain C. Enthoven, Ph.D
Marriner S. Eccles Professor of
Public and Private Management
Graduate School of Business
Stanford University

Lynn M. Etheredge
Chevy Chase, M.D.

Paul Freiman
Chairman, Syntex Corporation
and Pharmaceutical Manufacturers' Association

Jerome Grossman, M.D.
President
New England Medical Center

John Iglehart
Special Correspondent
The New England Journal of Medicine, and Editor, Health Affairs

Ted Kelly
President, Group Insurance
Operations, Aetna Life and Casualty

David Kendall
Legislative Director to
Congressman Michael Andrews
(D-TX)

The Hon. John Kitzhaber, M.D.
President, Oregon State Senate

Kermit Knudsen, M.D.
President
Scott & White Clinic
Chairman, American Group Practice Association

David Lawrence, M.D.
Chairman & CEO
Kaiser Foundation Health Plan. Inc.

William P. Link
President, Group Operations
The Prudential

John D. Moynahan, Jr.
Executive Vice President
Metropolitan Life Insurance Company

Glen Nelson, M.D.
Vice Chairman
Medtronic, Inc.

Marilyn Carlson Nelson
Senior Vice President of
Carlson Holdings

G. Robert O'Brien
Executive Vice President
Cigna Corporation

Thomas O. Pyle
Former President & CEO
Harvard Community Health Plan

Anand Raman
Legislative Assistant to
Congressman Jim Cooper (D-TN)

William L. Roper, M.D.
Director
Centers for Disease Control

William R. Roy, M.D., J.D.
Topeka, KS

Ray Scheppach, Ph.D
Executive Director
National Governors' Association

Carl Schramm
President
Health Insurance, Assn. of America

Thomas A. Scully
Director for Human Resources
Veterans and Labor
Office of Management and Budget

Michael Stocker, M.D.
Executive Vice President
U.S. Health Care

Barney Tresnowski
President
Blue Cross and Blue Shield Assn.

Robert Waller, M.D.
Chairman of the Board
Mayo Clinic
Rochester, MN

COMMENTARY: MEASURING THE CANDIDATES ON HEALTH CARE

THE standard I use to evaluate the candidates' positions on health care reform is the Jackson Hole Group initiative, a comprehensive proposal to remedy many sources of market failure and inequity in our present system, to foster an effective, decentralized market in the private sector, and to ensure everyone's access to it.[1,2] The Jackson Hole Group is an informal group of health profession and industry leaders and policy analysts who meet periodically in Jackson Hole, Wyoming. The group's proposal has five key elements, dealing with integrated financing and delivery of health care, managed competition, health insurance for small groups of workers and self-employed persons, establishment of a regulatory framework for health care, and universal health insurance.

INTEGRATED FINANCING AND DELIVERY

Much of the economic failure of our system can be ascribed to the traditional model of fee-for-service, solo medical practice and remote third-party payment. The incentives inherent in this model are inflationary. It creates a costly adversarial relation between provider and payer. It contains no force to match resources to needs. Financial separation of the components (for example, doctors and hospitals) blocks the rational allocation of resources throughout the system. There is no effective accountability for the cost or quality of care. This model must be replaced by integrated financing and delivery systems — health maintenance organizations (HMOs) and new partnerships among physicians, hospitals, and insurers — with per capita prepayment (i.e., global budgets set in advance in the marketplace) and with providers placed at risk for the cost of care and of poor quality, so that they are rewarded both for improving quality and for cutting costs. Such organizations should be publicly accountable for cost and quality. Favorable tax treatment and subsidies for other forms of health care financing should be phased out.

MANAGED COMPETITION

Only market forces can bring about such a change. So far, market forces have not contained the growth in costs to acceptable rates. Today's health care economy is dominated by cost-unconscious demand.[3] Employers typically pay the full price of a fee-for-service plan and offer little reward to employees for choosing the least expensive plan, thus creating no incentives for the health care system to be economical. The effects of this are exacerbated by the open-ended tax breaks for employer-paid health benefits, market segmentation, differences in health risks among groups, and lack of comparative information on the quality of care.

Each of these problems can be corrected by managed competition, a purchaser strategy based on informed, cost-conscious consumer choice, which is designed to reward with more subscribers those organizations that do the best job of improving quality and cutting costs. Employers must offer employees choices of health plans, including the most efficient, and they must make defined contributions that do not exceed the price of the lowest-priced plan, so that the lowest-priced plan can attract more customers by cutting its price. Coverage should be standardized to facilitate price comparison and reduce market segmentation. There should be compensatory payments for health plans that enroll a population with worse-than-average health risks. There must be a limit on tax-free employer contributions set at the cost of the lowest-priced plan of acceptable quality, so that people choosing a higher-priced plan must pay the extra cost with their own money, not the taxpayers'.

REFORM IN SMALL-GROUP INSURANCE

Roughly half of privately employed Americans work in groups of 100 or fewer employees or are self-employed. Such groups are too small to spread risk, achieve economies of scale in administration, acquire and process the information needed to make good decisions, and participate in managed competition. The lack of opportunity for individual choice in small groups makes it harder for efficient HMOs to capture that business.

These problems could be corrected by pooling hundreds of thousands of individual workers through Health Insurance Purchasing Cooperatives (HIPCs). Such cooperatives would contract with several HMOs and other qualified health plans to offer enrollees a price-competitive choice. They would manage competition (conduct the annual enrollment, standardize benefit packages, adjust premiums to compensate for differences in health risks, inform consumers, and so on), monitor the quality of care and compliance, and relieve participating employers of costly administrative burdens. Participating health plans would agree to accept all enrollees, at their community rate, with no exclusions for preexisting conditions or health status. HIPCs would be created by the states, with board members appointed by the governor or elected by participating employers.

For this plan to work, there must be powerful incentives for even healthy groups to join the pools. In the case of small employers, the exemption from taxation of employer contributions to employees' health care benefits should be conditional on their participation in an HIPC.

Regulatory Framework

Like financial markets, these health care markets need a regulatory framework that encourages competition. For example, we propose that a national health board decide, on the basis of science and values and not politics, which technological procedures should be included in covered benefits. We propose a board to set uniform standards for reporting health outcomes and to publish data for consumers on risk-adjusted outcomes. The proposed structure is analogous to the relation between the Securities and Exchange Commission, an independent federal agency, and the Financial Accounting Standards Board.

Universal Health Insurance

It should become possible to require that all Americans participate in a reformed market with appropriate subsidies to those who cannot afford coverage. Employers should be required to cover all full-time employees. Part-time employees, the self-employed, the unemployed, those who retire early, and all others not covered by government programs would have coverage purchased by public sponsors through HIPCs serving their area of residence.[2] The sources of revenue to pay for these purchases would include a payroll tax on all noncovered employment, a tax on adjusted gross income for those who are not covered and who escape the payroll tax (e.g., early retirees), increased revenue from the limit on tax-free employer contributions, and use of existing sources of funding for the care for the uninsured.

The Candidates for President

The candidates for president face a tough problem. Any serious reform proposal must be too complicated to explain in a campaign speech and must contain features that will antagonize powerful interest groups. So, both sides are reluctant to take clear positions until after the election. Furthermore, within both camps there is a variety of views.

President Bush

On the broadest issue — expanded government entitlement programs and price controls versus a reformed market system — President Bush's proposal points in the right direction, but his proposed remedies are not nearly strong enough. The length and comprehensiveness of "The President's Comprehensive Health Reform Program"[4] suggest that the administration recognizes that effective market reform will require many coordinated actions. What is missing so far are actions with teeth. Ineffective proposals for market reform risk discrediting the whole idea.

The administration professes a desire to encourage coordinated care (their term for HMOs and similar insurer–provider partnerships). Correcting the anti-HMO bias in Medicare payment methods and broadening the program to include a wider variety of managed-care systems would be helpful. But the administration has failed to propose the most powerful step government could take to encourage the growth of cost-effective HMOs and to motivate them to restrain growth in cost — that is, to place a limit on tax-free employer contributions to employee health care equal to the price of the lowest-priced plan in the area, and to require that tax-favored employer contributions must be a fixed amount (defined contribution). This is an essential foundation of effective market reform.

The Bush administration has patterned its proposals for small-group market reform on those of the National Association of Insurance Commissioners. Some of these reforms sound fine as far as they go, but they leave in place some of the worst anticompetitive features of the present failed market. They leave insurers plenty of room to defeat price competition by segmenting markets. They do not permit individual workers a choice among health plans. Moreover, they leave room for very wide variations in premiums among groups.

The administration would also encourage the development of health insurance networks (HINs), similar to the HIPCs proposed by the Jackson Hole Group but without the powerful incentives to join them and the territorial franchises needed to make them work. Purely voluntary arrangements would not work in this case. Market forces motivate pools of insured groups to underwrite or exclude groups with poor risks, thus defeating their larger social purpose. The incentives proposed by the Bush administration are not strong enough to overcome this factor.

The administration proposes a transferable tax credit, or voucher, for the poor. The implied declaration that, in the future, all poor people in America would be covered is most welcome. But more must be done; about two thirds of the uninsured are not poor (i.e., they do not have incomes below the federal poverty line). The administration does not explain how to pay for the tax credit, which would cost more than $20 billion a year. The best source of revenue would be a limit on tax-free employer contributions for health insurance.

If poor families are free to shop in the private sector for coverage, healthy people will be able to get cheap private insurance while the state gets the bad risks. It would be better to require the poor to use their credits to buy coverage through their local HIPC, so that their health risks would be spread widely. As for uninsured employed persons who are not poor, it would be a lot easier to require employers to cover their full-time employees if there were an effective small-group market reform with competitive community rates set through an HIPC.

The question for voters who would like to see an effective market reform is whether we can be confident that a reelected President Bush would carry through with the strong measures that are needed, especially if he has no electoral mandate for them.

Governor Clinton

Governor Clinton says that "we need a new approach that will control costs, improve quality, maintain choice, and cover everybody."[5] He would streamline the insurance system, guarantee benefits, limit cost increases, reduce bureaucracy, reduce increases in drug prices, reduce billing fraud, and more — all commendable goals. But he does not really explain how he would achieve them. He does not make clear whether he favors an overall strategy based on reformed incentives and organization in a decentralized private market system, or whether he prefers centralized top-down government control. There are words in his statement to please supporters of both options. He is preserving his options. Governor Clinton thus raises both my hopes and my fears.

My hope is that as president he would embrace the position of the Conservative Democratic Forum, a group of about 70 Democratic members of Congress whose leaders have declared their support for the Jackson Hole initiative and who are developing legislation to implement it. My fear is that he would favor legislation sponsored by liberal Democrats, known as "play-or-pay," that would achieve universal coverage by renaming Medicaid and expanding it to cover all those not covered through their employers. Employers would have a choice: cover employees with a private program meeting federal standards, or pay a payroll tax and cover them through the public program. A Federal Health Expenditure Board would set overall national expenditure goals and goals according to sector (for hospitals, physicians, and so forth). It would negotiate rates with providers, which would mean federal price controls.

Government price controls simply do not work, especially in a field as complex and dynamic as health care. Regulators cannot manage utilization and appropriateness of care by remote control in an adversarial relationship with doctors. Furthermore, this scheme would lock in the fee-for-service, remote-third-party payment model that is at the root of so many of our present problems. It would not reward the creation of more efficient systems of care.

The government would suffer the effects of adverse selection. Those most likely to choose the government insurance plan would be those with the lowest pay and the highest medical costs. So revenues would fall short, and costs would run over global budgets. If the government raised the payroll tax to compensate for these increased costs, the relatively healthy and better paid would be motivated to leave the public program. The likely outcome would be to limit the tax, under pressure from small business, and to add to the federal deficit. The scenario would be a replay of the fiscal disasters we are observing in the Federal Savings and Loan Insurance Corporation, the Federal Deposit Insurance Corporation, and Medicare Hospital Insurance.

Governor Clinton has worked hard to move his party back to a moderate position. The question for voters who would like to see market reform is this: In the absence of a clear campaign position, can we be confident he would side with the moderate wing of his party? Or would he find it expedient to turn health policy over to the liberal wing, in exchange for their support for the rest of his agenda?

I believe a postelection consensus will favor trying market reforms first. If they do not succeed, centralized controls will follow. In either case, however, market reforms would give us a more efficient and accountable health care system.

Stanford University
Stanford, CA 94305 ALAIN C. ENTHOVEN

References

1. Ellwood P, Enthoven A, Etheredge L. The Jackson Hole initiatives for a twenty-first century American health care system. Health Econ (in press).
2. Enthoven A, Kronick R. A consumer-choice health plan for the 1990s: universal health insurance in a system designed to promote quality and economy. N Engl J Med 1989;320:29-37, 94-101.
3. Enthoven A. How employers boost health costs. Wall Street Journal. January 24, 1992:A12.
4. The President's Comprehensive Health Reform Program. Washington, D.C.: The White House, February 6, 1992.
5. Bill Clinton's American Health Care Plan. Little Rock, Ark.: Bill Clinton for President Committee, 1992.

Hillary Clinton's Potent Brain Trust On Health Reform

Far from the capital, a once-obscure group provides the blueprint.

By ROBIN TONER

WASHINGTON

THE CLOCK is running on the Clinton Administration's task force on health care, which now has only two months to produce a comprehensive restructuring of a system that has resisted comprehensive restructuring for years. But Ira C. Magaziner, who is running the mammoth policy-making enterprise with First Lady Hillary Rodham Clinton, still found time last week to make the long trip to the Tetons.

There he met with a loose-knit group of experts that has become one of the most important influences in the shaping of the Clinton plan. Known as the Jackson Hole Group for the Wyoming ski town where its members meet, it has included over the past three years about 100 academics; executives from the insurance, hospital and pharmaceutical industries; physicians; representatives of business and assorted policy makers.

Although Mrs. Clinton did not attend the session, she demurred regretfully and respectfully. The Jackson Hole Group is, at the moment, hot — the leading proponent of "managed competition," an approach to health insurance that was embraced by President Clinton during last year's campaign and thus moved to the center of the policy debate.

To understand the shadowy fascination of the Jackson Hole Group, one must first understand this: An exercise in policy-making that affects virtually every major constituent, interest group and business is under way in Washington, and it is largely taking place in endless meetings of working groups behind closed doors. In such a blackout, deciphering the intellectual forces at work on Mrs. Clinton and her top advisers might hint at the outcome. While Mrs. Clinton and Mr. Magaziner have marshaled more than 300 experts to assemble the health reform proposal by May 1, the Jackson Hole Group has already provided much of the basic blueprint.

How It Works

Managed competition is still, as Mr. Clinton's political adviser James Carville puts it, a term that "no *person* has ever heard of, only intellectual forces." And it has its critics, including those who call it a kind of Insurance Industry Preservation Act and those who question whether it alone will truly control medical costs. But it has gained a wide following in recent years.

In theory, it would band employers and individuals into large cooperatives to purchase health insurance, giving small businesses and individuals the same bargaining power as big companies. On the other end, it would force doctors, hospitals and insurers to form partnerships that would compete for the cooperatives' business, each trying to offer the highest-quality but least-expensive health plan.

The thinking is that such competition — overseen by a National Health Board establishing standards for benefit plans — would hold down medical costs yet improve health care. As for Americans currently uninsured, contributions from employers and the Government would allow them to join a cooperative.

Two of the principal advocates of managed competition are Alain C. Enthoven, a professor of economics at Stanford University, who began formulating these ideas back in the 1970's, and Dr. Paul M. Ellwood, a pediatric neurologist from Minnesota who is widely considered a father of health maintenance organizations.

While the informal meetings at Dr. Ellwood's home in Jackson Hole have taken place for 20 years, they — and the concept of managed competition — received little attention until soaring medical costs forced policy makers on the state and national level to seriously consider change. The concept was set forth in 1991 in a formal document: "The 21st Century American Health System — Managed Competition: A Proposal for Public and Private Health Care Reform."

Around that time, various versions of managed competition began creeping into

Continued on Page 8

Continued from Page 1

the political process. The theory was embraced by a group of conservative Democrats on Capitol Hill, led by Representative Jim Cooper of Tennessee, by former Senator Paul E. Tsongas of Massachusetts, and ultimately by President Bush and Mr. Clinton. The editorial page of The New York Times also played an important role with a number of editorials in support of managed competition, according to longtime players in the debate.

The group and its proposal have many fans, who see it as a sweeping reform of the health-care system that is sensitive to American culture and sensibilities; the very name sounds like a muscular but orderly capitalism. It also has a strong political appeal for elected officials who fear that other widely discussed alternatives, including a Government-run system like Canada's, are too radical or too costly to sell to the voters.

The Disbelievers

The group and its ideas have legions of critics and skeptics. "If you get it down to sea level, it doesn't do anything, which is why everybody likes it," said Representative Pete Stark, the California Democrat who is chairman of the health subcommittee of the House Ways and Means Committee. "There's no new taxes needed, it provides universal access, and if you believe all that, that's somewhere between the tooth fairy and the chuckling oyster."

More specifically, many critics see the Jackson Hole philosophy as an attempt to stave off true reform and preserve the lucrative franchises of the establishments that dominate health care — especially the insurance industry. Dr. Steffie Woolhandler, an assistant professor of medicine at Harvard and a founder of Physicians for a National Health Program, a supporter of a Canadian-style system, says: "Managed competition is a last-ditch effort to preserve a role for the insurance industry in health care."

Dr. Ellwood says he was only trying to bring together all the players in the health-care system and sit them down in his living room to hunt for solutions. "The basic problem with the health industry is, here's this huge industry and there's no obvious leader," he said in an interview. "In order to get some sense of consensus, some sense of what could be accomplished, the device I used was to informally assemble leaders to focus on the problems."

Dr. Ellwood, who practiced medicine for 17 years, has been advising and consulting on health policy and planning for many years through the research group he founded, called InterStudy. Mr. Enthoven, a former economist with the Rand Corporation and an assistant Secretary of Defense under President Johnson, has also consulted and written extensively on health issues. Along with Lynn M. Etheredge, a Washington-based health-care consultant, those two are considered the principal architects of the Jackson Hole initiative.

The insurance industry and the medical profession are both well represented in the group, as is the pharmaceutical industry, which has been criticized by both Clintons lately.

Jackson Hole Group organizers are careful to note that not all the participants support the group's formal proposal. Mr. Enthoven said in an interview: "What was valuable is that we brought together people from many perspectives. We learned from each other."

Dr. Ellwood said the organizers "go to great lengths psychologically to make this meeting work." Participants dress casually and engage in opening ceremonies and skits, occasionally in frontier or Western attire. (Mr. Magaziner, reflecting Washington more than Wyoming, showed up in a suit.)

Last weekend's meeting was technical, detailed and focused on the practical problems of moving toward a system of managed competition, Dr. Ellwood said. Mr. Magaziner, who attended on Sunday, briefed the group and sought proposals on cost containment, Dr. Ellwood added.

The links go beyond that meeting. Mr. Enthoven and Mr. Etheredge are among the consultants to the Clinton task force, for example. (The culture of secrecy is such that the White House refuses to provide a full list of consultants brought in to aid in the effort.)

Jackson Hole leaders also briefed Mrs. Clinton a few weeks ago. "Clearly, the Jackson Hole group is seen as the intellectual brain trust for the managed competition model," said Bob Boorstin, the White House spokesman for the health-care task force. "Given that, they obviously played a very, very strong indirect role in what has evolved into the President's plan."

But, as Mr. Boorstin suggests, the President's plan will be the President's plan. The health-care task force is widely expected to propose some form of managed competition, but one with some kind of cap on overall medical spending. "We don't like it," Dr. Ellwood said, "mostly because we don't think it's practical. You don't get a market started by slapping price controls on it."

Is It Enough?

But if the Clinton Administration hopes to control medical costs and provide coverage to the more than 35 million Americans without health insurance, it badly needs savings from health-care reform, and quickly. And the Congressional Budget Office has suggested that managed competition — like other alternatives — will take substantial time to produce significant savings.

Helping to meld these imperatives into a coherent policy are Mr. Magaziner, senior White House domestic policy adviser, and Judith Feder, who is coordinating the operation in Health and Human Services. (Both denied requests for interviews through a White House spokesman.)

On the intellectual front, Paul Starr, the Princeton sociologist who won the Pulitzer Prize for his book "The Social Transformation of American Medicine," is closely watched for making the case for a grand compromise. He recently made such an attempt in an article in Health Affairs magazine with Walter A. Zelman, special deputy for health issues to California's Insurance Commissioner, John Garamendi.

Mr. Starr and Mr. Zelman, who are advising the task force, argued that a system combining managed competition with some form of spending limits is the answer.

In fact, many analysts suggested that if Mr. Clinton holds true to form, his health-care policy will almost certainly be the "third way" he so often seeks in truly polarized debates — not pure Jackson Hole, not total regulation, but something that seeks to meet the progressive goals of making health insurance more affordable and more widely available without utterly dismantling the American system.

For now, however, the Jackson Hole Group is engaging in a little pride of parentage. "We're acting like it's going to happen," said Dr. Ellwood in an interview this week, far from the Tetons, but just a few blocks from the Capitol. ■

CONSERVATIVE DEMOCRATIC FORUM PLAN

Conservative Democratic Forum Task Force on Health Care Reform. H.R. 5936: The Managed Competition Act of 1992 (Highlights). Washington, D.C.: CDF; 1992:1-8.

American Hospital Association. (October 19, 1992). CDF Serves Up Menu of Health-Plan Options for Consumers. *AHA News.* 28(42):5. [This is an interview with Congressman Jim Cooper (D. - Tenn.), who chairs the Conservative Democratic Forum's health care task force.]

H.R. 5936
The Managed Competition Act of 1992

Proposal of the Conservative Democratic Forum's
Task Force on Health Care Reform

HIGHLIGHTS

In order to allow consumers to shop wisely for health plans, the bill uses strong tax incentives to encourage providers and insurance companies to form health partnerships which will be publicly accountable for costs and quality. Large regional purchasing cooperatives will give individuals and small businesses the benefits of greater buying power. A national board will establish a uniform set of effective health benefits. In order to have tax-favored status, health plans will be required to offer those standard benefits, comply with insurance reforms and disclose information on medical outcomes, cost-effectiveness and consumer satisfaction.

• **Tax fairness:** Employers will be allowed to deduct basic health plan costs, but not the excess costs of policies which cover more than the basic benefits. Basic policies must require co-payments to make consumers cost-conscious, and must be provided through publicly accountable health plans. All individuals, including the self-employed, will be given a tax benefit for 100% of basic health plan costs.

• **Access to coverage:** Individuals and small businesses will be able to afford health coverage by joining Health Plan Purchasing Cooperatives, which will offer group rates with lower administrative costs. Individuals will choose from a menu of health plans, and their employers will choose the dollar amount, if any, they wish to contribute.

• **Health plan reform:** Health plans will not be allowed to exclude coverage of pre-existing conditions and will not be allowed to use "experience rating" to charge higher rates for individuals who have a history of higher medical expenses.

• **Access for low-income individuals:** A new federal program will pay health plan premiums for all people below 100% of the poverty level. Individuals and families between 100% and 200% of the poverty level will receive a federal subsidy for the purchase of a health plan. The federal program will also make most copayments for those below 200% of poverty. States will no longer have to finance Medicaid, and will gradually assume responsibility for long-term (e.g. nursing home) care for the poor.

• **Preventive health** will be key to the success of the new health partnerships. In addition, the bill significantly increases funding for early intervention, immunization and screening programs.

• **Malpractice reform** will reduce the costs of expensive litigation and the cost of defensive medicine.

• **Paperwork reduction**: Health plans will develop standards for claims forms and electronic transmission of data in accordance with federal goals.

• **Basic access:** To assist rural and other underserved areas, funding for Community and Migrant Health Centers and National Health Service Corps will be substantially increased.

SUMMARY

Managed Competition — The Heart of Cost Control

Providers, Insurance, and Patients — New Accountability

If costs are to be controlled, the government must encourage the market to fundamentally restructure the way health care is provided. In today's market, few providers have strong incentives to hold down costs: The more services they provide, they more they can bill insurance companies, and the more they are paid. Providers are not accountable for what they charge, and they are not accountable for medical outcomes.

Managed Competition Act: Through changes in the tax code, the bill strongly encourage providers and insurance companies to form Accountable Health Plans (AHPs) — improved and expanded versions of today's Health Maintenance Organizations, Preferred Provider Organizations, and other group practices. AHPs will be organized to compete on the basis of offering high-quality, low-cost care, and will offer insurance and health care as a single product. They will be responsible for looking after the total health of individuals.

AHPs will have to price their plans in a dramatically different way than they are priced today. In our current system, health plans can "cherry-pick" the healthiest individuals, and deny coverage or charge extremely high rates for others. Plans can also deny coverage for individuals with pre-existing medical conditions. Under our proposal, any plan engaging in those practices will lose their tax-favored status.

• AHPs must offer a standard health plan of federally-defined uniform, effective health benefits, and they will be publicly accountable for medical outcomes. They may offer more comprehensive plans, but employers and individuals who purchase those plans will receive a tax break only for the least costly package of basic benefits. AHPs must require copayments for medical services, except for preventive care.

• AHPs must require all of their providers to report medical outcomes in accordance with federal guidelines.

• AHPs will not be allowed to use experience rating, varying premiums based on how sick people have been and how many claims they have had in the past. AHPs will be allowed to vary premiums based only on geographic location, and to a limited degree based on age.

• AHP plans must enroll all individuals who apply for coverage (open enrollment), and will not be allowed to deny coverage for pre-existing medical conditions.

• AHPs will be allowed to contract for costly high-tech or specialized services and will be exempt from all state mandates on benefits and all state restrictions on managed care.

• An AHP may be set up by a very large business to provide coverage for its employees. It must meet all of the above rules, except for the requirement of open enrollment.

Tax Fairness Under Managed Competition

Current law provides two tax benefits for the purchase of health insurance:

• Most businesses are allowed to deduct the full cost of any health coverage they provide to their employees. This deduction is allowed for any kind of health plan, without limit.

• Individuals may exclude from their income any amount their employer pays toward health coverage. Like the business deduction, this tax exclusion is available for any kind of health plan policy with no dollar limit.

The federal revenue loss associated with these tax provisions exceeds $65 billion a year, making it the third largest federal health program after Medicare and Medicaid. And because these tax benefits grow with greater health care spending, they contribute to health inflation.

In addition, these benefits are not equitably distributed. Self-employed individuals and certain small businesses are only allowed to deduct 25% of the cost of health benefits. And individuals who buy coverage on their own get no tax benefit unless their health expenses exceed 7.5 percent of their income. *As a result, families earning more than $100,000 receive, on average, almost 30 times as much tax benefit as those with incomes of $10,000.*

Managed Competition Act: To encourage health plans to offer standard benefit plans so consumers can shop on the basis of price and quality, and to discourage inflationary "Rolls-Royce" health policies, which don't control costs, the bill caps tax deductibility at the cost of the lowest-price AHP plan (meeting minimum federal standards) in the area. Subject to this cap:

• Tax deductibility for the self-employed is increased to 100% of their AHP premium.

• Individuals who pay all or part of an AHP premium would be able to fully deduct their payments.

• If an individual or employer purchases coverage from a plan which is not a federally-qualified AHP, none of the amount paid is deductible.

Small Business and Individual Purchasing Power

Compared with large businesses, small businesses and individuals face two major disadvantages that discourage them from purchasing health coverage:

• As much as 40% of the premiums paid by small businesses and individuals goes toward administrative costs of health insurance (compared with less than 10% for large businesses).

• Small businesses do not have enough employees to spread the risk of insurance around, and if even one employee has high medical expenses, insurance can quickly become unaffordable. The problem is even worse for individuals.

<u>Managed Competition Act:</u> To make health coverage more available, all individuals, except for employees of very large businesses, would join a Health Plan Purchasing Cooperative (HPPC):

• HPPCs will be state chartered, not-for-profit organizations, with exclusive geographic territory (i.e. there will be one HPPC per region). States will have the option of establishing more than one HPPC in a state (e.g. one in a metropolitan area and one for the rest of the state).

• All businesses with fewer than 1,000 employees will join a HPPC, and states will have the option of requiring businesses of up to 10,000 employees to join.

• HPPCs will offer to each enrollee a menu of accountable health plans, including clear, standardized information for each plan on its price, quality and enrollee satisfaction. Each individual will be able to choose the health plan he or she prefers.

• HPPCs will collect all individual and small business employee premiums and distribute them to the accountable health plans. Using a federal risk-adjustment procedure, HPPCs will pay more to AHPs which have enrolled high-risk individuals and will reduce payment to AHPs which have enrolled low-risk individuals.

• HPPCs will eliminate the burden of COBRA health plan continuation coverage for businesses. If an individual loses his job, he can remain in the HPPC and pay premiums himself.

• HPPC administrative expenses will be financed by a small surcharge on individual premiums which should be dramatically less than today's administrative charges.

National Health Board and Accountability

Managed competition will work only if the market is carefully overseen and AHPs are held publicly accountable for the care they provide.

<u>Managed Competition Act:</u> An independent national health board will oversee the health market, much like the Securities and Exchange Commission oversees the financial market.

• The board will:
  - Establish and update the standard health benefits package, which must include the full range of clinically-effective treatments and preventive services
  - Establish standards for reporting prices, health outcomes, and measures consumer satisfaction
  - Develop factors for risk adjustment of AHP premiums
  - Provide for information on AHP quality to be distributed to consumers

• The board will function independently. Its recommendations on the basic benefits will be submitted to Congress and will have to be approved or rejected on an up-or-down vote.

• The board will be advised by expert industry boards which will focus on benefits and health plan standards (this will work in much the same way as the Federal Accounting Standards Board advises the SEC).

• Funding for the board will come from a small annual fee per enrolled member in AHPs.

Consumer Information

Accountable Health Plans will be required to report full information on the outcomes of treatments and the costs of their plan. Such information will include:

- The number of each procedure performed
- The cost of procedures
- The medical results (e.g. the proportion of patients who died, had complications, fully recovered, etc.)
- Patient satisfaction

This information will be given to consumers and employers to allow them to choose the most efficient, highest-quality providers. It will also be used by providers to help them change their practice styles. This new accountability is fundamentally different from the current practices of some managed-care groups, where doctors are second-guessed on a case-by-case basis.

Universal Access Under Managed Competition

Low-Income Access

Medicaid is the main program providing health services to the poor. The program is financed by both the federal government and the states, and covers both acute care (e.g. hospitals and physicians) and long-term care (e.g. nursing homes and home health care).

Medicaid has a complicated set of requirements for eligibility, and today covers fewer than half of the people below the poverty line. The criteria for coverage vary substantially from state to state. In general, eligibility for Medicaid is linked to eligibility for welfare, though pregnant women and children may receive Medicaid coverage even if their incomes are above the welfare cut-off.

Managed Competition Act: Medicaid is replaced with a new federal program which will help purchase coverage through AHPs for low-income individuals:

- All individuals and families with incomes below 200% of their state's poverty level will be members of a HPPC and will receive federal assistance for premiums and copayments. Eligibility for this new program will be separated from eligibility for welfare.

- Individuals and families with incomes below 100% of poverty will be eligible to join an AHP with no premium cost to them, and with nominal copayments. They will also receive assistance for certain items (e.g. eyeglasses or hearing aids) which might not be covered by the basic benefit package offered by AHPs.

- Individuals and families with incomes between 100% and 200% of poverty will be eligible to join an AHP, and will be responsible for paying a portion of the premium, based on a sliding scale. They will also have nominal copayments.

- Medicaid will be repealed, freeing up substantial state funds. The states will gradually assume responsibility for long-term care, with greater flexibility to try innovative approaches.

Access in Rural and Other Underserved Areas

Practitioners are scarce in many rural and other areas, so there are fewer opportunities for competition. The National Health Board will carefully monitor underserved areas to make sure there is sufficient competition. Like other AHPs, those in underserved areas will be allowed to contract for capital-intensive or high-tech services.

The bill will improve access to basic care for rural and inner-city residents through a $100 million increase in funding for Community and Migrant Health Centers, a $25 million increase in funding for the National Health Service Corps, and a $10 million increase in funding for Area Health Education Centers.

Other Provisions

Expansion of Preventive Health Services

Greater use of preventive care is key to health care cost-containment and a healthier nation. The bill encourages preventive care in a number of ways:

• Because they will be offering insurance and health care as one product, AHPs will have a strong financial incentive to keep their enrollees healthy.

• Preventive health care will be the only service for which no co-payment or deductible may be charged.

• The bill provide significantly increased funding for a variety of existing preventive health initiatives, including immunization grants, lead poisoning prevention, breast and cervical cancer screening, and early AIDS intervention. Increased funding will also be provided for the Office of Disease Prevention and Health Promotion and the Office of Smoking and Health.

• In addition, preventive services available under Medicare will be expanded to include annual mammography, certain immunizations and colorectal screening.

Malpractice Reform

Unnecessary litigation and defensive medicine have contributed to rising medical costs, and must be controlled as part of health care reform. In some regions of the country the high cost of liability insurance has not just driven up costs, but has reduced access to care, especially for high-risk services like obstetrics.

The bill makes substantial changes in the law, including limiting non-economic damages and reducing unreasonably long statutes of limitations. It supersedes state laws, except where they are more stringent than federal law. These changes will be combined with new efforts by AHPs to identify sub-standard providers.

Paperwork Reduction and Administrative Simplification

At least $5 billion in annual health care expenditures could be saved by reducing the paperwork required by the nation's 1,500 insurance companies with their multitude of forms. The bill would establish national goals for health plans to achieve efficiencies from standard claims forms and electronic transmission of data. The National Health Board would have the responsibility and authority to ensure that these goals are met.

Financing

The bill is budget-neutral. It contains complete financing for the Medicaid reforms and other provisions. The major sources of financing include: eliminating the limit on income which is subject to the Medicare HI tax (currently $130,200); capping deductibility of health plan expenses at the price of the most cost-effective AHP; and redirecting federal Medicaid spending.

September, 1992

MANAGED COMPETITION

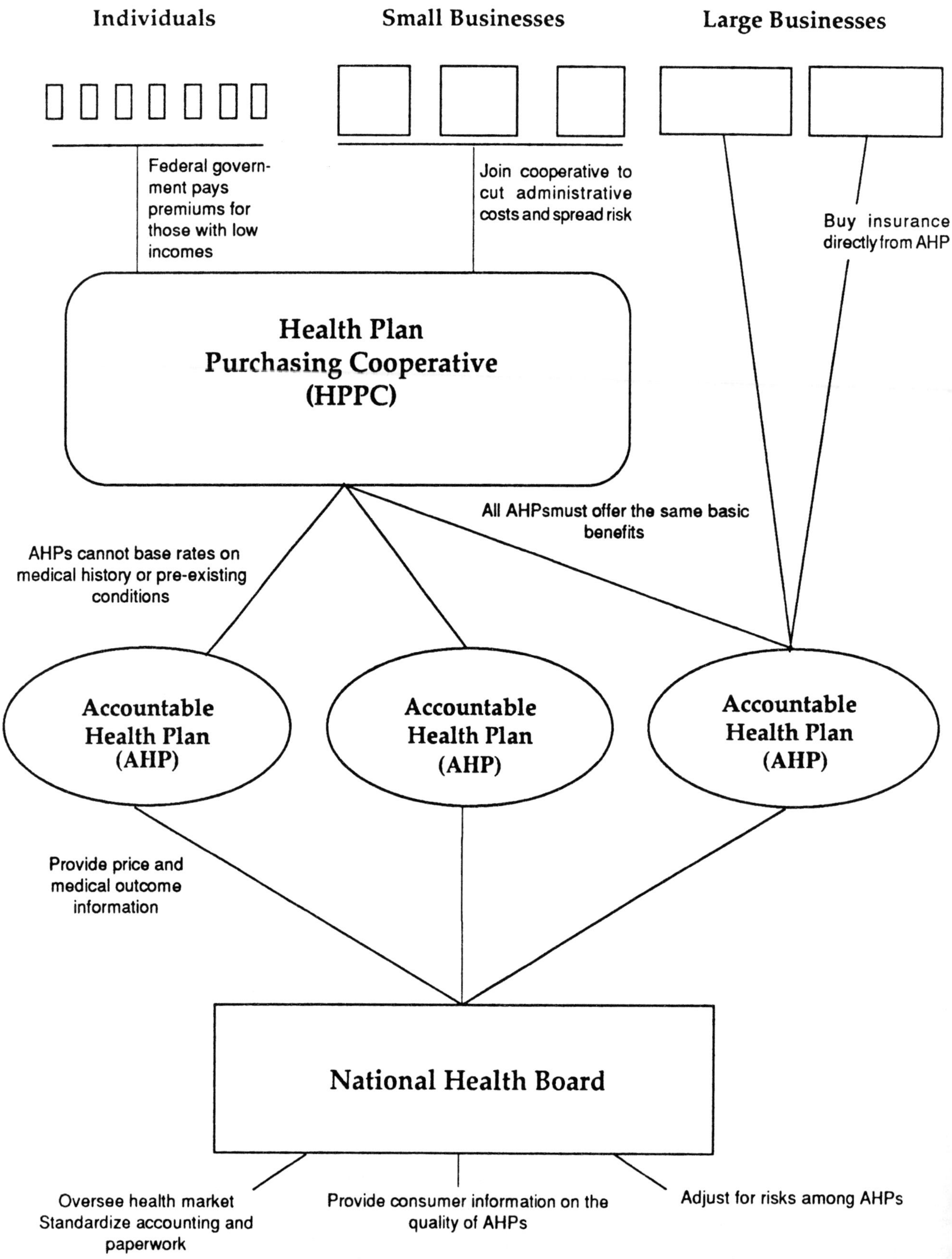

CDF serves up menu of health-plan options for consumers

Rep. Jim Cooper (D-TN) leads the Conservative Democratic Forum's (CDF) health care taskforce and is one of the architects of the CDF's Managed Competition Act of 1992, which was introduced last month. The plan aims to control costs through tax changes and system restructuring, and to provide universal access through Medicaid reform and insurance-purchasing cooperatives.

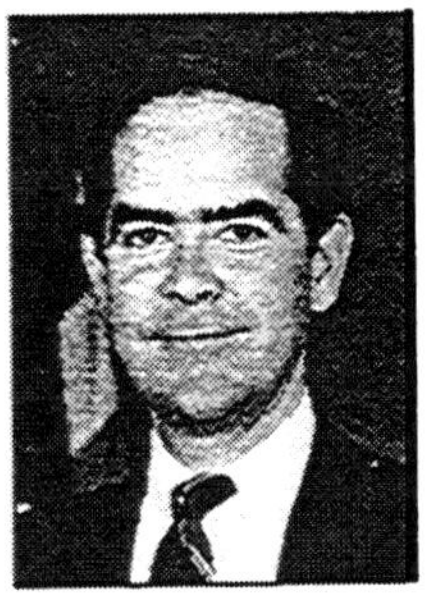

Cooper

To encourage consumers to shop wisely for health care plans, the bill uses strong tax incentives to encourage providers and insurers to form health partnerships, which would be publicly accountable for costs and quality. Under the bill, a national board would create an effective uniform health-benefits package. To enjoy tax-favored status, health care plans would have to offer the uniform package, comply with insurance reforms, and disclose information on medical outcomes and cost-effectiveness.

AHA News Staff Writer Christopher J. Gearon recently interviewed Cooper about the managed-competition approach to reform and the politics of reform.

Q How would the CDF plan work?

We would give all employees the same purchasing power in the health care market. We would try to set up provider/insurance groups that would offer employees the quality of medical care that you can find, for example, at the Mayo Clinic. That's the goal — setting up large purchasing groups and provider groups.

The actual mechanism: Give every employee in America an annual menu that contains local health care options, including basic health care plans, each with the same copayments and deductibles so they can compare them on the basis of price, quality and consumer satisfaction. The lowest cost plan would be fully deductible. The groups on the menu would be obligated to report their outcomes. They would be a combination of provider and insurance groups. You would buy health care as one product on an annual prepaid basis. Fee-for-service reimbursement would probably be discouraged. The third-party payment system would be hidden, if not fully eliminated.

We would repeal the Medicaid program and replace it with a 100 percent federal program for acute care, and we would shift responsibility for long-term care to the states.

Q What are the incentives for providers to join Accountable Health Partnerships (AHPs)?

Tax deductibility. If you want to have the government subsidize the provision of services, you have to form an AHP. Our idea basically is to take away luxury health care benefits and to broaden the availability of health benefits to all Americans. We would be allowing employees as well as employers to have the benefit of this tax deduction. It's one of the most overlooked parts of the system. We're talking about serious inequity, which could be remedied and also generate revenue for health care reform.

Q How much guidance or regulation does the plan lay out for providers and insurers to form AHPs?

There would be certain minimum standards to be met. Quality and solvency are the guidelines to make sure the plan could live up to its promises. You would have to offer a basic-benefits package.

There's near community rating; we would allow for variations on the basis of age, but very little else. [Small-market reforms are included.] What we're seeking is minimum government involvement but enough government involvement to make sure the marketplace works properly. For many of today's providers, this could result in a lessening of the backseat driving they're seeing.

Q So communities could determine how they want to set up an AHP?

Every state would have at least one Health Plan Purchasing Cooperative (HPPC), which is the menu-forming body. It's the cooperative made up of the owners of the various small businesses in the area. Most of the larger businesses don't need these purchasing groups that we are offering, but smaller businesses do. The HPPC is a key function. Each menu offering would have to qualify for tax deductibility, and that's going to be up to innovative providers, insurers, entrepreneurs, etc., to form these groups. They can include insurers, anything as long as they meet basic standards. The consumer only sees one annual fee as a uniform copayment or deductible for a basic-benefits package.

Q If the market has to decide what the average price is for a basic plan and include all of the currently uninsured, many of which pose bad risks for insurers, wouldn't this threaten the universal-access element of the plan?

There are a couple of ways to approach it. We're paying those costs today on the back end, and we could do it much more intelligently if we face it on the front end.

It is true for some young people that community rating looks like their premium goes up to pay for an older person. But we allow age variation in the premium. There are some cross subsidies in life that are worth preserving.

Q With so many members of Congress pledging not to raise taxes, how can this country ever hope to finance a comprehensive health care plan?

Considering that we have the greatest expansion of health care to the poor since the Great Society days, our plan is remarkably affordable. It should cost about $30 billion a year to the federal government. Some $10 billion can come from limiting tax deductibility, which is not a new tax — it's restructuring the current tax.

Another $12 billion can come from the Medicaid disproportionate-share program, which is refocusing Medicaid spending. An additional $5 billion to $8 billion could come from lifting the Medicare [hospital-insurance fund] tax-earning limit above $130,000. And there you have about $30 billion remarkably painlessly. The president's program is underfunded. The plan proposed by Rep. Pete Stark (D-CA) and Rep. Richard A. Gephardt (D-MO) has no real outreach. They claim systematic savings that will fund things, but we try to be up front and make sure our program will not add one penny to the federal deficit.

Q How would you explain to hospitals that you are going to cut their disproportionate-share payments when Medicaid already is underfunded?

The purpose of that program is to help hospitals who are unduly burdened with disproportionate numbers of medically indigent people. When you repeal Medicaid, as the plan does, and replace it with a program that helps everyone up to 200 percent of poverty, that's beyond the wildest dreams of any hospital administrator. Also, it compensates providers at private-pay levels. You're talking about obviating the Medicaid disproportionate-share program.

Q Why did the CDF introduce its proposal with three weeks remaining in the 102nd Congress?

We were dissatisfied with single-payer, play-or-pay, and with price-control proposals. It took a long time to draft the bill because it's the first time this approach has ever been drafted. We thought it was important to formally introduce it in this Congress so people could poke holes in it before the next Congress.

Q Speaking of the next administration, how would the CDF plan fare under a Bill Clinton or second Bush administration?

We see our proposal as being the basis for health care reform regardless of who wins the presidency because top advisers for both Bush and Clinton have endorsed the key elements of our plan. You can look at it from either perspective, but there is a moderate middle that is agreeing on these fundamental approaches.

Q How far could you go with global budgets and spending caps before you rip the heart out of managed competition?

It's theoretically possible to build on our low-bid system and then aggregate some national spending target from that. But that's a bottoms-up approach. It's the completely opposite from a top-down approach, in which some Washington bureaucrat says $800 billion is the right number for America and then tries to allocate that among the states.

To think there would be any enforcement or any discipline or any fairness in that type of system is rhetorical cost control. Price controls do not work, and we've got to learn that the big government approach is not the right solution.

AMERICAN ASSOCIATION OF RETIRED PERSONS PLAN

American Association of Retired Persons. Health Care America: The Draft Health Care Reform Proposal. Washington, D.C.: AARP; March 1992. [Pages i-vii, which constitute the Executive Summary, are reprinted here.]

HEALTH CARE AMERICA

March 1992

EXECUTIVE SUMMARY

INTRODUCTION

AARP's draft health care reform proposal, Health Care America, calls for the replacement of this country's fragmented health care system with a standardized, simplified system that would guarantee comprehensive health insurance, including coverage for long-term care, to all individuals. The centerpiece of the reformed system would be a strengthened, improved and expanded Medicare program; Medicaid would be eliminated. Under Health Care America, everyone would be eligible through the new Medicare program for a generous, nationally mandated package of medical benefits (i.e., acute/preventive/ transitional benefits) and long-term care benefits.* Individuals would obtain access to the full range of covered services using a standardized "smart card." In addition to ensuring access, the system would continue to foster choice, diversity, and innovation in the delivery of health services.

For the first time in our nation's history, cost containment would be achieved by means of a nationally established target for total annual national health expenditures. This spending target would be used to establish uniform reimbursement levels for health care providers; balance billing would be prohibited. Operating within the parameters of nationally established reimbursement rules and state-specific spending targets, states would retain sufficient administrative flexibility to address local needs. Undergirding--though separate from--the strategies to increase access and control costs would be a new, comprehensive, national program to assure a high level of quality throughout the health care system. Finally, Health Care America offers two alternative, broad-based financing options, each one adequate to generate the tax revenues needed to pay for the proposed restructuring of the health care system.

The medical and long-term care provisions of the reformed health care system have been discussed separately in this draft proposal in order to facilitate understanding of the proposal's various features. Nevertheless, a major goal of AARP's reform efforts is the creation of a continuum of medical and long-term care along which services would be provided, as needed, to people of all ages. The medical and long-term care provisions of this proposal are thus seen as part of a single, integrated system linked by: a common foundation in the new Medicare program; complementary benefit design and cost-sharing structures; shared financing; spending targets and other cost containment mechanisms; quality assurance programs; and the use of a "smart card" to gain access to a full range of services. (See Addendum I, "Summary of Proposed Changes in the Medicare Program, 1993.")

---

*Employers would be required to help pay for medical care coverage for workers and their nonworking dependents, and could discharge this responsibility by either paying a payroll tax to enroll them in the new Medicare program or by purchasing coverage for them privately. Any coverage provided privately would have to conform to, or exceed, the new Medicare program's standards. Employers would not be required to cover long-term care benefits, however.

Note: In order to facilitate a smooth transition to the proposed reformed health care system, it is intended that plan elements would be phased in over time. The details of the phase-in schedule have not yet been addressed.

I. Medical Care (i.e., Acute/Preventive/Transitional Care)

Coverage and Eligibility: All individuals would be eligible for coverage through a strengthened, improved, and expanded Medicare program. Employers would be required to help pay for acute/preventive/transitional care coverage for workers and their nonworking dependents by either paying a payroll tax to enroll them in the new Medicare program or purchasing coverage for them privately. Employers opting to purchase coverage privately would be required to pay at least 80 percent of the cost of coverage for these workers and their nonworking dependents. Additionally, the coverage purchased privately could not be less generous than that provided through the new Medicare program and would have to meet the same insurance, cost containment, and quality standards required of Medicare.

Benefits: Both the new Medicare program and all private, employer-based insurance plans would be required to provide coverage for a mandated, standard package of comprehensive acute, preventive, and transitional care benefits. This benefit package would consist of the current Medicare program's benefits, with added coverage for outpatient prescription drugs and prevention and screening services.

The standard benefit package would also cover screening and treatment for dental, vision, and hearing services/products for all children, as well as for all adults with incomes at or below 200 percent of poverty. All others would receive screening (but not treatment) coverage for these categories of care.

Individual/Family Premiums: Individuals and families enrolled in the new Medicare program would be responsible for a monthly premium that would replace the existing Medicare premium. The new premium could not exceed a specified percent of the community-rated, actuarial cost of coverage, adjusted by family size. Initially, the premium for an individual adult would be set at $50 per month ($600 per year) in 1993. Families with children would pay an additional $25 per month, regardless of the number of children.

Those covered by private, employer-based insurance would be responsible for up to 20 percent of the cost of the private insurance premium, depending on the employer's contribution. The premium schedule for private, employer-based coverage would also be based on family size.

Cost-sharing: Medicare's existing cost-sharing structure would be replaced with a new set of cost-sharing requirements that would apply to both public and private coverage. An annual plan deductible for medical care would be set at $200 for individuals and $400 for families. The standard copayment rate would be 10 percent, but there would be no copayment for inpatient hospital care, including inpatient psychiatric care, and hospice services. Prevention and screening services would be available to all without charge. Annual cost-sharing liability would be capped at $1500 for individuals and $3000 for families. Caps would be lower for, and thus provide greater protection to, those with annual incomes below 200% of the poverty threshold.

Low-income Protections: All persons with incomes at or below 200 percent of poverty, regardless of the source of their insurance coverage, would be eligible to apply for low-income protections against the cost of premiums, cost-sharing requirements, and taxes. Protections would take the form of sliding scale subsidies for those with incomes between 100 percent and 200 percent of the poverty level, and full subsidies for those with incomes below 100 percent of the poverty level.

Business Assistance/Small Group Insurance Reform: The proposal would offer an extra two-year phase-in period and temporary subsidies to (1) new businesses meeting certain payroll thresholds, and (2) existing businesses meeting the same payroll thresholds who have not offered employee coverage for at least a specified period of time. Additionally, the private, small group insurance market would be reformed to improve the availability and stability of coverage for small businesses. Pre-existing condition exclusions would be prohibited in all private insurance products.

Cost Containment: For the first time, the health care system would operate according to overall national and state spending targets that would be established by a federal body, the Federal Health Care Commission, but administered at the state level. Each state would be at risk for expenditures exceeding its spending target.

In addition, the new Medicare program would establish a rate-setting system for hospitals, physicians, and other major providers of health services/products. All payers for health services/products within the system, including the new Medicare program and private, employer-based insurance plans, would reimburse providers according to Medicare's payment methods and Medicare's rates. The net effect of setting provider reimbursement rates at Medicare levels in 1993 would be to reduce current average reimbursement rates by 5 percent. Balance billing by providers would be prohibited. Operating within the parameters established by the spending targets and reimbursement rules, states would retain sufficient administrative flexibility to address local needs.

The new Medicare program would also establish certain administrative rules and procedures that would simplify the entire system and reduce administrative costs, including: (1) a single, standardized, electronic system for claims processing and billing, and (2) standardization of insurance forms. All individuals would gain access to the system through the use of a standardized "smart card" that would allow for the tracking of individuals and families, as well as payments for services.

Additional cost containment strategies in the system would include the continued use of negotiated discounts with providers, organized delivery systems (e.g., HMOs and PPOs), utilization management, competition among providers and insurers, greater investment in outcomes research, and the development of clinical practice guidelines.

Quality of Care: An integral part of the reformed system would be a new, comprehensive, national quality assurance program. The program would be built around: (1) significant expansion of the scientific knowledge base in order to improve quality; (2) creation of a federally administered quality assurance system utilizing statewide quality assurance organizations; and (3) a comprehensive, national system of technology assessment.

The Health Care Delivery System:

(1) Organized Delivery Systems (ODSs): ODSs would be offered along with traditional insurance coverage in both the new Medicare program and the private sector. It is expected that as ODSs compete on the basis of price and quality of services, they would introduce innovative approaches to health care delivery.

(2) Public Health and Underserved Populations: The existing public health system would be focused and strengthened, particularly in its ability to carry out organized public health activities directed at community-level concerns and needs.

(3) Delivery System Reforms: A number of provisions -- primarily changes in local infrastructure such as provider supply and distribution -- would be aimed at remedying existing inequities in access to service by medically underserved populations in both rural and inner city locations.

(4) Health Promotion and Disease Prevention: Greater emphasis within the health care system would be placed on the potential benefits of health promotion and disease prevention activities. In general, this would be accomplished through the inclusion of a comprehensive set of preventive services in the standard benefits package and through enhanced health education and clinical outreach activities designed to address community-level concerns and needs.

(5) Public Outreach/Consumer Responsibility: Public education efforts, designed to give consumers the information they need in order to make responsible health-related decisions, would represent an important dimension of Health Care America. These efforts would include: national outreach campaigns (e.g., to educate individuals and families, especially those most likely to be uninformed, about their coverage); establishment of a National Center for Health Quality Information; and wide dissemination of information on quality and cost by the quality assurance system.

Malpractice Reform: The quality assurance component of Health Care America would include several provisions designed to address the serious problem of patient injury resulting from medical negligence, including: (1) the development and implementation of clinical practice guidelines; (2) a strong system of external review; (3) strengthening of internal quality assurance efforts; (4) improvements in current methods of provider accreditation and licensure; and (5) wider dissemination of provider performance data. In addition, Health Care America calls for the exploration and testing of promising alternatives to the existing system of professional tort liability, including a system of voluntary binding arbitration, mediation, and a "selective no-fault" system.

II. Long-term Care

Coverage and Eligibility: The goal of the long-term care program is to allow functionally and cognitively impaired persons of all ages to remain at home as long as possible, through the provision of a comprehensive range of home and community services that build upon the informal support of family and friends. The program also would cover nursing home care, when such care is required. These services would be provided through the new Medicare program.

Eligibility for long-term care benefits under the new Medicare program would be based solely on the need for care, not income, as determined by a Care Coordination Agency (CCA), a public or private non-profit organization that would be prohibited from having proprietary interests in the provision of services. No asset test would be required. Eligibility would be extended to individuals who need human assistance with two activities of daily living, as well as to those needing constant supervision, either because of cognitive impairment or behavior that is disruptive, dangerous, or difficult to manage. Children (under age 18) would be eligible if unable to perform an age-appropriate activity of daily living.

Benefits/Income Protections: The program would provide care in the home, in the community, or in a nursing home. The unmet long-term care needs of people living in the community would be covered under the proposal. Clients in the home and community would be responsible for a 20 percent copayment. Residents in nursing homes would receive coverage during the entire length of their nursing home stays. They would be responsible for a room and board copayment not to exceed 35 percent of the average cost of nursing home care.

All long-term care clients would benefit from certain financial protections: (1) copayment liability for both nursing home and home and community services would be limited; (2) nursing home residents would be allowed to keep a personal needs allowance of $100 per month, indexed to the general inflation rate (CPI); and (3) spouses and dependents in the community would receive protection against impoverishment.

<u>Administration</u>: The financing and service delivery system relating to long-term care would be fully integrated with the medical care component of the new Medicare program. The Federal Health Care Commission, charged with responsibility for recommending to the Congress national spending targets for medical care, would do the same for long-term care. As on the medical care side, the Commission would then derive individual long-term care spending targets for the states. The new Medicare program would determine reimbursement methods for various types of service providers, set national base reimbursement rates and maximum rates for providers, develop operational guidelines for states to follow relating to provider licensure and certification, promulgate standards for CCAs and care coordinators, and develop a uniform assessment tool. States would administer the program within these federal guidelines.

<u>Eligibility Assessment/Care Coordination</u>: States would certify and contract with CCAs to assess applicants' eligibility for services, collect financial information from people who seek income protection, and provide ongoing care coordination services. The CCAs would use a standard assessment tool to determine a person's level of impairment. The care coordinator would be responsible for authorizing and coordinating the mix of services necessary to address a client's unmet needs and for monitoring the quality and use of services. The client would be able to select both a care coordinator and providers of long-term care services.

<u>Cost Containment and Provider Reimbursement</u>: Cost containment features would include state spending targets, set at the national level, and the use of specified reimbursement methodologies for providers, again set by the federal government. States would retain some flexibility to develop alternative reimbursement methods for long-term care providers. States would be at risk for the costs exceeding state expenditure targets. CCAs also would operate within fixed budgets, based on the number of clients and their disability levels.

<u>Quality Assessment/Assurance</u>: The new Federal Health Care Quality Agency would develop regulations for assuring the quality of the assessment and care coordination functions of CCAs, nursing facility services, and home and community care. Quality Assurance Organizations (QAOs) at the state level would use federal standards to monitor CCAs' services to clients. QAOs would also run appeals procedures for CCA clients and maintain easily accessible public information about providers.

<u>Education and Research</u>: The government would play a major role in educating the public about long-term care benefits. The federal government would also fund or oversee research and demonstration projects that focus on such areas as cost containment, quality assurance, and service delivery.

III. Financing

Overview: Health Care America would be financed from five major sources: (1) existing federal revenues from Medicare, Medicaid, and other programs; (2) existing state spending; (3) an 8 percent payroll tax on employers electing to enroll their workers in the new Medicare program; (4) premiums paid by those enrolled in the new Medicare program; and (5) new taxes. It is estimated that the proposed health care system, including both medical care (i.e., acute/preventive/transitional care) and long-term coverage, would require approximately $112 billion in new federal tax revenues in 1993. Most of the new tax revenue would come from one (but not both) of two tax options which are discussed below:

1. New Tax Revenues

a. Income Tax Option: A 3 percent tax on income above $15,000 for singles and $20,000 for joint filers. Income would be defined as the sum of: adjusted gross income; gross Social Security benefits including all benefits not currently taxed; contributions to IRAs, 401K plans, and Keogh plans; and tax-exempt interest.

OR

Value-added Tax (VAT) Option: A 5 percent value-added tax, with exemptions for food, housing, and medical care.

b. Additional Tax Revenue Sources: Additional tax revenue would come from the following sources: (1) a 5 percent surtax on corporate income; (2) a doubling of the current tax rates on cigarettes and alcohol; and (3) raising of estate tax rates to their pre-1981 levels.

c. Tax Credits for Low-Income People: To reduce the burden of taxes and health care costs on low-income people, tax credits would be available for individuals filing tax returns. The credit would be refundable for those with no federal income tax liability.

2. State Contributions: Health Care America would capture and maintain most of the revenue currently raised by the states to finance their own health and long-term care expenditures, including state expenditures for the Medicaid program. State contributions would be adjusted annually for inflation and for differences in needs, capacity, and effort across states.

3. Trust Funds: All revenues would flow into a single trust fund designated as the Medicare Trust Fund, but the fund would have a number of separate accounts to allow for tracking (1) program income by source and (2) disbursements by beneficiary population and services category.

PRESIDENT CLINTON'S PLAN

Magaziner I. Memorandum for the First Lady, *et al.* Preliminary Work Plan for the Interagency Health Care Taskforce. Washington, D.C.; January 26, 1993. [The cover letter and page 1-12 of this memorandum are reprinted here.]

President Clinton. Clinton-Gore on Affordable, Quality Health Care. Little Rock: Clinton/Gore Campaign Headquarters; September 24, 1992. [campaign statement]

THE WHITE HOUSE

WASHINGTON

January 26, 1993

MEMORANDUM FOR THE FIRST LADY AND CHAIRPERSON, HEALTH CARE TASK FORCE
THE SECRETARY OF DEFENSE
THE SECRETARY OF THE TREASURY
THE SECRETARY OF COMMERCE
THE SECRETARY OF LABOR
THE SECRETARY FOR HEALTH AND HUMAN SERVICES
THE SECRETARY OF VETERANS AFFAIRS
DIRECTOR, OFFICE OF MANAGEMENT AND BUDGET
THE CHIEF OF STAFF
ASSISTANT TO THE PRESIDENT AND CHIEF OF STAFF FOR THE FIRST LADY
ASSISTANT TO THE PRESIDENT FOR DOMESTIC POLICY
ASSISTANT TO THE PRESIDENT FOR ECONOMIC POLICY
ASSISTANT TO THE PRESIDENT AND DIRECTOR OF COMMUNICATIONS
ASSISTANT TO THE PRESIDENT AND DIRECTOR FOR LEGISLATIVE AFFAIRS
ASSISTANT TO THE PRESIDENT AND DIRECTOR OF PUBLIC LIAISON
ASSISTANT TO THE PRESIDENT AND DIRECTOR FOR INTERGOVERNMENTAL AFFAIRS

FROM: IRA MAGAZINER
Senior Adviser for Policy Development

SUBJECT: Health Care Task Force

Attached is a draft work plan for the Health Care Task Force. Please review it and send your comments with your Task Force designee. The first meeting of the Task Force Working Group will be held on Wednesday, January 27, at 2:00 p.m. in Room 213 of the Old Executive Office Building.

Please designate someone as your official representative to this working group and ask them to attend the meeting. Your designee should be prepared to spend a significant portion of their time on this effort over the next 100 days.

Please also review the staffing chart (exhibit 3) of the draft work plan and identify people from within your department who can be assigned full-time to the Task Force for the next 100 days (longer for the outreach and coordination teams and for policy team leaders). We must fully staff up by early next week if we are to meet our schedule.

I know that you are all very busy and that some of you are still learning your departments. However, our schedule is very tight, as the President has committed publicly to the 100-day deadline for submitting comprehensive health care legislation.

We will phone you Tuesday afternoon or Wednesday morning to ask for the name of your designee.

We need your help to fulfill this commitment.

Attachment

PRELIMINARY WORK PLAN FOR THE INTERAGENCY HEALTH CARE TASKFORCE

BACKGROUND

The United States is in the midst of a health care crisis.

Health care costs are high and growing rapidly (14 percent of GDP in 1992, expected to reach at least 18 percent by 2000). Rising health care costs are placing a tremendous burden on individuals, businesses, and governments and are erasing gains in living standards.

Rising costs are also causing firms to drop or cut health care benefits and preventing people with pre-existing conditions or serious medical needs from getting insurance. At least 35 million people do not have insurance; many others have inadequate coverage; still others are at risk of losing coverage.

To meet the objectives of controlling costs and ensuring universal access, we must move immediately to restructure the nation's health care system.

The Campaign Health Care Plan

The health care plan outlined by President Clinton during his campaign contained the following principles for providing universal access to affordable, high quality health care for all Americans.

- A National Health Board would set a standard comprehensive benefits package for all Americans.

- All employers would be required to pay a percentage (perhaps 75-80 percent) of the cost of a standard plan for their employees and dependents. Hence most people would continue to have largely employer-financed coverage. The federal government would assist small companies in the early years so that this requirement would not cause undue hardship.

- State-based Health Insurance Purchasing Cooperatives (HIPCs) would manage competition among private health care plans on behalf of at least small businesses and individuals who lack negotiating clout. Businesses not included in HIPCs would negotiate with providers to offer the basic package directly to their employees, much as they do today.

- Specifically, these HIPCs would negotiate premiums, distribute information and marketing materials to consumers, and risk-adjust premiums to prevent adverse selection. Consumers would choose among these plans during an open enrollment period.

- The unemployed and other non-workers would be entitled to buy a plan on a subsidized basis through the HIPCs.

By building on our existing employer-based system, this scheme would minimize the disruption and public cost associated with expanded access. It favors consumer choice and private provider competition in allocating health services.

The plan (often described as managed competition with global budgets), would provide a new market structure within which competition could work to ensure efficient care delivery and control costs.

- Insurance reforms (standard benefits, no medical underwriting, community rates) would provide individuals freer choice of plans. HIPCs and large companies would drive tough bargains with insurers eager to sign up the consumers they represent.

- The reforms would stimulate competition on price and quality among insurers; prevent risk selection and encourage insurers to promote efficiency.

- Consumers would be given incentives to choose efficient plans. This could be done through mechanisms such as: requiring consumers buying more expensive plans to pay for added costs above a "benchmark" premium, rather than employers; or taxing these added payments if made by companies for employees.

- Insurers would be held responsible for controlling costs. They would likely replace uncontrolled fee-for-service systems with new payment mechanisms (e.g., capitated payments, salaried doctors). These systems would likely hold providers accountable for managing the volume and quality of care.

While this competition and consumer incentives would likely slow the growth of health costs, global budgets, enforced by the National Health Board, would guarantee results.

- Per capita state budgets would put a limit on HIPC spending, limiting premiums if competitive bidding falls short. The budgets also would limit premium costs outside HIPCs. The budgets would be set to bring health care inflation in line with overall economic growth over time.

- States where competition among plans is not possible or desired may regulate provider fees in order to meet the budget.

<u>Likely Criticisms</u>

Any comprehensive health reform plan will be controversial. Some criticisms would apply to any plan; others are specific to the type of managed competition with global budgets proposed by President Clinton. Criticisms are likely to center on the following arguments:

1. Cost containment would be ineffective and have perverse results.

   - Little evidence exists that managed care networks will produce efficiencies and thus deliver the cost containment we require; the result will be reliance on existing perverse behaviors (e.g., risk selection, claims denials) to meet global ceilings.

- Limiting spending on health care through global budgets will lead to service rationing, and interfere with quality improvements and consumers' traditional freedom to spend.

2. Universal coverage would involve redistribution of income and disrupt satisfactory arrangements for many Americans. The result would be to increase rather than reduce many Americans' costs of care.

- Community rating of insurance premiums would raise costs for currently insured populations who are young, male and healthy.

- "Recapture" or other taxes needed to apply private savings toward access would tax healthy currently insured people.

- Taxation of benefits above the nationally mandated package would put a burden on some working middle class families.

- Requirements to purchase coverage would lower disposable incomes for individuals who have gone without health insurance.

3. The plan would be cumbersome:

- Consumers would have to deal with new and unfamiliar agencies ("purchasing cooperatives") and choose from among plans they feel ill-equipped to evaluate.

- Unanticipated barriers to service would be erected when people are sick.

- Unanticipated financial obligations would be imposed on people who wanted to use providers not included in their plan.

4. Many small businesses may fiercely resist the proposal.

- Even with subsidies for low-wage or newly insuring employers, our plan would impose premium requirements that small business groups and other critics will challenge as:

  - A "payroll tax".

  - A threat to current jobs.

  - A threat to small business development and job creation.

In designing our reforms, we must take cognizance of these potential criticisms. We need to allow states flexibility to use alternative models that may make sense for them.

In developing the reform strategy, we will work closely with Congress and the health care community to ensure that we are effectively addressing their policy and political concerns.

This work plan is preliminary. It will be revised many times as we progress.

WORK MODULES

The goal of the interagency taskforce is to prepare comprehensive health care reform legislation in the next 100 days. This will require detailed policy work and a significant outreach effort. This preliminary work plan dimensions the work to be done.

POLICY ANALYSIS

There are at least seven areas of analysis necessary to form the comprehensive health care reform package.

1. Defining the structure for the new American health care system proposed in the campaign -- Managed Competition Within a Budget.

2. Planning the phase-in of guaranteed universal health insurance under the new system.

3. Defining options by which health care cost increases can be controlled during the next few years as the new system phases in.

4. Developing ways for the federal government to finance the new system, capturing private health care savings to cover universal access and possibly contribute to deficit reduction.

5. Devising programs to make short-term improvements in preventive care and in care for underserved populations.

6. Defining programs for improving long-term care.

7. Analyzing the economic impact of current health care policy versus our proposed policies.

1. Managed Competition Within a Budget

The model that President-elect Clinton has proposed for health care in the United States does not exist anywhere in practice. The campaign proposal, while sensible conceptually, needs significant definition. Some of the key questions which must be answered are:

- What constitutes a reasonable guaranteed benefits package? If the chosen package is too thin, a multi-tier health care system will develop based on income; if it is too comprehensive, cost increases may be difficult to control.

- How should budgets and the associated premium caps be set? Who should set them? How should they differ by state? Should there be different capitations based on the health status of individuals and how should they be determined? Should there be a reinsurance system and how should it work? How should rates of increase be determined from year to year?

- How should a state global budget be set and enforced? How can the plan discourage the evolution of an elite system which "busts the budget?" How should taxation for benefits above the guaranteed package be implemented?

- How will the state purchasing cooperatives work? Will certain companies be required to participate? Will Medicaid be folded in? Will individual choice of insurance plans be preserved through the HIPC?

- How will states monitor the solvency and reliability of insurers and enforce community rating? How will states guarantee competition while preventing "fly-by-night" insurers from adversely affecting consumers? How will states be sure that insurers are not finding new ways to compete through underwriting?

- How will quality of care be measured and improved? How will quality be ensured without burdensome micromanagement of health care processes? How can the system move towards meaningful outcome measurements? How can "best practice" information be collected and disseminated efficiently? How can we be sure that cost control does not lead to lower quality care?

- How will administrative savings be realized? How do we create universal quality and reimbursement forms? How do we create an efficient patient information system? How do we reconcile the desire of different health care insurers to control costs and utilization in their own way with the need for simplification of provider paperwork?

- How will the malpractice system work? What review mechanisms will be built into health networks themselves? Under what circumstances will lawsuits be tolerated? Will there be caps on awards? How will malpractice insurance be sold?

- What restrictions, if any, will be placed on the type of relationship which can exist between insurer and provider? Will providers be free to affiliate with multiple insurers? Will hospitals be permitted to deny use rights to physicians not participating in affiliated plans of that hospital?

- How will drug price increases be controlled? Will this be done nationally? How can we ensure that innovation is not stifled?

- Will states be permitted to fold their workers compensation health care systems into the new health care system? How would this work?

- How will the employer mandates be enforced? Will companies be required to cover part-time employees? What will happen to current retiree commitments? How will seasonal employees or employees on layoff be handled? Will individual insurance memberships be portable?

- To what extent will insurers be permitted to offer packages which differ from the nationally guaranteed package? If they can, how can complexity and its extra costs be avoided?

- How will the national and state boards be constituted? How can we assure that they will be representative bodies? How will their activities be limited by law? Do we envision the boards or legislatures or some other mechanisms as agents of system change?

- How much flexibility will states be given to operate systems other than managed competition as long as they stay within the global budget? Will a small state be allowed to operate a Canadian-style single payer model system if it chooses?

- Can doctors, hospitals and nursing homes opt out of the system entirely and work on a fee-for-service or own insurance basis and be free of spending caps? If so, then might we be creating an elite system for those who can afford to pay more? If not, then are we denying people basic freedoms?

- How will we ensure an adequate supply of primary care professionals for the new system?

- What will be the underlying ethical guidelines for the system? Will rationing be explicitly condoned or prohibited for certain tests and procedures? Will living wills or other similar mechanisms be required or encouraged? Will ethical review panels be required for provider or insurer groups, etc.

- How should the DOD and VA systems be integrated with the new national health care system?

These are only a small number of the key questions which will need answering about the new system we will be creating. The transition team has done a good job of exploring answers to some of these and other related questions, but a tremendous amount of work is yet to be done.

The issues raised by these question can be addressed by the following work modules:

- The Benefits Package
- Budgets and Caps and How they will function
- Insurance Reforms, Organization of the HIPC and state oversight of Health Networks
- Health Care Quality Assurance
- Administrative savings, Reimbursement Systems, and Patient Information Systems
- Malpractice Reform

- Drug Price Controls
- Organization of Employer Mandates and Subsidies to Employers
- Organization and Mandate for the National Board
- Ethical Guidelines for the System
- Integration of VA and DOD Health Care
- Health Care Workforce Development

2. Controlling System Cost Increases in the Short Run

Comprehensive reform of the health care system will require time to implement. However, the current upward trajectory for health care costs suggest that actions must be taken more quickly to control costs in order not to imperil economic progress.

There are no easy options. We must explore the options which do exist and draw up proposals to control the costs of health care while a new system is being instituted. The President may or may not choose to adopt such measures, but if he does, they should be part of the comprehensive bill.

Relatively little work has been done by the transition team on this topic. Some options which should be explored are:

- Various means to institute cost controls.
- Ways to extend Medicare rate regulation to private insurance systems or to institute some other form of all payer rate regulation.
- Ways to accelerate the move to managed competition within a budget.
- Ways to introduce global budgets or caps soon even if managed competition takes more time to phase-in.
- Ways to elicit voluntary controls from the health care industry.
- Ways to provide incentives for states and private entities to manage care more efficiently.
- Ways to use tax incentives or penalties to influence utilization and price of health care services.
- Other means not yet identified to control costs.

Any policy option we choose would likely be temporary, and so phase-in and phase-out mechanisms must be created for each option.

Each of these options is complex and will lead inevitably to a series of unintended consequences. Our analysis must explore detailed options for implementation to identify risks and to design "fall back" mechanisms as appropriate.

In addition to economic and cost analyses, we should conduct extensive legal and political analysis of each of these options since most will require regulatory legislation and congressional approval against fierce lobbying.

3. Phasing-in Universal Coverage

The transition team and most Democratic policy analysts associated with the campaign have done much work in this area. As a result, there is a comprehensive body of analysis upon which to build this part of our work.

Embedded in all of this work, however, are a series of assumptions which represent policy choices. Most access proposals include assumptions on increasing Medicaid reimbursement schedules, extending subsidies to people between 100 percent and 200 percent of the poverty level, subsidizing small companies as they begin covering their employees, etc. These must be decoded and separated into discrete pieces for proper decision making.

Access proposals also include crucial assumptions on cost and utilization of care by those now uninsured and underinsured and about how the insurance market will change as access is phased-in. These assumptions must be examined so that a range of possible cost outcomes can be projected and risk properly evaluated.

Cost savings realized from universal access should be calculated and weighed against the extra costs associated with greater utilization. These calculations can only be made in ranges, but we must understand the boundaries of potential impacts.

Finally, we should create a model which will allow us to analyze alternatives for phasing-in universal coverage with implications for population served, cost to the system, budget impacts for states and the federal government, demographics, demand for providers in under-served neighborhoods, etc.

Depending on definitions and program structure, universal access could mean $30 billion or $90 billion of additional annual expenditure by the government by 1997. Despite a good start, we have a great deal more work to do to choose our program design and schedule.

4. Federal Financing

As we design both the short- and long-term programs, we should develop options for recapturing some private sector savings for funding universal access and possibly for deficit reduction.

Most system savings under almost any set of policy options will be generated in the private sector. We must decide what level of recapture we want to affect. Then we must choose among a number of options on how to do it. Some possibilities are:

- Allowing insurance premiums to go up somewhat faster than intended and taxing the premiums.

- Raising a corporate tax to capture part of the savings corporations will realize from slower premium growth.

- Taxing benefit plans offering coverage above a certain level.

- Reducing uncompensated care payments.

- Instituting higher taxes on alcoholic beverages, tobacco products, pollutants, guns or other products which contribute to health problems.

- Creating a tax on non-critical service usage.

- About 20 other alternatives.

These recapture mechanisms are crucial to realizing positive effects from health care reform for the federal budget. They will be complex to design economically as they must be efficient and equitable.

They also will be hard to design politically. We will need to crate program designs which link private sector savings to the capture mechanisms and which link the capture mechanisms to funding of universal care. Methods of linkage will be part of the formulation of each option.

Finally, we will need CBO scoreable revenue estimates for each of the options we develop.

5. Short-term Improvements

There are many relatively inexpensive extensions of care which we can recommend to be implemented immediately. These will be both good health policy and will also assist us in designing a package with broad appeal.

Some possibilities include:

- Immunization programs.

- Enhanced funding for community health centers in disadvantaged communities.

- An AIDS program.

- More funds for women's health research.

- Increased assistance to pregnant women and young children now receiving inadequate care.

- Preventative health programs.

- A dozen others from campaign documents and reports of "think tanks."

We should create a detailed analysis of each measure which would include:

- Demonstration of need for the program.
- Population to be served.
- Precedent for the program, if any, in states, cities or other countries.
- Implementation mechanisms which maximize total program dollars spent for consumer benefit, not for administration.
- Total costs under a variety of program options.
- Likely supporters and opponents of the program.
- Those who will benefit and those who will be penalized by the program.
- Former legislative proposals which resemble the proposal.

We should follow a common format so that we can weigh the advisability and impact of each of these programs against one another, should we not be able to propose them all.

6. Long-term Care

While fully funding long-term care would be costly, a comprehensive health reform package without some provisions for addressing long-term care problems may be flawed economically, socially and politically.

We should research and present a series of long-term care options, some of which address full phase-in of long-term care insurance and others of which provide shorter-term, less expensive means of addressing problems now experienced by the frail elderly and disabled.

Some include:

- Establishment of a contributory insurance scheme for people to pre-fund long-term care. This could include tax incentives and/or mandates for individuals to contribute or raises in social security taxes or cuts in COLAs with diverted funds used entirely for long-term care, or a variety of other options.
- Increased access to home care as an alternative to nursing home and hospital care including waivers to allow funding for homemaker services.
- Increased funding for community senior centers to enhance their ability to provide health, transportation and food services for neighborhood elderly.

- Increased drug covrage under Med"are.

- The AARP, Gray Panthers and The Roosevelt Group have a number of other proposals on the table for enhancing long-term care. We should analyze them and prepare to include some in our deliberations, should the President choose to do so.

7. Economic Impact

Since any major health reform is almost by definition also a major economic program, we should analyze the economic effects of current policy as well as the effects of our recommended policies.

This analysis should include:

- A definition of the current impact of the health sector on the economy and anticipated impacts if current trends continue.

- An analysis regarding the transition issues as we move from the current situation to the one contemplated by the reforms. In particular, we should consider such issues as the nature and impact of efforts to reduce the rate of growth of health costs; and the form and significance of efforts to transfer cost savings. In general public policy has not considered transitional issues and effects with sufficient care. With a program this big, we should try.

- A definition of all the distributional tradeoffs that will occur so that we can answer "who is better off and worse off" questions that normally accompany budget or tax changes.

- A description of the economy that will result as a consequence of the reforms.

This analysis should include the effects of growing health care costs on GDP growth, personal income growth, wages, the cost levels of U.S. companies, corporate profits, etc. This analysis will also be useful for the public campaign the President might have to lead if one of the more active cost control options is followed.

Finally, as President Clinton asked, the analysis should include a comparative presentation of why U.S. costs are so much higher than costs of our major competitor nations. This will be useful both for our background planning and for the public campaign.

[SUBSEQUENT MATERIAL OMITTED]

Clinton • Gore on Affordable, Quality Health Care

We can't afford four more years without a president with a plan and the will to guarantee affordable, quality health care for every American. The American health care system costs too much and does not work. It leaves 60 million Americans without adequate health insurance and bankrupts our families, our businesses, and our federal budget. Instead of putting people first, Washington favors the insurance companies the drug companies, and the health care bureaucracies. They are strangling the most advanced health care system in the world.

And working Americans are paying the price. Since 1980, the average cost of individual health insurance rose from $1000 to $3000 a year. Today health care costs are the number one cause of labor disputes, bankruptcies, and growth in the federal deficit. People can't change jobs because insurance companies will deny them coverage because of "pre-existing conditions." Small businesses are caught between going broke and doing right by their employees. Working men and women are forced to pay more while their employers cover less.

Health care should be a right, not a privilege. And it can be. We are going to preserve what's best in our system: your family's right to choose who provides care and coverage, American innovation and technology, and the world's best private doctors and hospitals. But we will take on the bureaucracies and corportate interests to make health care accessible to every American.

The United States is the only advanced country in the world without a national health care plan. In the first year of a Clinton/Gore Administration, that will change. We will send a national health care plan to Congress, and we will fight to pass it. No American family should have to go from the doctor's office to the poorhouse.

The Clinton/Gore Plan

Cap national spending to control health care costs

Take on the insurance industry

Stop drug price gouging

Establish a core benefits package

Develop health networks

Guarantee universal coverage

Health care should be a right, not a privilege. And it can be: America has the potential to provide the world's best, most advanced and cost-effective health care. What we need are leaders willing to take on the insurance companies, the drug companies, and the health care bureaucracies and bring health care costs down.

Cap national spending to control health care costs

• Create a health standards board made up of consumers, providers, business, labor and government. The health standards board will establish an annual health budget for the nation to limit both public and private expenditures.
• Crack down on billing fraud and eliminate incentives that invite abuse.

Take on the insurance industry

• Ban underwriting practices that waste billions trying to discover which patients are bad risks; prohibit companies from denying coverage to individuals with pre-existing conditions.
• Protect small businesses through "community rating," which requires insurers to spread risks evenly among all companies.
• Shut down the "paper hospital" and replace expensive and complex financial forms and accounting procedures with a simplified, streamlined billing system with one claim form. Under the current system, 1,500 companies waste millions of dollars processing 1,500 sets of forms.
• Work to provide everyone with "smart cards" coded with personal medical information.

Stop drug price gouging

• Eliminate tax breaks for drug companies that raise their prices faster than Americans' incomes rise to protect American consumers and bring down prescription drug prices.
• Discourage drug companies from spending more on marketing than on research and development — because saving lives must come before making money.

Establish a core benefits package

• Through the health standards board, guarantee a basic health benefits package that includes ambulatory physician care, inpatient hospital care, prescription drugs, and basic mental health services. The package will also include expanded preventive treatments such as pre-natal care, mammograms, and routine health screenings.
• Allow consumers to choose where they receive care to ensure a better fit between provider strengths and consumer needs.
• Expand Medicare for elderly and disabled Americans to include more long-term care; place special emphasis on home- and community-based care, and make funding flexible so that those who need care can decide what serves them best.

America is the only advanced nation in the world without a national health plan. During the first year of my administration, we'll send a national health plan to Congress. We will make sure that every American has access to quality, affordable health care.

Develop health networks

• Give consumers access to a variety of local health networks — made up of insurers, hospitals, clinics and doctors — to end the costly duplication of services and encourage the shared use of key technologies.
• Allocate to networks a fixed amount of money for each consumer, the networks the necessary incentive to control costs.

Guarantee universal coverage

• Guarantee every American a core benefits package set by the health standards board either through their employer or by buying into a high-quality public program. No one will be cut off, cancelled, denied or forced to accept inferior care.
• Limit costs for small employers by allowing them to group together and form larger groups to purchase less costly health insurance, or to buy into the public program if it is the cheapest option.
• Phase in business responsibilities, covering employees through the public program until the transition is complete.
• Improve preventive and primary care through community-based health solutions. A successful health plan must provide all Americans with adequate access to health facilities. The Clinton/Gore plan will expand school-based clinics and community health centers in medically under-served areas.

THE RECORD

Giving children a healthier future

• Bill Clinton provided outspoken support for school-based health clinics. The state now funds 21 such clinics reaching thousands of Arkansas children who wouldn't otherwise have access to health care. Clinic services range from health screenings to immunizations to education.
• Increased Early Periodic Screenings, Diagnosis and Treatment (EPSDT) screenings by more than 2,000 percent.
• Helped reduce the Arkansas infant mortality rate by 43 percent. Arkansas' infant mortality rate dropped from 20 percent above the national average in 1978 to virtual parity in 1990.
• Introduced the Healthy Beginnings/Nurse Midwife Program to provide low-income women in East Arkansas with access to comprehensive maternity care.
• Established the "Good Beginnings" program, which took advantage of new federal regulations to provide basic health services to more low-income women and their children; Arkansas was the first state to launch such a program.
• Proposed and passed a "Health Care Access Law" designed, among other things, to provide universal health coverage for all Arkansas children under age 16, regardless of family income. The law emphasizes preventive and primary care.

• Senator Gore was the principal sponsor of the Infant Formula Act to improve nutrition and safety standards.

Providing better care and more choice for the elderly

• Bill Clinton established the ElderChoices program to allow the state Department of Human Services to give senior citizens alternatives to nursing home care — including personal and home health care, adult day-care services, and more — with funds formerly available only for nursing home care.
• Imposed strict regulations on nursing homes in his first term, before strict federal regulations were implemented, and has since strengthened these regulations.
• Initiated a broad range of cost-effective in-home health care and supportive services for people recovering from serious or chronic illnesses, or who require assistance with daily living activities, to avoid institutionalization.
• Increased funding for in-home services from $2.4 million in fiscal year 1981 to a budgeted $38 million for 1992-93.

• Senator Gore led the fight for the "Medigap" law to protect seniors from buying worthless insurance coverage.
• Sponsored a law establishing Alzheimer's treatment centers.
• Senator Gore was a leader in the fight to make generic drugs more available and reduce the cost of prescription drugs.

Responding to the AIDS crisis
• As chairman of the National Governors' Association, Governor Clinton formed the first working group of governors to develop an AIDS policy. Clinton was a moving force in the creation of an AIDS action plan adopted by the Governors' Association, which called for education and prevention efforts at the local, state and federal levels.
• Established the AIDS Advisory Committee for Arkansas, which makes recommendations on HIV policy and program services.
• Developed confidential AIDS testing in all 75 Arkansas counties.

• Al Gore supported funding for Ryan White AIDS programs, including research and education.
• Voted to provide emergency relief to metropolitan areas hardest hit by AIDS.
• Promoted development of a full range of services including in-home assistance such as chore services, personal care, home nursing care, and home delivered meals, and community-based services such as transportation, respite care, and friendly visiting.

Improving the health of all Americans
• Strengthened the Arkansas State Employees Health Insurance Program. Between 1982 and

1991, Arkansas' contribution increased by 335 percent while the state employees' premium for family coverage grew by only 89 percent. Because the program is self-insured, it does not pay premium taxes or produce a profit. Currently, for every $1 collected, 97 cents are paid in claims and only 3 cents in administrative fees. The $200 yearly deductible, 80/20 co-payment scheme and $5,000 Stop-Loss provision provide some of the best coverage in the nation to current and retired public employees.

• Proposed and passed a "bare bones" health insurance coverage program, which will allow employers who have not provided employee health insurance for the previous 12 months to offer a package without some services usually thought to increase costs for employers and employees.

• Developed key programs to improve rural health: the Rural Physician Recruitment and Retention Program encourages physicians to locate and practice family medicine in small Arkansas communities; Rural Medical Practice Student Loans and Scholarships provide support for medical students agreeing to practice in rural communities.

• Enacted a 1989 law requiring the Director of the Department of Health to establish and administer quality standards for X-ray facilities conducting mammography.

• Appointed Dr. Joycelyn Elders State Health Department Director. She has received the National Governors' Assocation Distinguished Service Award, the National Endowment of the Arts' Mary Futrell Award for Creative Leadership in Women's Rights, and the American Medical Association's Dr. Nathan Davis Award.

• In August 1992, Arkansas was one of twelve states which received funding as part of the Robert Wood Johnson Foundation's State Initiatives in Health Care Financing Reform Programs. Arkansas was chosen for its innovative approach to increase health insurance coverage to residents and to contain the escalating costs of health care.

• Senator Gore conducted hearings that led to the passage of the National Organ Transplant Act, which Gore also helped write. The Act established a national network to match organ donors and recipients.

•Led efforts to establish and expand the National Bone Marrow Donor Registry, which now lists more than 200,000 potential donors.

• Co-sponsored legislation to help strengthen rural hospitals.

• Wrote and steered to passage the Cigarette Labeling Act to require stronger warning labels on the health effects of smoking.

• Gore authored and helped enact into law the Trauma Core Revitalization Act, which makes grants to hospital trauma centers incurring substantial uncompensated costs in providing trauma care in areas with high rates of crime related drug trafficking.

STARK PLAN

U.S. House of Representatives. H.R. 200 - Health Care Cost Containment and Reform Act of 1993. Washington, D.C.; Committee on Ways and Means:1993. [Pages 1-18 are reprinted here.]

SUMMARY OF

THE HEALTH CARE COST CONTAINMENT AND REFORM ACT OF 1993

January 5, 1993

TITLE I: COST CONTAINMENT

Subtitle A.--National Health Budget

1. National Health Expenditure Budget

A national health expenditure budget would be set by statute for total national spending for health services in each year, beginning with 1995.

In general, the national health expenditures budget for each year would be based on the national health expenditure budget for the preceding year, increased by the sum of the five-year moving average of the annual rate of growth in the gross domestic product (GDP) plus an adjustment factor.

The national health expenditures budget would reduce the rate by which health spending growth exceeded the rate of growth in nominal GDP by one percentage point each year. Health spending growth would phase down to the rate of growth in GDP by 1999.

To achieve this result, health spending would equal the rate of growth in the GDP plus 3.7 percent in 1995, GDP plus 2.7 percent in 1996, GDP plus 1.7 percent in 1997, GDP plus 0.7 percent in 1998, and GDP plus 0 percent thereafter.

Under these growth limits, health care expenditures are estimated to stabilize at slightly more than 15% of the GDP in 1999.

Expenditures covered by the national health expenditures budget would include payments for health services from all payers, including direct patient out-of-pocket payments.

Other expenditures excluded from the budget would include: non-operating revenues for personal comfort items, research funds, facility and services of the Department of Veterans Affairs, the Department of Defense, and the Indian Health Service.

The national health expenditure budget would be divided into two sectors: a Medicare sector and a non-Medicare sector. Each sector would be subject to the same annual limits on growth.

2. Classes of Services within the Budget

The Medicare and non-Medicare national budget secotrs would each be divided into separate "classes" of services. The classes would initially be specified as: inpatient hospital services, outpatient hospital services, diagnostic services, physician services, home health services, rehabilitation services including physical and occupational therapy, durable medical equipment, prescription drugs, nursing facility services, and mental health services.

The Secretary would publish a proposed specification of the classes by April 1, 1994, and final specifications by July 1, 1994. Once established, the classes could be changed only by statute. The Secretary would periodically submit a report to Congress recommending changes in the classes.

ProPAC and PhysPRC would submit recommendations to Congress on the specifications of the classes, and on the Secretary's proposed classes.

3. Allocation of the Health Budgets by Class of Service

In general, the Medicare and non-Medicare national health expenditure budgets would annually be allocated to each class of health services in order to provide for the establishment of maximum payment rates for each type of service.

The initial allocation of the budgets to the classes would be based on the historic allocation of health care spending to each class, within each budget sector. The Secretary would establish and publish the initial allocations, but, except as specifically provided in this bill, could not subsequently change the allocations.

In order to determine the allocation by class of service, the Secretary, after determining the amount attributable to each class in each sector in the base year of 1993, would trend spending for each class to 1994, based upon the historic rate of growth within each class.

The resulting amount for each class would be compared to the sum of the estimated amounts for all classes within each sector, and the percentage of the sum attributable to each class would be determined. That percentage would then be applied to the Medicare and non-Medicare national health expenditure budgets respectively to determine the 1995 budget for each class.

In subsequent years, the allocation to each class and sector would be equal to the amount allocated during the preceding year, increased by the historic rate of growth for the class within each sector, expressed as a percentage of the sum of the resulting amounts for all classes. The percentages so determined would then be applied to the Medicare and non-Medicare national health expenditure budgets respectively for the year to determine the budget for each class for the year.

The trend factors used to allocate the national health expenditure budget would be estimated based on the historic rates of growth for each class over the five-year period ending with 1993.

ProPAC and PhysPRC annually would review and submit recommendations to the Congress on the allocation of health expenditures to the different classes of health services.

In determining the allocations of the Medicare and non-Medicare national health expenditure budgets and the trends in spending by class of service, the Secretary would compute and apply the budget allocations and historic growth trends separately to expenditures for services covered by Medicare and to all other expenditures.

4. Adjustments for Changes in Medicare Benefits

With respect to the changes in benefits under the Medicare program provided in Title IV of this bill, the Secretary would be permitted to change the Medicare and non-Medicare health expenditure budgets, allocations and trend factors to reflect the shift of the benefits from the non-Medicare to Medicare sectors of the national health expenditure budget.

5. National Health Expenditures Reporting System

The Secretary would establish a national health expenditure reporting system for the purposes of: establishing the national health expenditure budgets; allocating budgets among classes of services; determining maximum payment rates; and monitoring State provider payment control systems. Providers of health services, including health maintenance organizations would be required to report such information as the Secretary specifies in regulation. To the extent possible, the reporting system would use existing data systems.

Subtitle B.--State Provider Payment Control Systems

1. Establishment of State Programs

States could establish payment programs for hospital and/or for physician services or for all services. The maximum rates of payment established by the Secretary would not apply to providers in States with approved programs.

The State would be required to provide assurances to the Secretary that the expenditures for services covered under the State program would not exceed expenditures if the maximum payment rates applied in the State. The Secretary would be required to reply to an application of a State to operate a program within ninety days of receipt, or the program would be deemed to be approved. States currently operating a statewide hospital payment program under Medicare would be deemed to be approved under this provision for purposes of operating a hospital payment program.

2. Standards for State Programs

The State program would be required to cover all payers and provide for equitable treatment of payers, although payment differentials between Medicare, Medicaid, and private payers would be authorized. States could provide for negotiated rates for HMOs, but could specify minimum payment rates for all payers. The State program would be required to be operated directly by the State or by a public authority. The State would be required to assure that operation of the program would not impair access for those patients unable to pay, or pay the full amount, for services or for those patients expected to require unusually costly treatment.

3. Termination of State Programs

The Secretary could terminate a State program if, during a rolling three-year period, aggregate expenditures, or Medicare expenditures, for the types of services covered under the program exceeded the expenditures which would have occurred if the State program were not in effect. If the State program provided for negotiated rates for HMOs, expenditures associated with HMOs would not be taken into account.

To recoup any excess spending in the State, the Secretary could provide for continuation of the State program with a lower limit, or for a reduction in the Federal maximum payment rates in subsequent years.

4. Use of Medicare Savings

If the Secretary determined that a State program produced savings to the Medicare program over a period of three consecutive years, the Secretary would pay the savings attributable to the first year of that period to the State in the following year.

Subtitle C.--Maximum Payment Rates for Services Not Subject to State Provider Payment Control Systems or Provided by Staff or Group Model Health Maintenance Organizations

Part 1-Establishment and Application of Maximum Payment Rates

1. Exemption for Services Subject to Approved State Provider Payment Control Systems or Provided by Staff or Group Model Health Maintenance OrganizationsT

Services provided in States with approved State provider payment control systems would not be subject to either the maximum payment rates established under this Subtitle, or to the reductions in Medicare as provided under this Subtitle.

Services provided by group or staff model HMOs would also be exempt from the maximum payment rate system.

2. Process

The Secretary would set maximum payment rates for each type of health service for non-Medicare services at levels estimated not to exceed the share of the non-Medicare national health expenditure budget for the relevant class. Rates would generally be set using Medicare methods.

The maximum payment rates determined by the Secretary would not apply to providers in states with an approved State provider payment control system or to providers associated with staff and group model health maintenance organizations. The budget allocation for each class used in determining the maximum payment rates would be adjusted to reflect services provided within each class that are exempt from the system of maximum payment rates.

The maximum payment rates determined by the Secretary would be the maximum which providers could charge for services payable by insurers, other than Medicare, or by individuals. Providers could agree to accept less than the maximum payment rates, such as in the case of Preferred Provider Organizations (PPOs), but could not increase charges to make up any shortfall resulting from agreeing to accept amounts less than the maximum payment rates.

Civil money penalties equal to three times the excess amount charged would be imposed on providers who charged in excess of the maximum payment amounts.

Part 2-Methodologies for Determining Maximum Rates

1. Hospital Services

(a) General Rule for Hospital Payment. -- The maximum payment rates for inpatient hospital services would be determined based upon an average payment per admission adjusted for case mix using diagnosis-related groups (DRGs).

The Secretary would determine a standardized amount for non-Medicare patients which would be based upon current average payments made by private payers. This would produce an average payment set at approximately 125% of costs.

Rates would be set separately for hospitals in large urban areas and for all other hospitals. New DRGs would be developed as necessary for the under-65 population, and new weights would be developed for all DRGs to reflect different resource consumption patterns among this population.

In determining the standardized amount, the Secretary would include revenues associated with services provided on an outpatient basis during the three days immediately prior to a hospital admission if the services are related to the admission.

A standard hospital benefit package would be defined to facilitate DRG reimbursement. The Secretary would develop a table of adjustment factors to reflect the actuarial differences between the standard benefit package and other benefit packages.

(b) Adjustments to Hospital Payments. -- A series of adjustments would be made to the standardized amounts. Payment rates would be adjusted: (i) by geographic area for wages and for non-labor input prices; (ii) for the higher costs of teaching hospitals; (iii) for the costs of capital; and, (iv) for certain high-cost or long length-of-stay cases known as outliers.

Payment rates would be adjusted on a hospital-specific basis for the level of uncompensated care, and for the Medicaid payment level in a State.

Payments would also be adjusted for direct medical education costs based on the number of FTE residents. The adjustment would be based on a modification of the current Medicare methodology that would encourage training of primary care physicians.

Specifically, in determining the number of FTE residents under Medicare and for the purposes of determining the maximum payment rates, primary care residents in family practice, general internal medicine and general pediatrics would be counted as 1.1 FTE resident. Other non-primary care residents in internal medicine and pediatrics would be counted as 1.0 FTE. Other non-primary care residents would be counted as 0.9 FTE during their first 3 years of residency. Other non-primary care residents beyond the initial three years of training in any specialty would be counted as 0.8 FTE.

Positions in general internal medicine would be designated by the Secretary as meeting criteria set by regulations following application by a hospital.

(c) Exempt Hospital Payments. -- Hospitals currently exempt from the prospective payment system under Medicare would not be paid using the DRG-based payment method. These hospitals would be paid using a rate-of-increase limit until prospective methods were developed. In developing a prospective payment system for children's hospitals, the Secretary would be required to meet certain requirements.

2. Physician and Other Professional Medical Services

In general, the maximum payment rates would be determined using a resource-based relative value scale (RB RVS) for physician and other professional medical services following the methodology established under Medicare.

The Secretary would establish and publish new relative value units for services not currently covered under Medicare.

The maximum payment rates for services would be determined by establishing a maximum conversion factor which, when multiplied by the relative value units of services estimated to be provided, would result in expenditures equal to the proportion of the budget allocated to this class during the year.

The maximum payment rates would include allowed extra-billing, determined based on the limits applicable under Medicare. In addition, the maximum rates would be adjusted geographically in the same manner as physician services under Medicare.

3. Other Services

Maximum payment rates for other ambulatory services would be determined using the methodologies established for such services under Medicare.

(a) Outpatient Hospital and Other Services Reimbursed on a Cost-related Basis under Medicare.--Outpatient hospital fees and fees for other cost-related services under Medicare would be set by limits on a year to year basis, pending development of prospective payment systems.

(b) Clinical laboratories fees.--Maximum payment rates would be set using the Medicare laboratory fee schedule. All services covered by a third party payer would be directly billed to the insurer.

(c) Durable Medical Equipment.--Maximum rates for durable medical equipment would be set based on Medicare policies and rates.

(d) Prescription Drugs.--The methodology for establishing the maximum payment rates for prescription drugs would follow the methodology for limiting Medicare payment for prescription drugs (as provided in this bill.)

(e) Dialysis Services.--The methodology for establishing the maximum payment rates for renal dialysis and related services would follow the Medicare methodologies for payments for such services.

(f) Other Services.--The maximum payment rates for other services paid on a reasonable charge basis under Medicare would be based on the methodologies used in establishing such limits. Such limits could be based on prevailing charge limits or fee schedules, as provided under Medicare.

(f) Development of Prospective Payment Methodologies. --The Secretary would, within 3 years of enactment, develop prospective payment methodologies for setting maximum payment rates for services for which an appropriate methodology does not exist currently under Medicare.

4. Conforming Medicare Payment Rates to Medicare Health Expenditure Allocations

Rates under the Medicare program would be determined based upon existing provisions of Medicare law and would be reduced as needed to assure that Medicare payments to providers conform to the Medicare national health expenditure budget.

TITLE II. MANAGED CARE AND MANAGED COMPETITION

Subtitle A.--Managed Care

1. Authorization for Health Care Plans to Pay Less Than Maximum Payment Rates

All health care plans would be free to negotiate rates below those set under the maximum payment rates

2. Staff and Group Model HMOs Exempted from Maximum Payment Rates

Qualified staff and group model HMOs would not be required to pay for services using the maximum payment rates. The overall budget and other payment policies would take expenditures by qualified HMOs into account but rates would not apply to these plans.

Qualified staff and group model HMOs would be those plans with a contract with Medicare under section 1876 of the Social Security Act or a qualified HMO under Title XIII of the Public Health Service Act for which ninety percent of the services are provided through members of the staff of the organization or through a medical group or groups.

3. Assistance for Establishment and Initial Operation of Staff and Group Model HMOs

$25 million in grants would be made available as grants to support the development and initial operation of staff and group model HMOs. Grants could be used for market surveys, initial enrollment activities, working capital, physician recruitment, and acquisition of buildings and equipment

4. Incentives for Expansion of Qualified HMOs

Mandatory "dual choice" requirements would be retained and expanded to "multiple choice." If requested by an HMO serving an area, an employer would be required to make the HMO available to employees as an option under the employer's health benefits, if any. Marketing materials for qualified HMOs would be provided to every employee of every company in the service area.

5 Preemption of State laws

State laws that mandate that any "willing provider" be allowed to participate in qualified HMOs would be pre-empted. This would allow network and other plans to enroll only those providers willing to manage health resources according to the plan of the HMO.

6. Increase in Payments to Medicare HMOs

Medicare payments to risk contract HMOs would be adjusted for the lack of enrollment in HMOs of beneficiaries where Medicare is the secondary payer.

7. GAO Study on HMO expansion

GAO would study and recommend additional measures to encourage the development and expansion of qualified HMOs.

Subtitle B.--Managed Competition

1. Establishment of Health Plan Purchasing Cooperatives

Health Plan Purchasing Cooperatives (HPPCs) would be established in each State for each HPPC area. Grants would be available to States to assist in the planning, development, and initial operation of HPPCs. The grant period could not exceed five years and total amount of assistance could not exceed $5 million. $150 million would be authorized for the five-year period beginning with 1994.

Each HPPC would be established pursuant to a specific State law authorizing its organization and operation. Each HPPC would be a not-for-profit public benefit corporation with its board appointed by the Governor of the State, pursuant to the State's Administrative Procedure Act.

States could provide for division of the State into more than one HPPC area so long as all portions of each Metropolitan Statistical Area (MSA) in a State were within the same HPPC area, and every portion of the State was within a HPPC area. One or more contiguous States could provide for the establishment of an interstate HPPC area, provided that the interstate HPPC included all portions of an MSA. If a State did not establish a HPPC for an area, the Secretary could establish a HPPC in that area.

2. Responsibilities of Health Plan Purchasing Cooperatives

HPPCs would have the following responsibilities: (i) to enter into agreements with qualified Health Maintenance Organizations (HMOs) and other qualified health plans that provide services in the HPPC area; (ii) to enter into agreements with employers in the HPPC area to provide comparable health insurance benefits to employees of participating employers; (iii) to enroll employees of participating employers with qualified health plans; (iv) to provide information to each employee of participating employers regarding health benefits available from each qualified health plan; (v) to enroll individuals purchasing health coverage directly on behalf of themselves or their immediate family; (vi) to receive and forward premiums; and (vii) to provide for coordination with other HPPCs. Participation in a HPPC by employers and employees would be voluntary.

Within one year after its establishment, a HPPC would be required to inventory and to inform all small employers in the HPPC area, including employers in rural areas, of the health benefits available through the HPPC. Small employers would be those with 100 employees or less. The HPPC could provide benefits to other employers and directly to individuals, at the option of the HPPC.

3. Operation of HPPCs

Health plans provided through HPPCs would generally be qualified HMOs providing services in the HPPC area. The Secretary could qualify other types of plans of they met additional standards relating to physician incentives payments, living wills, and beneficiary grievance procedures. Each such qualified health plan would meet the insurance standards established under this bill.

Each health plan would provide for an open enrollment process for employees of participating employers and other for individuals. HPPCs could impose a minimum participation requirement regarding the percentage of employees who receive health benefits on participating employers.

4. HPPC Core Benefit Packages

Each health plan would be required to provide a core benefit package that meets defined national standards. In addition a health plan could make available incremental benefit packages, but would be required to price such benefit packages separately from the core benefit package.

The core group of benefits would generally follow Medicare benefits. Benefits would include unlimited inpatient hospital coverage without spell-of-illness restrictions, outpatient hospital services, physician services, clinical laboratory and radiology, and other services with a single deductible of $300 per individual/$600 per family and an out-of-pocket limit of $2,500 per individual and $3,000 per family; and maternity, well-child and prevention benefits without cost-sharing.

The core benefit packages would not be required to include benefits or services mandated by States in addition to the benefits included in the core benefit package.

In the case of HMOs, nominal copayments and deductibles for benefits would be consistent with those specified pursuant to Title XIII of the Public Health Service Act.

5. HPPC Agreements with Employers

HPPCs would enter into agreements with participating employers to provide health insurance benefits to employees. Agreements would provide for payment by employers of the HPPC premiums for the core benefit package plus any additional incremental benefits for which the employer has chosen to be responsible. Participation in a HPPC by employers would be voluntary.

The employer would provide the HPPC with the names, names of dependents, addresses, and other identifying information required by the HPPC, for each employee, including part-time and seasonal employees.

6. Premiums for HPPC Health Plans

HPPCs would receive payments from employers and individuals participating in the HPPC. The payments would, in the case of employers, be the community-rated group premium, or in the case of individuals, be the community-rated individual premium, of each HMO or other qualified health plan in the HPPC area. An additional amount would be added in each case to the annual premium as a standard percentage overhead charge to provide revenues equal to the annual budget for the HPPC. The overhead percentage could not exceed five percentage points.

Each HPPC would make available to employers participating in the HPPC, and each such employer would make available to employees, information in comparative form on the benefits provided by HMOs and on outcomes and enrollee satisfaction for each plan based on information contained in the annual outcomes and enrollee satisfaction report described below.

Each HPPC would coordinate its activities with other HPPCs. Each HPPC would provide information about HMOs providing services in its area to other HPPCs which request the information. HPPCs would provide health benefits to employees who reside in the HPPC area but whose employer's place of business is outside of the area. Such services would be provided in coordination with the HPPC for the area in which the principal place of business of the employer is located

Subtitle C.--National Patient Outcomes and Enrollee Satisfaction Reporting Program

1. National patient outcomes program

The Secretary would establish a national patient outcomes data base. In order to collect uniform information on outcomes, the Secretary would define tbe data to be collected and establish reporting requirements for the routine collection of such data. All HMOs, other health benefit plans and providers would begin reporting such data by January 1, 1996.

The Secretary would publish and distribute an annual report on patient outcomes, including data on individual providers.

2 Enrollee satisfaction with health plans

The Secretary would establish a national data base on enrollee satisfaction with health benefit plans, including self-insured plans.

The Secretary would develop and publish a standard enrollee satisfaction survey instrument to be used by health plans. By January 1, 1996, all health plans would report data on enrollee satisfaction to the Secretary on an annual basis.

The Secretary would publish and distribute an annual report on enrollee satisfaction with health plans.

3. Research and demonstrations

The Secretary would provide for research and demonstration projects concerning new methods for collecting and analyzing outcome and enrollee satisfaction data, and the use of outcomes information systems by health maintenance organizations, health benefit plans, and providers of health care services. The Secretary may also provide for research and demonstration projects concerning the collection and analysis of indicators of system performannce, including health status of communities served, prevention of illness, and capacity of delivery systems with respect to integrated health care delivery systems. The bill provides for an authorization of $20 million annually for fiscal years 1994 through 1998.

Subtitle D.--Study of Universal Health Insurance Coverage

1. Study

A study of the costs and benefits of universal health insurance coverage and cost containment would (i) analyze options for establishing universal coverage and (ii) assess the effectiveness of alternative strategies for controlling costs under such plans. The study would be conducted by the Congressional Budget Office with assistance from the staff of the Joint Committee on Taxation. The CBO would submit a report by January 1, 1994 to the Committees on Ways and Means and on Energy and Commerce of the House and the Committee on Finance of the Senate.

TITLE III. HEALTH SYSTEM REFORMS

Subtitle A.--Health Insurance Reform

1. Anti-discrimination and Anti-Job Lock Requirements

(a) Anti-discrimination Requirements.--Health insurance for all employer groups, including self-insured groups, could not deny coverage to any eligible group or individual member of an eligible group based on health status, claims experience, receipt of health care, medical history, or lack of evidence of insurability or medical condition. The same requirement would apply to insurance offered to individuals.

For insurance offered through Taft-Hartley Trusts, the plan could restrict membership to those eligible under the terms of the Trust, but could not deny coverage to any person otherwise eligible.

Health insurance premiums paid by members of employer groups could not be adjusted for an individual's medical status.

(b) Anti-job-lock and Pre-existing Conditions.--Any worker changing jobs with less than a three-month break in insurance coverage, including coverage under COBRA, could not have a new exclusion period applied. Pre-existing condition exclusions would otherwise be limited to six months. Pre-existing conditions limits could not be applied to new-borns.

2. Requirements for Insured Health Plans

(a) Open-enrollment.--Health insurers, other than self-insured groups and Taft-Hartley Trusts, would be required to provide year-round open enrollment for groups and individuals.

Insurers offering coverage through an association or multiple employer arrangement could restrict membership in that plan to the members of the association or arrangement. To qualify for this restriction, the association or arrangement would have to be formed for a purpose other than the purchase of health insurance.

Health Maintenance Organizations would be required to offer open enrollment, but only up to the capacity of the plan to absorb new members.

(b) Guaranteed Renewability of Coverage.--Insurers would be required to guarantee renewability of coverage, and could only refuse to renew coverage due to nonpayment of premiums and to fraud. Plans would be required to provide notice of the terms of renewal at least thirty days prior to the expiration of the plan, and could not charge higher renewal rates. Plans would be required to provide coverage for twelve-month periods.

(c) Community Rating.--Health insurers would be required to set family and individual premiums for coverage purchased by employer groups based upon community rates. Insurers would also be required to set premiums for insurance purchased directly by individuals on a community basis, but individual rates could be set differently from group rates. The limits on community rating would be phased in over three years in equal increments. For purposes of this provision, a community could be no smaller than a Metropolitan Statistical Area (MSA).

(d) Payment of Commissions.--A plan could not pay premiums to agents based upon the claims experience of a group.

3. Limits on Self-insurance.

(a) Limits on Small Employer Self-insurance. -- The bill would provide that employers with 100 full-time employees or less would be prohibited from self-insuring.

(b) Limits on MEWAs. -- Multiple Employer Welfare Arrangements (MEWAs) and similar multiple employer plans would be prohibited from self-insuring. Such groups could provide health insurance, but only to the extent that the plans met all applicable standards as health insurers in each State.

4. Continuation Coverage Offered by Universities.

The bill would pre-empt State laws that prohibit universities from offering graduating students health insurance.

5. Enforcement

(a) Federal standards. -- The standards would be established in regulations by the Secretary of Health and Human Services (HHS), and enforced by HHS with sanctions applied by the Department of the Treasury, based upon determinations of the Secretary of HHS.

(b) State certification. -- The Secretary of HHS could delegate authority to State governments meeting Federal standards to certify and supervise these requirements, although sanction authority would remain with the Federal government.

(c) Sanctions. -- The sanctions would be Federal excise taxes which would be imposed on insurers and employers (in the case of self-insured plans) which violate the standards. The excise tax would not be otherwise tax deductible.

[SUBSEQUENT MATERIAL OMITTED]

SHORTELL PLAN

Shortell SM. (1992). A Model for State Health Care Reform. *Health Affairs.* 11:108-125.

A MODEL FOR STATE HEALTH CARE REFORM

by Stephen M. Shortell

Prologue: *One of the major challenges facing U.S. health system reformers is finding a way to repair the shortcomings of the system while maintaining the cherished American values of autonomy, pluralism, and choice. For this reason, many believe that looking to health systems such as Canada's or Great Britain's—which reflect the centralized nature of their respective governments—as models for reform has only limited usefulness. Our population is vast and diverse; we value individual over collective endeavor; and we prefer local problem solving to federal mandates. Any health system reforms that are to succeed must accommodate these unique aspects of American culture and politics. In this paper, Stephen Shortell proposes an approach to health system reform built on these assumptions. His model, called health promotion and accountability regions (HPARs), are, in his words, "common incentive structures for managing population-based care." The HPARs, organized as public/private partnerships at the state level, "serve as an organizational cornerstone around which health care reform might be implemented," he explains. The model includes both basic benefit packages and financing options, linking the functions of planning, insurance, payment, delivery, and evaluation. Shortell is the A.C. Buehler Distinguished Professor of Health Services Management and professor of organization behavior in the Department of Organization Behavior of Northwestern University's J.L. Kellogg Graduate School of Management in Evanston, Illinois, where he is also a member of the Center for Health Services and Policy Research. He holds a doctoral degree in the behavioral sciences from the University of Chicago. Shortell is senior author of the award-winning book* Strategic Choices for America's Hospitals: Managing Change in Turbulent Times *and is a member of the National Academy of Sciences' Institute of Medicine.*

The United States differs fundamentally from such countries as Great Britain and Canada in its preference for a greater degree of autonomy, choice, and pluralism in all domestic matters. This is accentuated by a diverse population scattered across fifty states. Americans generally favor local problem solving and control over federally mandated approaches, even though local approaches are not always more effective. Thus, health care reform that features a prominent role for the federal government is not likely to be Americans' first choice; we are likely to make better progress by focusing on reforms at the state and local levels, where health care is actually delivered.[1]

Toward this end, I outline here an approach for state health care reform, upon which subsequent federal initiatives might be structured. It is intended as a prototype and framework to guide current efforts rather than as an idea that can be readily implemented as proposed. The concept can be adapted to fit local situations and circumstances. The central notion involves the creation of state health authorities called "health promotion and accountability regions," or HPARs. HPARs are common incentive structures for managing population-based care. Key aspects of the concept include population-based health status needs assessment; an established set of benefits; a global budget; multiple payers but a single paymaster or "funnel;" negotiated contracts with integrated insurer/ provider delivery organizations (health plans); and payment based on both clinical and fiscal accountability.

Key features of the HPARs are as follows: (1) The HPARs are created by state legislatures to serve as the focus for the development and implementation of health policy for the state. More populous states would likely have several HPARs or sub-HPARs within them.

(2) HPARs would be governed by a board composed of around twenty members with at least two representatives from each of the following groups: hospitals, physicians, insurers, employers, labor, government, and consumers. Each group would submit a list of qualified nominees who would then be appointed by the state department of health (or equivalent governmental entity). Additional representatives might be drawn from nursing, other health professional groups, long-term care providers, and others as determined by each HPAR. Each HPAR would have the option of forming additional consumer/citizen advisory panels as deemed useful.

(3) Each HPAR would be run by an executive director assisted by a technical staff trained in clinical epidemiology, statistics, planning and evaluation, and relevant social science disciplines. The executive director would report directly to the HPAR board.

(4) The main responsibilities of the HPARs would be to set health care policy for the region; establish health care goals and specific targets

to be achieved based on an established health benefit package and epidemiological assessment of the health care needs of the population; determine the premiums, resources, and associated budget required to meet those needs; enter into a series of negotiated contracts with health plans to deliver care; and monitor and hold the health plans accountable, according to predetermined clinical and fiscal performance criteria.

(5) Operating within the HPAR's overall policies and goals, each health plan (insurer/provider entity) would be free to develop its own innovative approaches for delivering cost-effective, high-quality care to its enrollees. Health plans would compete with each other for contracts based on the value (cost/quality) each plan can provide.

HPARs emphasize the development of health care budgets based on a health benefit package and the needs of populations served. All relevant parties contribute to the design of the benefit package, needs assessment, and budget determination. Trade-offs must be made and priorities established in advance. The result is the development of shared incentives for all parties to keep people healthy and to provide the most cost-effective care when needed. Incentives are created for hospitals, physicians, other providers, and insurers to form health plans that negotiate contracts with HPARs to care for defined population groups.

Elaborating The Basic Features

HPARs are organized as public/private partnerships at the state level for purposes of linking planning, insurance, payment, delivery, and evaluation responsibilities. They would be responsible for seeing that health services are delivered to people in a defined geographic region and represent a forum for structuring discussion and negotiation among all of the relevant stakeholders. In this respect, they would be similar to the German sickness funds, which negotiate with regional provider units, and to the concept of regional payer/provider groups.[2] HPARs would extend these approaches, however, in regard to planning and accountability features related to the allocation of resources based on the population's health care needs, established benefits, and payment of providers based on value-added performance criteria (Exhibit 1).

The process begins with a needs assessment of the population, which, along with citizens' preferences, helps to determine the benefit package. The needs assessment is based on experience, current data, and selective new data collection.[3] It is important that the benefit package be comprehensive enough to meet the needs of the majority of the region's population both for reasons of equity and to assure that the incentives for providing cost-effective care under a global budget work.[4] In most states, the benefit package would include inpatient and outpatient hospital

Exhibit 1
The Health Promotion And Accountability Region (HPAR) Model

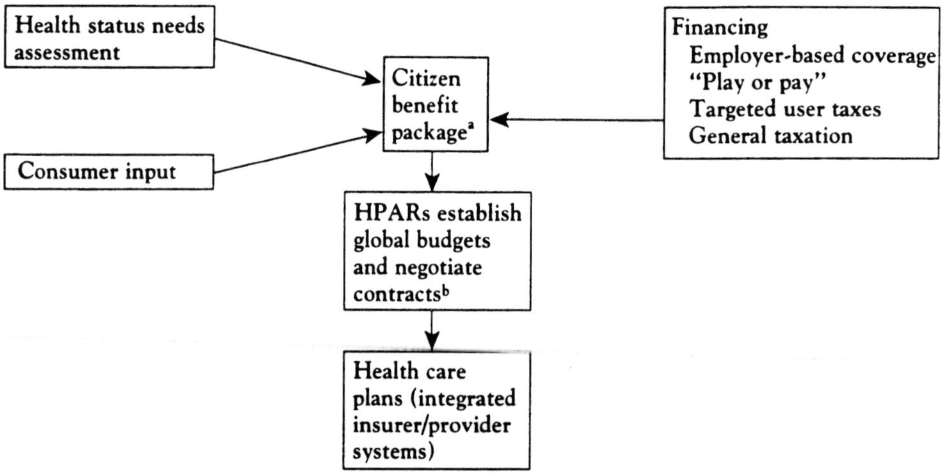

[a] Under federal legislation, this could become a basic health plan for all Americans.
[b] Under federal legislation, the federal government would be responsible for legislation directing the states to create HPARs for the administration of the basic health plan for all Americans and for encouraging use of the HPAR to organize all health care services in a state or given area.

care, emergency treatment, physician services, preventive diagnostic and screening services, prenatal and well-baby care, and perhaps selected mental health, dental, and vision care. Provision would also be made for home, nursing home, and related long-term care services.

The benefit package would have multiple sources of financing but would be anchored to the tradition of employer-based insurance. As in several current recommendations, employers would be required to provide health insurance coverage or contribute to a public plan. Copayments, deductibles, and premium-sharing arrangements would be income-related, based on a sliding scale, with out-of-pocket limits in the neighborhood of $2,500 to $3,500 per family per year. Tax incentives and coalitions would help small employers to participate in this "play-or-pay" approach. Citizens not covered through their employer would be covered through the state health plan with revenues derived from employees selecting the "pay" approach; from targeted user taxes (for example, alcohol and cigarettes); and from general tax revenues as needed.[5] It is important to note that the benefit package would be identical whether one receives benefits through an employer or through the state.

Based on the needs assessment, the benefit package, and its own cultural values, each HPAR would develop a mission statement and health plan for its region and translate these into annual operating goals and objectives. The emphasis would be on promoting the health of the population served and not solely on the treatment of illness—hence the term *health promotion and accountability region*.[6] Based on the data, the HPARs would establish premiums for the benefit package and the overall level of resources required to meet assessed needs. While the benefit package would remain the same for everyone, several different premium levels could be established for different population subgroups based on their health status. Groups with greater needs would have higher premium levels. This then would become the region's health care budget for the year and would represent a locally determined expenditure cap reflecting the region's mission and health care objectives.

All insurers doing business within the state would be required to offer the benefit package at or below the established premium with recommended provisions for income-related copayments, deductibles, and premium sharing, as previously noted. Since the premiums would already be risk-rated according to the needs of the population, there would be no need for insurers or plans to exclude the less healthy or otherwise avoid risk based on consumers' health status.[7] Since all insurers would be offering the same benefits for essentially the same premiums, their financial success would depend on their ability to control costs. This, in turn, would create incentives for insurers to join with organized delivery systems to form integrated health plans. Each HPAR would control the premium dollars flowing to it from the various payment sources.

Operating within this overall budget, the HPARs would then negotiate contracts with each health plan for those segments of the population the plan chooses to serve. Premiums based on health status and benefits would constitute capitated managed care accounts that might be thought of as "health fund" (as opposed to the German "sickness fund") arrangements between the HPARs and the health plans. HPARs would also be free to contract directly with certain specialized facilities and providers that may not be part of a regionally integrated insurer/provider entity or that may operate across geographic market boundaries.

To reduce the administrative costs associated with multiple health care plans, all plans would be asked to adopt a common claims processing and billing system and use common language in explaining benefits to potential enrollees. The health care plans that delivered services within their defined budgets would be rewarded by being allowed to keep a significant percentage of the savings (for example, 50–75 percent) and would position themselves as "preferred providers" in the following year's negotiations.[8] To balance the incentives for fiscal responsibility, each HPAR would also establish criteria for clinical accountability based on the growing body of research on patient outcomes, clinical practice guidelines, patient satisfaction, and continuous quality improvement approaches. Payment thus would be based not only on financial performance but also on the quality of care provided and outcomes achieved.

The HPARs would also play an important role in disseminating health promotion information to the public, along with feedback on health plan performance. The individual health plans, of course, would have additional incentives to share such information as part of their interest in maintaining and expanding their enrollee base.

Each of the major interest groups (hospitals, physicians, insurers, government, business, labor, consumers, and others) would be represented on the HPAR boards and thus would have a say in the overall policy-setting process. Each also would have a specific role to play. Hospitals, physicians, and insurers would have incentives to form health plans and develop proposals for HPAR funding. They also would have a role in assuring that quality standards were met and that efforts were made to continuously improve quality. The employer's role, in addition to participation in the play-or-pay financing approach, would be to provide feedback to the health care plans regarding enrollees' experience. A similar role would exist for consumers and unions from their perspectives as individual and collective recipients of care.

Local initiative and collaboration. A major challenge is the extent to which states have the necessary leadership, commitment, and expertise to make HPARs work. Encouragement can be taken from examples such as the Rochester (New York) Area Hospital Corporation, Michigan's interest in creating integrated regional health care delivery systems, and the development of models in California for increasing access while assuring greater accountability.[9] In Rochester, leadership from the business community (chiefly, Eastman Kodak and IBM), combined with leadership from the Blue Cross/Blue Shield Association and local hospitals, has resulted in several experiments in providing more cost-effective care. In Michigan, the Greater Detroit Area Health Council developed a plan based on integrated regional health systems providing care to defined service areas. In California, a Blue Ribbon Committee of the California Association of Hospitals and Health Systems developed a proposal featuring (1) establishment of a basic health care benefit package funded from multiple sources; (2) creation of a statewide Health Care Commission to negotiate and monitor contracts with health plans and oversee the health care trust fund; and (3) initiation of reforms in health insurance underwriting to accept all groups with guaranteed renewal unless the health plan demonstrates a lack of delivery capacity. The California proposal as yet lacks sufficient consensus to proceed, but momentum continues to build.[10]

Opportunities to incorporate HPAR features into states with all-payer models (such as in New Jersey and Maryland) also exist. Nonetheless, lack of leadership by major interest groups represents a major challenge. For example, Illinois's recent effort to create a more accountable and coordinated delivery system involving the city, county, and state governments faltered due to lack of concerted political leadership.[11] In Massachusetts, downturns in the state's economy along with transitions in state leadership threaten proposed reforms. In many areas of the country, the situation may need to get worse before the private and public sectors are moved to explore creative cooperative approaches.

Decentralized fiscal accountability. Many are opposed to expenditure caps or global budgets because they fear that the needs and preferences of local citizens will not be taken into account; that economic concerns will dominate over quality concerns; and that the autonomy of health professional interest groups will be curtailed. A major feature of the HPAR concept is the determination of local needs and preferences initially based on use of sociodemographic data and past utilization and supplemented over time by the growing body of research on patient outcomes and patient satisfaction and by the development of clinical practice guidelines. The actuarial experience of Blue Cross/Blue Shield, other insurance carriers, and existing integrated insurance/delivery organizations such as Kaiser Permanente can be drawn on in this process.[12] Nonetheless, because the task of linking resources to needs is complex, a mechanism is needed for reinsurance to cover unanticipated events such as natural disasters or underestimates of utilization. One approach would be the development of medical/reinsurance futures contracts, which would allow each HPAR the opportunity to hedge its underestimates.[13]

Provisions must also be made for portability of benefits across states. The benefit/premium package one receives at the beginning of the year would serve as the standard for that year. Year-end adjustment or "settlement of accounts" (similar to Blue Cross/Blue Shield's interplan bank) could be established, in which HPARs would pay each other for services used by those who are members of their population at the beginning of the year but who relocate and use services in another region.[14]

The defined areawide health budgets provide the context for totally "managing" care. As John Wennberg has noted, "The key to the preservation of fee-for-service markets . . . is not the micro-management of the doctor-patient relationship but the management of capacity and budgets."[15] The approach also addresses the concerns of corporate executives such as Bill Ferguson of NYNEX: "If managed care is going to work, . . . it will have to be used by everyone, everywhere. Otherwise, provider costs will merely be passed over and around the managed plans."[16]

The HPAR concept also supports the Health Insurance Association of America's (HIAA's) judgment that "cost containment cannot be achieved if the delivery and financing system places no constraints on providers or consumers, and imposes no penalty for unnecessarily costly use of medical resources, and provides no rewards for making efficient choices."[17] HIAA advocates managed care delivery systems that retain elements of privately based insurance that encourage innovation and promote flexibility—principles inherent in the HPAR concept.

Clinical accountability. Proposals based primarily on cost containment criteria are no longer politically acceptable.[18] Equal if not greater emphasis must be given to the quality of services provided, to patient outcomes achieved, and to the health status of the population. Incentives must be established and performance rewarded for the delivery of services that take into account both economic/efficiency criteria and clinical accountability/health promotion criteria.

This ability to hold health plans clinically accountable is a major feature of the HPAR concept. While major knowledge gaps remain, it is becoming increasingly possible to assess patient treatment outcomes using functional health status, patient satisfaction, and related measures. The application of continuous quality improvement and statistical quality control principles, while currently unevaluated, may also hold promise.[19] Clinical practice guidelines and patient outcomes research need to be integrated into a continuous quality improvement paradigm. Local and regional hospital/health systems operating within the HPARs can serve as important laboratories for experimentation in this undertaking.[20] Ultimately, each HPAR might create a quality improvement award similar to the Baldrige Award given in industry.[21] HPAR technical staff and other groups such as the Joint Commission on Accreditation of Health Care Organizations could work with providers in promoting quality improvement consistent with the Pepper Commission's call for organizations that "have skills in data integration and analysis, quality assessment and quality assurance."[22]

Related Issues And Approaches

Beyond the basic elements of the HPAR concept, consideration needs to be given to the payment of capital (particularly in regard to the adoption of new technology), medical and health professions education expenses, antitrust and professional liability reform, and the need for a more adequate supply and distribution of primary care physicians and other health professionals.

Paying for new technology and capital improvements. A major factor behind the rising cost of U.S. health care is new technology. There is little evidence suggesting that having more technology is adding value measured on cost-effectiveness criteria. In fact, most new technology does not replace existing technology but is simply added to the overall technological arsenal, and thus further increases costs. Since our nation prizes innovation and technological progress, we are unlikely to adopt incentives that retard such growth. But we may be willing to establish a process by which new technology is more efficiently and effectively allocated to maximize its impact on outcomes. This, of course, was the general intent of health planning legislation in the 1970s, which created the health system agencies that oversee the certificate of need process. This process, however, was not linked to the establishment of overall area budgets based on health status needs and an established benefit package, nor was it tied into an overall strategic health plan for a state or region.

Toward this end, I recommend that capital expenses associated with new technology and physical plant be incorporated into each HPAR's budget, based on three criteria: (1) an assessment of the physical plant capability and technological adequacy of facilities in the area relative to the demands on the delivery system; (2) the experience and ability of institutions and providers to use the technology; and (3) the emerging health status needs of the population. Incorporating payment for new technology and overall capital replacement as part of the HPAR's responsibility assures that technological and service capacity will be linked to the state/region's strategic health plan. It also provides incentives for institutions and providers to take a broader geographical perspective in the allocation of capital resources.[23] Each HPAR would designate one or more research-oriented medical centers in its region to serve as the initial testing ground for assessing the efficacy, appropriateness, and effectiveness of selected new technology. Based on these assessments, the technology might remain centralized in the major regional medical centers and teaching hospitals, particularly when sufficient volume is needed to achieve better patient outcomes. Selected technologies might also be diffused to other area institutions and providers, based on their likely ability to use the technology and on patient access criteria. Preference should be given to institutions and providers willing to share technology. Grappling with the economic, social, and ethical dimensions of technology adoption and diffusion will be one of the HPARs' major challenges.

Paying for health professions education. Health professions educational costs would also be incorporated into each HPAR's budget. Educational budgets would be based on linking the current and anticipated health personnel needs of the region with the epidemiologically determined health care needs and estimates of cost-effective demand for services. Appropriate adjustments would have to be made for universities that serve as national rather than state or regional resource pools.

Antitrust reform. The HPAR concept provides incentives for concentration of institutions, providers, and insurers into more closely integrated organizations for financing and delivering health care. This would require changes in or reinterpretations of antitrust law as applied to health care. The HPARs' clinical and fiscal accountability criteria could be used to assess the benefit to the community of particular organizational linkages.

Professional liability reform. Any proposal for restructuring the delivery system must deal with professional liability reform. Given HPARs' inherent clinical accountability criteria and standards, Congress might feel more comfortable setting limits on compensation. But beyond limits, incentives should be developed to reward more cost-effective providers. For example, the HPAR might provide malpractice coverage for all physicians practicing within the region based on the average case-mix-adjusted risk for that physician in his or her specialty.[24] Physicians with higher-than-average adjusted risk for their specialty would be eligible for HPAR-purchased liability insurance but would have to contribute the difference between the average specialty premium and the premium applicable to them. This approach would permit economies of scale in liability insurance; avoid rewarding providers with higher-than-average liability cost; and reduce the incentive to practice defensive medicine.

Supply and distribution of primary care physicians. The need for a greater supply and more equitable distribution of primary care physicians, nurses, occupational therapists, physical therapists, pharmacists, and other health professionals is an issue that exists apart from the HPAR concept but can be influenced by it. Increasingly, physicians and other health care professionals are complaining about the frustrations of providing care within a morass of counterproductive regulations, perceived inadequate resources, and lack of strategic direction. HPARs, which promote integrated financing and delivery of care, operate within a strategic health plan, and focus on a defined population, can provide a context and work setting for efficient, effective use of health personnel. These arrangements are likely to provide more satisfactory professional career opportunities. HPARs could also lobby state legislatures for changes in licensing laws to permit more flexible use of personnel, the development of multiskilled practitioners, and experimentation with new ways of delivering patient care.

Existing approaches similar to HPAR. Most of the components of the HPAR concept are not new. What is new is bringing them together when advances in health services research, growing consolidation of institutions and providers into regional health systems, and broader-based public concern over cost, access, and quality may make the "bundling" of the components workable.

For example, the HPAR concept builds on some of the positive elements of the American Hospital Association's (AHA's) Perloff Report issued over twenty years ago.[25] The Area-Wide Health Care Corporations proposed by the AHA at that time are equivalent to the integrated insurer/provider health care plans of the HPARs. The significant growth of hospital/health systems over the past twenty years, coupled with advances in health services research and information systems to permit greater clinical and fiscal accountability, make the Area-Wide Health Care Corporation concept much more viable today than in 1970.[26] In fact, the recent AHA proposal for health care reform emphasizes the importance of integrated payment/delivery organizations charged with the responsibility of maintaining the health status of defined populations.[27] Also, as noted, HPARs incorporate some of the capital expense evaluation features of the health system agencies of the 1970s; however, unlike those agencies, HPARs are responsible overall for creating, implementing, and evaluating health policy and for meeting budgetary targets.

The HPAR concept also shares some similarities with Canada's use of area budgets and its somewhat more restrictive approach to technology diffusion.[28] But there are more differences than similarities. First, Canada does not use multiple payers, whereas the HPAR concept retains the concept of multiple payers (although a single funnel) through the combined insurer/provider health plan entities. Second, Canada does not allocate resources based on the defined health status needs of the population—a central feature of the HPAR concept. Third, Canada does not reward providers based on performance against clinical guidelines, the achievement of desirable patient outcomes, and patient satisfaction, as proposed by the HPAR concept. Finally, the Canadian system does not encourage local competition or innovation among providers as does the HPAR concept.[29] The HPAR concept is a compromise in which autonomy, choice, and pluralism are balanced against the need for greater clinical and fiscal accountability in providing increased access to health care services for more Americans.

Advantages Of HPARs

A number of criteria have been proposed for evaluating health plan reforms: (1) development of a health benefit package for all Americans; (2) development of budgets and allocations of resources based on locally determined needs; (3) preservation of some degree of strategic choice for insurers and providers and individual choice for consumers; (4) payment based on defined clinical and fiscal accountability criteria; and (5) political feasibility that merges the interests of the important stakeholders.[30] HPARs meet all of these criteria.

Citizen benefit package. HPARs would provide an organizational mechanism for implementation of health benefit plans for all citizens within each state and, perhaps eventually, a basic health plan for all Americans. The HPARs, along with the health plans, would be responsible for ensuring that the benefits were adequately communicated to citizens and for monitoring plans' clinical and fiscal performance.

Needs-based budgeting. Allocating resources based on defined needs and benefits keeps insurers from enrolling only better risks, as currently occurs with the emphasis on experience rating. HPARs would establish an overall areawide health care budget based on community rating of the entire population in the area. But, at the same time, allowance would be made for different premium structures to recognize the likely higher utilization needs of the less healthy population segments, thus removing disincentives for health plans (insurer/provider combinations) to provide care for these individuals. All revenues from all payer sources would flow through the HPARs, thus assuring accountability against the established budget. Existing research suggests that efforts to contain health care costs have been most successful when payers' efforts have been coordinated.[31]

Preservation of choice. HPARs would also promote some degree of autonomy for the insurer/provider health plans and choices for consumers. Some plans may be organized around staff- or group-model health maintenance organizations (HMOs), while others may remain in more loosely defined provider networks. Some hospital and physician groups may move toward a more vertically integrated delivery system organized around multispecialty group practices, while others may work through more traditional arrangements. Plans would be free to choose how individual providers are paid, with options ranging from salaried relationships to more traditional fee-for-service arrangements.

The HPARs are likely to stimulate considerable experimentation in the development of coordinated continuums of care that link regional teaching medical centers with community hospitals and multispecialty group practices, nursing homes, rehabilitation facilities, home health care agencies, adult day health care centers, and related services. In most areas of the country, consumers would be able to choose among the different health care plans based on various service quality, technical quality, and cost features. As part of the negotiated contracts, each health plan would be required to provide basic fiscal and clinical accountability performance data, which would be disseminated to purchasers and consumers by the HPARs, in addition to individual marketing efforts that the plans themselves might undertake. Those plans perceived to add greater value are likely to be more frequently selected by large and small purchasers alike.

Clinical and fiscal accountability. A major advantage of the HPAR concept is its built-in criteria for clinical and fiscal accountability. Incentives to contain costs and use resources efficiently are balanced against concerns of undertreatment that might harm patients. This would be accomplished through use of practice guidelines and outcome measures (functional health status, achieved treatment objectives, and patient satisfaction) in assessing plan performance. Plans do not win just by controlling costs, but by adding value—that is, for a given level of cost, achieving better outcomes and consumer satisfaction or, conversely, for a given level of outcomes and satisfaction, doing it for less.

The ability to pay plans based on their clinical performance will evolve slowly, as much remains to be learned regarding what clinical and organizational practices are more strongly associated with positive patient outcomes.[32] Nonetheless, pioneering experiments are under way. One notable experiment is Blue Cross/Blue Shield of Minnesota's development of a system to pay thirty-two of the state's largest hospitals based on illness-outcome groups.[33] Those with higher-than-expected adverse outcome rates will be at financial risk for the excess cost associated with such treatment. Those with lower-than-expected adverse outcome rates will gain. Implementation of the HPAR concept will go a long way toward stimulating additional such efforts and incorporating the results of patient outcomes research into operational settings. This may result in eliminating costly clinical and organizational practices that are actually harmful or of no value to patients while identifying new practices and interventions that provide demonstrable value.

Political feasibility. The litmus test for the HPAR concept is in its political feasibility. The HPAR concept would force the major players at the state and local levels to work with each other and negotiate among themselves the benefits to be included in the health plan and the trade-offs under which they wish to live. When dollars to be allocated for health care conflict with other state priorities, the HPAR would provide the possibility of a "health industry" perspective, as opposed to the splintering that often now prevails and that enables a state to play one group off against another.

Hospitals, physicians, and other providers would benefit from the elimination of uncompensated care and from the increased, predetermined level of resources to provide patient care. They would have the freedom to enter into alliances with insurers to form health care plans for purposes of negotiating with the HPARs to serve populations of interest. They would have incentives to maintain and enhance the health status of populations, which would encourage creative and innovative health maintenance and promotion strategies. In addition, physicians would benefit from the malpractice liability reforms and from having formal, ongoing input into health policy making. Insurers would maintain an important role through their linkages with provider delivery systems in negotiating contracts with the HPARs. They also would benefit from removal of the disincentives for covering sicker populations and, like the other groups, would have an institutionalized and ongoing voice in the policy process. Employers, government, and other payers would benefit from the elimination of indirectly subsidizing the cost of uncompensated care and from the inherent incentives for cost-effective provision of care.

Consumers themselves stand to gain the most, as all citizens would be provided a basic package of benefits along with income-related cost sharing to encourage prudent use and a delivery system structure in which all providers and components of the system face common incentives for providing cost-effective care. The public would also benefit from the competition between health care plans as they vie for potential enrollee groups based on criteria of service quality, technical quality, and cost. HPARs would create an environment in which community-based health care efforts could flourish.

Some Major Questions

Several major questions remain to be addressed. These include (1) whether the HPARs will add value; (2) whether the various interest groups can find sufficient common ground to generate a platform for leadership; and (3) how best to encourage experimentation.

Will HPARs add value? It is estimated that 22 percent of U.S. health care expenditures are administrative costs, amounting to $132 billion in 1989.[34] The administrative cost of a system organized around approximately sixty HPARs will inevitably be higher than the more centralized approaches of Canada and the United Kingdom.[35] Employers and other payers (and ultimately the American taxpayer) must accept this tradeoff in return for maintaining some autonomy, pluralism, and choice. However, the added administrative costs associated with the HPAR staff and boards should be more than offset by the common billing and claims processing associated with the single "funnel" approach to managing the flow of dollars. The likely consolidation of insurers and the development of integrated insurer/provider plans should result in additional savings. Most importantly, economic incentives for all parties to promote health and to provide the most cost-effective care should provide needed economic discipline to the system. Since managing care is a cornerstone of HPARs, some estimate of cost savings may be gleaned from the experience of such organizations as Kaiser Permanente.[36]

Whether or not such savings are likely to be one-time only as states adopt HPAR approaches will depend largely on the year-to-year performance of the health plans and on the negotiations between HPARs and plans. Of particular significance will be the decisions made regarding the adoption and use of new technology. The HPARs would provide a forum in which all interested parties could examine and manage the pace and extent of diffusion of new technology—perhaps the most important factor fueling the continued escalation of health care costs.

A platform for leadership. The key stumbling block to meaningful health care reform may not be financing but the threat of losing professional, managerial, and ultimately economic control. It is not whether we can raise the dollars or how that responsibility (or burden) should be shared, but, rather, who gets to manage the resources and who determines how they should be allocated.

For decades, the various interest groups have argued over the relative purity of their motives for justifying their portion of the pie. The nature of these debates is changing in the face of an accumulating data and information base on what constitutes cost-effective treatment practices, cost-effective hospitals and health plans, well-designed benefit packages, clearly written insurance plans, and key factors associated with patient satisfaction. HPARs would bring all relevant parties together with a common information base and incentive structure to enable more informed judgments. Because HPARs would be backed by state authority, interested parties could not walk away from the challenge of establishing and evaluating priorities. The "pain" would be shared, and different views on how best to serve patient interests would have to be reconciled. All would gain by supporting the most cost-effective ways of restoring, maintaining, and enhancing the health status of the populations served.

Each party must give up some autonomy to maintain other freedoms and influences. For example, hospitals that perform poorly and those that lack desired technology may be threatened by the HPAR approach to payment and technology acquisition. But recent surveys indicate a growing willingness of hospital executives to acknowledge the need for some fundamental reforms. One survey found that 53 percent are willing to accept global budgets; 62 percent are willing to accept more stringent limits on spending for new capacity; 53 percent are willing to accept a significant reduction in the number of hospital beds; and 51 percent are willing to accept stricter limits on spending for costly technology.[17]

Many physicians may resist the incentives to consolidate into larger groups and, in turn, to link with hospitals and insurers in an integrated delivery system able to provide more cost-effective care under global budgets. Nonetheless, in the survey previously noted, 54 percent of responding physicians indicated that they would accept a fixed global budget if the flexibility of fee-for-service reimbursement were retained.

Insurers may perceive that they have the most to lose, because the benefit packages and premium structures would be largely established by the HPARs. The incentive to work together with provider delivery units to form integrated health plans also means some loss of autonomy for insurers. Significant consolidation is likely to occur among insurers, with perhaps five or six major insurer/delivery system combinations emerging in many states. But the winners would play a key role in the negotiating process and in serving as the financial conduits for forming partnerships with the local delivery systems. This would allow them to play a much more meaningful role than if they simply served as fiscal intermediaries under a federally administered health system.

Encouraging experimentation. The fact that most of the current experimentation and innovation in health care reform is taking place at the state level provides a favorable climate for the HPAR concept. Since it is a state/region-level concept, considering reform at this level would be easier than would attempting to graft it onto health policy reforms at the federal level. It contains stronger incentives and accountability for cost containment than most of the current proposals and much greater sensitivity to local needs and preferences than do centralized federal proposals.

HPAR demonstration programs should be initiated in states with a reputation for progressive health care legislation, a history of experimentation and innovation in health care delivery, or experience in all-payer payment. They should only be placed in states with the technical and analytical capacity required to support a resource needs–based approach to delivery and accountability. Experience gained in these states could be used to gradually phase in the concept in all states, perhaps over a period of five years. Freedom and flexibility should be promoted so that the states can mold the concept to fit their needs. The federal government could play a useful role by providing technical assistance grants to the states for initial HPAR development work, emphasizing the exchange of information and consultation among states with varying degrees of experience. There will be differences in the ability to assess needs, to balance different interests, to encourage the formation of integrated provider/insurer health plans, and to develop the clinical information infrastructure for purposes of performance-based payment. But once a state-level health policy-making authority composed of the relevant interest groups exists, incentives are created to make rapid progress on all of these issues.

The existence of a diversity of managed care systems throughout the country is encouraging as well. The Kaiser Permanente approach contains most of the elements of the HPAR concept. It links hospitals and physicians in providing health care to defined populations, operating within a fixed budget that is based on estimates of the health care use of the population served. The Mayo Clinic and the Henry Ford Health System offer models of linkages between hospitals and largely salaried physicians that negotiate with purchasers to deliver cost-effective care across the continuum of care. Humana's Hospital-Group Insurance represents a different approach whereby group health insurance plans link enrollees to fee-for-service physicians who are largely affiliated with Humana hospitals operating in defined geographic markets.

Conclusion

Ensuring financial accessibility to health care services for all Americans is the morally and socially responsible thing to do. But it is only part of what is needed if all Americans are to receive better value for the resources invested in their health care. Improvements in financial accessibility must be accompanied by changes in the organization of the delivery system; otherwise, we are simply adding more cost to the system without knowing what we are getting for our investment.

While sentiment is growing for the development of a basic health plan for all Americans, it may be prudent first to gain experience from state-level efforts to define benefit packages for citizens based on the epidemiologically determined health care needs and preferences of the population and a matching of resources to those needs and preferences.

Deborah Steelman, chair of the Social Security Commission Advisory Panel, recently noted that "everybody says we need a public-private partnership. But no one is willing to define that."[15] The HPAR concept defines a public/private partnership model in which each party plays a key interdependent role. It provides incentives for all of the interest groups or "dominoes" to move in the same direction. It provides a focus for more concerted leadership by directly appealing to the interests of key stakeholder groups. It provides an organizational mechanism and framework for moving from inertia to action.

I am grateful to Martin Barkin, Wayne Lerner, Walter J. McNerney, Douglas S. Peters, Suzanne Mulstein, William C. Richardson, the California Association of Catholic Hospitals, members of the Health Care Policy Issues seminar group, the Sisters of Providence Health System, and anonymous reviewers for their comments on an earlier draft of this paper. Recognition is also due the Agency for Health Care Policy and Research and The Robert Wood Johnson Foundation for support of the original research from which the HPAR concept evolved. This acknowledgment is not meant to imply that the above individuals or groups agree with all aspects of the proposal, nor does it constitute a formal endorsement of the HPAR concept.

NOTES

1. While the Pepper Commission made a major contribution to the health care reform debate, one reason for its report's lack of political appeal was its emphasis on a federally administered program. Emphasis on federal oversight is also a feature of the Senate Democratic health reform proposal sponsored by Sen. George Mitchell (D-ME); the Kennedy-Waxman proposal; and a proposal by Rep. Dan Rostenkowski (D-IL).
2. B.L. Kirkman-Liff, "Physician Payment and Cost-Containment Strategies in West Germany: Suggestions for Medicare Reform," *Journal of Health Policy, Politics and Law* (Spring 1990): 69–99; J.K. Iglehart, "Germany's Health Care System" (first of two parts), *The New England Journal of Medicine* 324 (1991): 503–508; and S. Altman, presentation at Estes Park Conference, "Market Warfare: Hospitals and Physicians in a Competitive Environment" (Kona, Hawaii, 10 January 1990).
3. Examples of data that can be used include those derived from the National Health Interview Survey, National Ambulatory Medical Care Survey, and Health Care Expenditure Survey; the data collected by the Health Care Financing Administration on use of services by Medicare beneficiaries; and growing research on health status and patient outcomes conducted by the Agency for Health Care Policy and Research. The actuarial expertise and experience of the various insurers can also be put to use.
4. For some examples and specific proposals, see Basic Health Benefits for All Americans Act (S. 768, H.R. 1845), sponsored by Sen. Edward M. Kennedy (D-MA); J. Kitzhaber, Oregon Basic Health Services Act, S.B. 27, 65th Oregon Legislative Assembly (1989); A.C. Monheit and P.F. Short, "Mandating Health Coverage for Working Americans," *Health Affairs* (Winter 1989): 22–38; G.R. Wilensky, "Viable Strategies for Dealing with the Uninsured," *Health Affairs* (Spring 1987): 33–46; and D. Chollet, "Minimum Health Insurance Benefits," in *Improving Health Policy and Management: The Baxter Health Policy Review*, ed. S.M. Shortell and U.E. Reinhardt (Ann Arbor: Health Administration Press, 1992).
5. W.G. Manning et al., "The Taxes of Sin: Do Smokers and Drinkers Pay Their Way?" *Journal of the American Medical Association* 261 (1989): 1604–1609.
6. See M.A. Stoto, R. Behrens, and C. Rosemont, eds., *Healthy People 2000: Citizens Chart the Course* (Washington, D.C.: National Academy Press, 1990); and U.S. Public Health Service, Office of Disease Prevention and Health Promotion, U.S. Department of Health and Human Services, "Strategies for Promoting Health for Specific Populations," *Journal of Public Health Policy* 8 (1987): 369–423. See also the health care goals spelled out in the Oregon Basic Health Services Act.
7. A. Enthoven and R. Kronick, "A Consumer-Choice Health Plan for the 1990s: Universal Health Insurance in a System Designed to Promote Quality and Economy," *The New England Journal of Medicine* 320 (1989): 29–37.
8. The residual savings not returned to the health plans would go to HPARs to support staff planning and evaluation and to provide funds for reinsurance pools that could be used to buy future contracts to hedge unanticipated losses. See J. Hayes, "Hedging Opportunities in Health Care," *Healthcare Strategic Management* (March 1990): 12–14.
9. S.C. Hartman and D.B. Mukamel, "How Might a Low-Cost Hospital System Look? Lessons from the Rochester Experience," *Medical Care* 27 (1989): 234–243; Greater Detroit Area Health Council, *Restructuring the Health Care Delivery System*, GDHC Planning Report (2 November 1989), 1–25; California Association of Catholic Hospitals, *Health Council for Resource Equity: A Proposal to Address Emerging Issues in California's Health Care System* (July 1989), 1–10; and California Association of Hospitals and Health Systems, *California Health Program*, Revised Blue Ribbon Committee Report (27 November 1990).
10. California Association of Catholic Hospitals, "Would a Public Utility for Health Care

Assure a Public Good?" (February 1991).

11. A joint effort on the part of the city of Chicago, Cook County, and the state of Illinois to provide health care for the poor is temporarily stalled due to lack of political leadership. The plan called for creation of a Cook County Health Council responsible for advising existing city and county health boards and eventually assuming more accountability. The report also recommended that fourteen "corridors of care" be created, each with an advisory board. These corridors would coordinate services in their areas and set up partnerships between clinics and hospitals in each corridor. For further details, see *Report of the Chicago and Cook County Health Care Summit: Chicago and Cook County Health Care Action Plan*, vol. 1, Executive Summary (April 1990), 1–39.
12. Such estimates can be made using census tract data on age, sex, education, income, and ethnicity and aggregating to broader geographical levels.
13. Hayes, "Hedging Opportunities in Health Care."
14. *Policy Perspectives: Blue Cross and Blue Shield Association Position Summaries* (Chicago: Blue Cross and Blue Shield Association, July 1991), 8.
15. J.E. Wennberg, "Outcomes Research, Cost Containment, and the Fear of Health Care Rationing," *The New England Journal of Medicine* 323 (1990): 1204.
16. W.C. Ferguson, "A National Health Policy?" *Federation of American Health Systems Review* (May/June 1990): 31.
17. Health Insurance Association of America, *The Health Insurance Industry Strategy for Containing Health Care Costs* (Washington, D.C.: HIAA, February 1990), *ix*.
18. Even if cost containment–based proposals were initially acceptable in the case of The Robert Wood Johnson Foundation's Community Program for Affordable Health Care (CPAHC), evidence suggests the lack of sufficient incentives for a concerted impact. See L.D. Brown and C. McLaughlin, "Constraining Costs at the Community Level: A Critique," *Health Affairs* (Winter 1990): 5–28.
19. D.M. Berwick, A.B. Godfrey, and J. Roessner, *Curing Health Care* (San Francisco: Jossey-Bass, 1990); and M.E. Walton, *The Deming Management Method* (New York: Putnam Publishing Group, 1986).
20. One such experiment is emerging among five Rochester-area hospitals that have agreed to establish norms and share data to meet continuous quality improvement objectives.
21. U.S. Department of Commerce and National Institute of Standards and Technology, *Malcolm Baldrige National Quality Award: 1990 Application Guidelines* (Gaithersburg, Md., 1990).
22. The Pepper Commission, *Recommendations to the Congress* (Washington, D.C.: U.S. Government Printing Office, 2 March 1990), 9.
23. D.W. Young, "Privatizing Health Care: Caveat Emptor," *International Journal of Health Planning and Management* (October/December 1990): 237–270.
24. Such an approach is being examined in Michigan. See *Michigan Health Plan: Universal Health Security*, Report of the Governor's Task Force on Access to Health Care, The Academic Consortium of Michigan (31 August 1989), 9.
25. *Ameriplan: A Proposal for the Delivery and Financing of Health Services in the United States*, Report of a Special Committee on the Provision of Health Services (Chicago: American Hospital Association, 1970).
26. S.M. Shortell, E.M. Morrison, and B. Friedman, *Strategic Choices for America's Hospitals: Managing Change in Turbulent Times* (San Francisco: Jossey-Bass, 1990).
27. *A National Health Care Strategy: A Plan for Change* (Chicago: AHA, 4 February 1991).
28. J.K. Iglehart, "Canada's Healthcare System Faces Its Problems," *The New England Journal of Medicine* 322 (1990): 526–528; and A.C. Linton, "The Canadian Health Care System: A Canadian Physician's Perspective," *The New England Journal of Medicine* 322 (1990): 197–199.
29. The HPAR concept also expands the health system agencies' responsibilities estab-

lished by the Health Planning and Resource Development Act of 1974, while providing for much broader policy-making input by greater numbers of relevant stakeholders.

30. S.M. Shortell and W.J. McNerney, "Criteria and Guidelines for Reforming the U.S. Health Care System," *The New England Journal of Medicine* 322 (1990): 463–467; and E.R. Brown, "Principles for a National Health Program: A Framework for Analysis and Development," *The Milbank Quarterly* 66 (1988): 573–617.
31. K. Thorpe, "Health Care Cost Containment: Results and Lessons from the Past Twenty Years," in *Improving Health Policy and Management*, ed. Shortell and Reinhardt.
32. A.M. Epstein, "The Outcome Movement—Will It Get Us Where We Want to Go?" *The New England Journal of Medicine* 323 (1990): 266–270.
33. B. Hutchinson, *Minnesota IOG-based Reimbursement System* (St. Paul, Minn.: Blue Cross and Blue Shield of Minnesota, March 1991).
34. J. Meyer, S. Silow-Carroll, and S. Sullivan, *Critical Choices: Confronting the Cost of American Health Care*, Report to the National Committee for Quality Health Care (Washington, D.C., 1990).
35. S. Woolhandler and D.U. Himmelstein, "The Deteriorating Administrative Efficiency of the U.S. Health Care System," *The New England Journal of Medicine* 324 (1991): 1253–1258.
36. *How California Wastes At Least $10 Billion in Health Care Dollars Each Year* (San Francisco: Health Access, April 1991).
37. L. Wagner, "Executives Ready to Sacrifice for Reform," *Modern Healthcare* (11 February 1991): 28.
38 D.G. Goodwin, "Speaking English! An Interview with Deborah Steelman," *Federation of American Health Systems Review* (May/June 1990): 37.

AMERICAN COLLEGE OF PHYSICIANS PLAN

Scott HD, Shapiro HB. (1992). Universal Insurance for American Health Care. *Ann Intern Med.* 117(6): 511-519.

POSITION PAPER

Reprinted from ANNALS OF INTERNAL MEDICINE Vol. 117; No. 6, 15 September 1992
Printed in U.S.A.

Universal Insurance for American Health Care

A Proposal of the American College of Physicians*

America urgently needs comprehensive health care reform. The American College of Physicians (ACP) believes that universal access to care can be achieved only through system-wide reform in the organization and financing of health care (1). This paper outlines our proposal for a national policy to achieve that reform.

Overview

As a professional society of physicians whose goal is excellence in medicine, we see a system failing all who are a part of it—patients, physicians and other health professionals, purchasers, and insurers. Most of the problems have been well documented: over 35 million Americans without health coverage, excessive utilization of high technology coexisting with substandard care, astonishing increases in spending without commensurate gains in health status, acute care promoted at the expense of preventive services and technology-based care at the expense of primary care. As practitioners, we feel the fear of uninsured and underinsured patients at the prospect of severe illness, and appreciate the dilemma of those locked into jobs just to keep health coverage. We confront every day the crushing bureaucracy of a system that diverts time, energy, and resources from patient care, frustrating the ability of physicians and patients to deal with illness.

Three aspects of the health care system appear particularly troubling. First, it promotes inequity and conflict between its private and public components. Costs are shifted from one component to the other, public programs lacking a powerful constituency are underfunded, and the total system suffers from unwieldy administrative complexity and cost. Second, benefit packages consist of circumscribed lists of covered services that reflect more the needs of payers than those of the patients. Third, cost-control efforts have failed to make the system affordable and have imposed an intrusive regulatory burden on both patients and physicians.

The College would correct these problems through a universal health insurance system covering everyone living in this country. Our design for a reformed system addresses the major problems through four elements:

- *Assuring Access to Care:* We propose a universal insurance system that relies on employer and publicly sponsored insurance plans. All public programs for health care would be consolidated, and everyone would be guaranteed coverage, funded through a combination of private premiums and public revenues.
- *Assuring High-Quality and Comprehensive Health Care:* We propose that all medically effective services be covered when they are appropriate for a particular patient.
- *Promoting Innovation and Excellence:* We propose measures to enhance the crucial institutional underpinnings that sustain excellence in medical care—research, education, and medical information management.
- *Controlling Costs:* We propose a national health care budget with a mixture of centralized and decentralized mechanisms to influence the price, volume, supply, and demand for health care services.

The ACP plan envisions substantial change, including insurance reform, limitations on spending, fee negotiations, and new structures such as a national health care commission representing all sectors of society. At the same time, the College's plan would incorporate elements of our current system that are valued by patients and providers—for example, a pluralistic approach that would accommodate fee-for-service and managed-care options, but a role for government that is circumscribed.

The College has developed this plan after extensive consultation, including input from a network of 4500 ACP members and from many organizations, review of other proposals, and examination of health care systems of other nations. Careful transition will be essential, but the nation must move forward quickly to adopt and implement a comprehensive plan.

Assuring Access to Care

The College proposes a plan for universal insurance, through a mixture of private and public financing, in which everyone living in the United States would be insured. Covered benefits would be the same for everyone: all medically effective and appropriate care. Public plans serving specific segments of the population would be eliminated.

We envision an integrated system in which employer-sponsored and publicly sponsored insurance plans would offer practice arrangements ranging from traditional fee-for-service to various organized delivery systems. Patients and providers would perceive no difference between health care in employer-sponsored and publicly sponsored plans; only the source of financing would be different.

Other proposals have suggested separate systems of care: private insurance through employers, public coverage for the unemployed, and continuing entitlement

* This paper, authored by H. Denman Scott, MD, MPH, and Howard B. Shapiro, PhD, was developed for the Health and Public Policy Committee: Clifton R. Cleaveland, MD, *Chair*; Cecil O. Samuelson, Jr., MD, *Vice-Chair*; Christine K. Cassel, MD; David J. Gullen, MD; Harold C. Sox, Jr., MD; Quentin D. Young, MD; Robert A. Berenson, MD; John M. Eisenberg, MD; Woodrow A. Myers, Jr., MD; Steven A. Schroeder, MD; and Gerald E. Thomson, MD. Approved by the Board of Regents on 10 July 1992.

programs for others (Medicare, Veterans Affairs, and other programs). Separate public and private systems perpetuate inequitable access to care, both because people in some public plans have only "minimum" benefits, in contrast to full benefits in most private plans, and because public programs are likely to be underfunded. Separate systems also perpetuate complex, overlapping, and costly administrative bureaucracies.

Some proposals rely on single-payer or centralized government approaches—basically a Medicare program for all. Government may be efficient at some functions, like collecting taxes and writing checks, but it is not well suited to administer and oversee the complicated set of interactions in the health care system. Nor would centralized control promote the variety of approaches to health care delivery that a private, insurance-based system fosters.

Employer-Sponsored Insurance

In the ACP plan, employers would have an option: They may sponsor insurance for employees up to 60 years of age and their dependents (including part-time employees) or pay a tax so that those employees can enroll in a publicly sponsored insurance plan. To encourage employers to sponsor plans, we propose three steps to make coverage more affordable and premiums more predictable:

- phase out employer responsibility for retirees and shift them into publicly sponsored plans;
- switch employees into publicly sponsored plans at 60 years of age; and
- provide payment for all catastrophic costs (over $50 000 per year per person) through publicly financed coverage.

These measures would remove the most expensive patients from employer-sponsored plans. The intent is to make premiums equal to or less than the payroll tax that would otherwise be required, encouraging employers to continue or initiate coverage. This addresses a criticism of those "play or pay" plans in which the premium cost to "play" is so much higher than the tax to "pay" that employers would terminate coverage and transfer employees to the public program—eventually leading to a single public system.

Employers who sponsor insurance would choose among private plans that meet national guidelines. The minimum employer contribution to the premium would be 50%, with the employee paying the rest, although the employer may choose to fund a larger proportion of the premium.

Publicly Sponsored Insurance

Everyone not covered by employer-sponsored insurance would enroll in a publicly sponsored plan. This group would include: employees whose employers choose not to offer plans, employees over 60 years of age, retirees, and the unemployed and those outside the labor market. The current array of federal and state entitlement programs created for specific groups would be replaced by the publicly sponsored insurance plans, which would provide benefits identical to those in employer-sponsored plans.

Funding for publicly sponsored plans would come from:

- payroll taxes from employers and employees in companies not sponsoring insurance;
- income-related premiums, collected through the tax system, for retirees and people not working but with incomes greater than the poverty level and for employees over 60 years of age in firms sponsoring insurance;
- increased alcohol and cigarette taxes; and
- general tax revenues.

The general revenues will be necessary to support premiums for low-income and unemployed people who pay no or reduced premiums, to pay for catastrophic coverage, and to cover costs for the elderly beyond premium revenues. We believe these expenditures are properly the responsibility of the public.

Our catastrophic costs program would be not only a public payment mechanism for costs in excess of $50 000 per year but would also be a stimulus to development of high-cost case management techniques, reliance on centers of excellence, and cost-efficient care. Our goal is to encourage smart decision making to govern allocation of resources.

The ACP approach to publicly sponsored insurance would strengthen the constituency of public programs. By including employees and dependents from companies not sponsoring insurance, retirees, and anyone facing catastrophic costs, the publicly sponsored plans would have strong backing under this proposal. Every person would have a stake in the system.

Insurance Plans and Insurance Reform

We believe an insurance-based system offers the best means of fostering a wide range of practice arrangements to suit the needs and preferences of patients and providers. This does not mean we approve of how private insurers have handled coverage in the past. We propose substantial reforms to alter their practices. We also believe system administration is best handled at the decentralized level, under national criteria.

Insurance plans would not compete on the basis of benefits offered, because all plans would cover all effective and appropriate care. They would not compete by underpricing reimbursement to providers, because there would be uniform rates for all payers. And they would not compete by excluding sick people.

Insurance plans would compete on the basis of *premium price* and *value* offered to employer and public purchasers. By better administration and other efficiencies, a plan could offer a lower premium. Another plan might market itself as providing better value at the same or even a higher price—for example, by organizing a group of providers it believes provides higher quality care. Traditional indemnity plans reimbursing fee-for-service providers could continue under this approach and might compete by offering greater value—for example, unrestricted choice of providers. Insurers might also compete by offering benefits beyond those covered, although under the benefits process outlined below, we do not see much of a market for that option.

Our plan should reinforce the movement of physicians and hospitals, as well as purchasers and payers, to organize more effective and efficient delivery systems to enhance their competitiveness. There would be strong incentives to develop criteria for quality of care, measure outcomes, and help practitioners provide effective and efficient care.

Competition among insurers would be channeled in this positive direction through reforms to eliminate the current risk-avoidance practice of insurers. Insurers would be required to accept all applicants. There would be no exclusions of coverage due to health problems ("preexisting" conditions). Experience rating (premiums calculated on the health status of the group), which has made rates unaffordable for many small groups, would be eliminated in favor of adjusted community rating (premiums that reflect the health status of the entire community) for all employers.

Finally, with insurance for all medically effective and appropriate services, individual state health benefit mandates would be eliminated.

Underserved People

Even with extension of health insurance to all, there would likely remain underserved people, including the poor, minorities, and rural populations. Providing insurance coverage is insufficient if the barrier to care is lack of nearby physicians and health care facilities. People in inner cities and remote rural areas as well as migrant workers will need more than an insurance plan. We therefore support an expansion of the public health system, including community health centers, local health departments, and the National Health Service Corps, and other ways to deal with geographic maldistribution of health care workers and facilities. Education reforms and related incentives are essential for producing providers to meet the needs of the underserved.

Fiscal, professional, and lifestyle incentives will be necessary to attract and retain health professionals in underserved areas. Capital will be necessary to develop or upgrade facilities and equipment. More effective integration of health services will be required, including efficient transportation and communication. Telephone and computer-based links and mobile clinics may help to deliver care to patients in sparsely populated areas. Strategies must consider cultural differences that influence how care can be delivered effectively.

Assuring High-Quality and Comprehensive Health Care

The College proposes a patient-oriented benefits determination process. Under our plan, a national health care commission would be responsible for determining covered benefits—with the requirement that all medically effective services be covered—and setting and allocating budgets. The commission would have representation from patients, physicians and other health professionals, employers, insurers, government, and other key sectors of society.

All effective and appropriate health services would be covered under all publicly sponsored and employer-sponsored plans. The scope of benefits covered would be based on medical effectiveness research and expert consensus. We would further ensure high-quality care by promoting practice guidelines, creating a scientifically reasoned system of quality assurance, and redefining malpractice protection.

Benefits Determination

For determining benefits, we propose a cascading process structured around three questions of increasing specificity to the patient.

1. Is a service medically effective?

2. Is the service medically appropriate for a particular group of patients or set of clinical circumstances?

3. Is the service appropriate and of value to a particular patient?

Effectiveness

The question of whether a service is medically effective is answered by research or expert consensus. Effectiveness extends along a continuum from clearly ineffective, to unknown/unproven but promising, to somewhat/sometimes effective, to clearly effective care. Decisions at the extreme are clear, but decisions become complex for interventions in the middle range. Greatly expanded efforts in medical effectiveness research will be essential to ensure that clinical decisions would be based increasingly on scientific data and less on individual opinion. Meanwhile, we recognize that there are procedures and therapies that clinical consensus would deem effective but that have not been scientifically evaluated. Such interventions should not be excluded from coverage while their effectiveness is being measured, but measurement should be expedited.

Services that would be assessed for effectiveness would represent all aspects of health care: preventive care; primary care; medical, surgical, and psychiatric care both in-hospital and in outpatient facilities; ambulatory mental health and substance abuse care; oral health; rehabilitative services; and prescription drugs. The *medical care* needs of patients in home-care programs and nursing homes will also be included.

The national health care commission would be responsible for determining covered benefits and for establishing the global budget. Should rationing of care become necessary, this mechanism would allow decisions to be explicit and apply to everyone, in contrast to the rationing now done tacitly through the allocation of resources, and largely affecting the poor. These decisions will confront the commission clearly with the trade-offs between expanding medical technologies and limited resources.

The commission's proposals on what services would be covered would not be subject to selective change by Congress. Congress could reject the entire package, but not add, delete, or modify individual items.

Appropriateness According to Guidelines

For services deemed effective, the next step would be to determine the appropriateness of the service under practice guidelines developed by the clinical community. Guidelines may indicate that a particular procedure is effective for some patients but ineffective for others. As an example, annual screening mammography is effective and indicated routinely for women in their 50s but not in their 30s.

Practice guidelines should be professionally developed and viewed primarily as a means for assisting physicians and patients in making appropriate clinical decisions. They will also help correct over- and underutilization. It is important they not be viewed as a cost-control mechanism.

Guideline development is a science in its infancy. The College has committed our resources to developing guidelines, and we call for increased public and private funding. For the present, guidelines should be applied judiciously, with reliance more on those for which there is strong scientific evidence and less on those for which there is controversy or insufficient evidence.

When practice guidelines are available, they would be tied to the profiling of practice patterns to determine if a physician is generally following the criteria for clinically appropriate use of services. "Generally following" is the key phrase: Oversight would look at patterns, not at individual case decisions. If a practice pattern consistently deviated from guidelines, there would be reason to challenge payment for services. If guidelines are not available, practice profiles would allow comparison with community norms.

Appropriateness for an Individual Patient

Clinical guidelines may not always apply to a specific patient, because guidelines are usually more general and apply to patient groupings. Individual patients may have unique characteristics not covered by the guidelines. A physician may decide, in consultation with the patient, that it is reasonable not to follow the guidelines. This decision will reflect individual clinical circumstances and the personal values of the patient. After the physician provides a service that is medically effective and appropriate for the patient, reimbursement would be made. There would be no questioning of decision making or denial of reimbursement. Payment could be challenged only retrospectively, and only if the physician's practice pattern, indicated through profiling, consistently departed from guidelines.

Other Considerations

To promote innovation, the benefits determination process must accommodate experimental procedures, tests, and therapies. We propose that experimental diagnostic and therapeutic services be evaluated for clinical effectiveness. Insurance plans would cover experimental services if both the physician and patient agree to participate in a formal, scientific evaluation sanctioned by the national health care commission.

We believe the process we have described would provide reimbursement for all appropriate services. Some patients, however, will want services beyond those covered. Others will want amenities such as a hospital suite. Under our proposal, people can pay for these services out-of-pocket or through supplemental insurance, but those expenditures would not be tax-deductible or included in the national health care budget.

Quality Assurance and Utilization Management

An essential element of systemic reform is restructuring the external oversight of quality of care. We believe physicians will accept the constraints necessary in a reformed system, particularly to control costs, if there is an end to the overwhelming regulatory intrusion that dominates practice today.

The goal of assuring quality has been displaced by the imperative of utilization management—a set of techniques designed primarily to drive down costs. Part of this trend has been the transfer of many of these review activities from the traditional setting of quality assessment (the clinical service, the hospital, the organized group practice) to the purview of insurance carriers, Professional Review Organizations, and a rapidly growing number of proprietary groups. These reviewers have relied mainly on time-consuming and intrusive case-by-case reviews. Review criteria are often unspecified and left to the judgment of the reviewer. The techniques are labor intensive, costly, and have not been shown to improve quality of care. Rather, they have intruded excessively into the daily clinical decisions of most physicians, and contributed to mounting frustration and dissatisfaction within the profession and among patients.

The College believes the primary locus of quality assurance must be returned to the medical profession and to health institutions. Clinicians should be responsible for providing high-quality, cost-effective care, and be held accountable for efficient use of resources. Concepts of continuous improvement should underlie this responsibility.

Under the proposed national health care budget, medical organizations would have the responsibility and incentive to monitor practice patterns because those would affect the resources available to the organization and the community. We envision a process tied to the second stage of the benefit determination process described earlier. Practice guidelines are used at this stage to determine the appropriateness of providing services in particular clinical circumstances. Profiling would indicate whether the overall pattern of a physician's decisions falls within the guidelines. Profiles would be relayed from the insurance plans to hospitals, organized delivery systems, and professional organizations so that they can identify outliers, determine reasons for the deviation, and help the practitioner make appropriate changes.

Malpractice Reform

The nation must restore the medical liability system to its proper role: compensation for patients injured by substandard care. We propose substantial reforms of liability determination, as well as stronger efforts by the profession and licensing authorities to monitor physicians and correct problems.

The College has been committed to improving the competence of practitioners, through writing practice guidelines (2) and developing criteria to establish skill levels for procedures (3). Professional standards help identify good care. Continuing education keeps practitioners current in basic and clinical science and will help physicians meet the important new requirement of periodic specialty board recertification.

The profession must take greater responsibility for monitoring itself. Physicians must identify colleagues who are impaired or show evidence of deficiencies, correct problems, or, if necessary, limit the practice of those impaired physicians. Licensing boards must have the resources and the authority to enforce standards. Data on quality of care will be essential to these efforts. Federal and state governments, insurers, accrediting agencies, institutions, and the profession must agree on indicators for monitoring quality of care.

Significant tort reforms are necessary to defuse the malpractice crisis and begin the retreat from the defensive medicine so ingrained in physicians' patterns of thinking. Tort reforms may not have a dramatic impact, but they are a necessary beginning to restructuring the entire process of liability determination. For various constitutional and political reasons, most states have been unable to enact meaningful tort reform. The malpractice crisis is a national problem that demands a national solution. Congress can and must take steps immediately to pass legislation that preempts state tort law for malpractice, with the following reforms:

- a cap on awards for non-economic damages (so-called "pain and suffering" awards);
- the elimination of suits seeking full damages from all parties (joint and several liability);
- an offset of awards if there are collateral sources of recovery (insurance, workers' compensation, and so forth);
- a penalty for frivolous lawsuits;
- modifications to the statute of limitations; and
- limits on attorney contingency fees.

Also, it should be noted that universal coverage would eliminate costly awards for future medical care.

We reaffirm that the profession must set and enforce standards for physicians who serve as expert witnesses (4). The testimony of these physicians should be subject to ongoing peer review.

Although the jury trial is an ingrained part of dispute resolution in the United States, we question whether it is the best method to achieve the goals of the malpractice system: identifying substandard care and compensating injured patients. The College has been a founding member of the AMA/Specialty Society Medical Liability Project, which formulated an innovative administrative process for liability determination (5). There would be administrative review and appeal, with final determination by a state board. This model deserves serious testing, supported by adequate federal funding. We also support testing alternatives, such as pre-trial screening panels, to eliminate claims not likely to have merit in court, and mandatory arbitration, in which parties to a dispute are bound by the decision of an arbitrator.

Promoting Innovation and Excellence

The American health care system must foster innovation and excellence in medical education, research, and data-based decision making. The College proposes adequate and dedicated financial support for each of these components of the "infrastructure" necessary for the delivery of high-quality medical care.

Medical Education

Reform of medical education is necessary to encourage and enable more students to become generalist physicians, to provide specialty care efficiently, and to prepare physicians to manage patients under the constraints of a health care budget.

A critical element of education reform is that all payers, both public and private, be required to contribute a fixed percentage of health expenditures to graduate education. In addition, appropriate mechanisms to finance training in ambulatory care settings must be developed.

Financial incentives could be used to achieve a balance of generalists and specialists. Financing of graduate medical education might be limited to the number of years required for residency training in general internal medicine, family practice, and general pediatrics. Payments per resident could be weighted for the training of generalists. Reduced or interest-free loans could be granted, or loan repayments deferred, only for residents training to be generalists. Loans might be partially or entirely forgiven for generalists practicing in underserved areas. Increased federal and state grants could be provided to support residency programs for generalists. Other, nonfinancial methods may be required, including capping the number of slots for nongeneralist training, and limiting the accreditation of new programs.

The nation must broaden opportunities for medical education. The government should supplement funding of undergraduate medical education to allow minorities and lower income students greater access. Funding is an increasingly urgent problem; three fourths of graduating medical students have debts, with an average of over $50 000 (6).

Optimal health care requires that physicians educate themselves actively throughout their careers. A new and more effective health care system will require even higher standards of physician competence. Thus, a design for greatly improved continuing medical education, including more meaningful curricula, more effective learning methods, better integration with guidelines, and other quality improvement techniques, as well as expanded, stable funding, should be included in planning for a new health care system.

Biomedical and Health Services Research

A major virtue of the U.S. health care system is its capacity to be innovative—in diagnosis and treatment and in delivering and evaluating care. Sustained investment in basic and applied research is essential to improve the health of the American people. To assure continued vigor in biomedical, clinical, and health services research, the College supports 1) regular increases in appropriations for the National Institutes of Health and 2) a percentage set-aside from total health care expenditures (for example, one quarter of one percent) to secure predictable funding for clinical and health services research.

Medical Information Management

The College is committed to informed, data-based decision making. This philosophy underlies health care reform. Informed decision making requires data systems to support excellence, not only in medical practice, but also in planning, policy development, and system administration.

To understand the dynamics of medical care and variations in use of hospitals and technologies, a reformed system must adopt common diagnostic and procedural codes, common indicators of quality of care, and a common data set. Unique identifiers for hospitals, physicians, and health plans would need to be standardized for statistical profiling to be meaningful and for evaluations of care. In addition, population-based data are essential to promote the effective distribution of health resources (manpower, technology, and facilities).

Controlling Costs

The United States cannot afford, and will not achieve, universal access to care without controlling costs, and costs cannot be controlled without system-wide reform. We must limit total health care spending, through a national health care budget and a matrix of national and local controls on the price, supply, and demand for health services. An effective strategy must incorporate both expenditure control and cost control. For expenditure control to be meaningful, participants must have tools to reduce costs; for example, if a community or a hospital is to achieve an expenditure target, it will have to identify and eliminate redundant capacity such as competing MRI units. Our proposals would influence forces that determine the cost and utilization of services.

We recognize that these proposals raise politically and procedurally difficult issues. It will take time and care to work out the details. But no plan for reform can succeed without substantial efforts to control spending.

National Health Care Budget

At the heart of the College's proposals to control costs is the recognition that the health care system must operate within financial limits. We must adopt a national health care budget—a ceiling on total health expenditures, sometimes referred to as a "global" budget. A national budget would take into account changing health needs of the population (including aging), new technology, and general inflation. What the budget should be is uncertain now, but we start with the assumption that the current level of spending, projected to be more than $800 billion in 1992, is enough to provide health care for everyone (7). This level reflects all the waste of the current system: administrative costs estimated by some in excess of 20% of spending, unnecessary utilization, duplicative facilities and equipment, overpriced care, and so on.

The national health care commission would recommend to Congress a health care budget for the nation, covering public and private spending and capital outlays. The commission, in consultation with state authorities, would develop a budget for each state based on its population and disease burden. The overall budget and state allocations would be updated periodically, based on changes in the variables that determine the need for health care and its true costs. In turn, states may choose to allocate funds to regional authorities within the state.

Providing good care within the constraint of fixed income is the underlying principle of the managed care industry (8). Other countries have shown that fee-for-service arrangements can operate within a budget, through negotiations over fees (9-12). Implementation of a national health care budget would be a forceful incentive for all providers, patients, and payers to begin to make decisions reflecting the need to operate within limits. The budget would give the authority to the planning process necessary to allocate resources.

Managing Price: Insurer-Provider Negotiations

States would be required to establish mechanisms for the employer-sponsored and publicly sponsored insurance plans to negotiate fees with physicians, hospitals, and other providers. Using systematic, research-based methods of valuing services, such as the resource-based relative value scale (RBRVS) for physicians and diagnosis-related groups (DRGs) for hospitals, insurers and providers would negotiate and agree on conversion factors to set yearly fee schedules. Uniform rates would apply under all plans within states or sub-state regions; all payers would pay the same price for the same service. Qualified managed care organizations, such as prepaid group practices, would negotiate an overall budget with all insurers based on enrollment, age distribution of enrollees, and expected morbidity; they could develop their own compensation packages for health care professionals. Organized delivery systems would negotiate budgets for institutions and practitioners within the system, to be allocated to providers under their financial arrangements. To permit these negotiations, antitrust restrictions must be revised.

The health care budget would encourage trends such as regionalized services integrated vertically and horizontally, primary care networks, multilocation group practices, and new organizational and financial relationships between hospitals and their medical staffs, all of which should improve quality and reduce costs. Because operating under a budget is normally part of these arrangements, the transition to a national budget should be eased.

Payments under the various fee schedules, when multiplied by expected utilization of services, could not exceed the state's allocation under the national health care budget. A state health care agency would monitor utilization patterns by service category and study variations from predicted use. To stay within the state's allocation, the state (or regional agencies within the state) would have the authority to change the conversion factor for all providers and suppliers of medical services.

If a state's health care expenditures exceed its budget allocation, even after corrections to the conversion factor, health care spending would not come to a halt. Expenditures that cannot be attributed to unanticipated illnesses would trigger reductions in fee schedules or other remedial action for the following year. The budget is a device to introduce fiscal discipline and evaluate whether expenditures reflect expectations and goals; it is not a mechanism to cut necessary care.

Implementing the global health care budget will require extraordinary cooperation among providers. Physicians, hospitals, and other provider groups would have to work out who would represent them in negotiations and how they would relate to each other. They would also have to create a climate of clinical decision making in which the profession does not tolerate unnecessary care. The important impact of the global budget would be its incentive to eliminate unnecessary expense at all levels of the health system. It would promote cooperation among providers and others to figure out how best to meet the community's needs—an element largely missing in an open-ended system that encourages excessive care and generation of unlimited revenue.

The fee schedules negotiated between insurers and providers would be the total payment for services. Making reimbursement fair in a reformed system would eliminate the need for any additional charge to the patient, or "balance bill" (the amount above what the fee schedule allows).

Managing Supply: Regulatory Approaches

Market forces have not led to appropriate distribution of health resources—manpower, technology, and facilities. Hospitals a short distance apart establish duplicative high-technology services. Running competing, partially utilized services is inefficient and leads to pressure to use the service regardless of clinical need. Freestanding outpatient facilities generate business to try to maximize revenue, and weaken hospitals by skimming away many of the patients having lucrative procedures, while hospitals must maintain their facilities. Many elements of health care have become a business and have adopted a business mentality, and traditional goals of community service have become endangered. The problem is not limited to hospitals or freestanding facilities. Physicians are attracted to specialties where they are not needed, in areas already oversupplied. There is a growing critical shortage of primary care and generalist physicians and providers and facilities in rural and inner city areas.

We conceptualize two levels of regulation: a "macro" level having to do with the capacity, supply or inputs to the system—basically the limits within which care is delivered; and a "micro" level—the physician-patient encounter. The College believes there is an appropriate role for regulation at the macro level, governing the supply of health resources. Government can have substantial impact on costs, in a nonintrusive way, by regulating these "inputs" to the health care system: physician supply and specialization, technology, and capital investment. Micro-level regulation of the physician-patient encounter has failed and would be eliminated under our plan.

We propose that, under federal guidelines, states and communities establish targets for the supply of health resources, expressed, for example, in terms of the distribution and concentration of physicians and other health professionals, beds, and major technologies. Setting these targets would require careful planning and attention to national resources such as teaching hospitals and specialized centers. Enforcing them would require that the targets be linked to the payment system.

The nation must develop a national health manpower policy. Of special urgency is the need to increase the number of primary care and generalist physicians. This shift will be necessary to provide for the millions of people who will gain access to care, as well as to ensure that care is cost efficient. The output of training programs must change from the current distribution of 35% generalists and 65% specialists to a balance in the profession as a whole. To achieve this goal would require major changes in how the country educates medical students and residents and how they would be paid once they move into practice. Fees must be substantially augmented for the evaluation and management services that form the core of practice for generalists, and for physicians practicing in underserved areas.

Managing Demand

Demand for services can be dampened by promoting individual responsibility. Patients must view good health as a lifelong endeavor, beginning with early prenatal care and maintained through careful habits and appropriate preventive care. Physicians must educate their patients about their diseases and the public about the benefits of health promotion and disease prevention, and funding must be available for these initiatives. In the long run, full insurance coverage for preventive services will do much to promote health and control spending.

Patients and families must understand that, in some circumstances, a diagnostic or therapeutic intervention is futile. Understanding is best accomplished in the context of a long-standing, doctor-patient relationship in which the patient is fully included in the decision-making process. The profession and public health authorities must teach patients more about reasonable expectations.

Research (13) and the experience of our members support the conclusion that a co-payment (typically, a flat payment or a percentage of the allowed fee) required of the patient discourages unnecessary services. For low-income people, however, co-payment may also discourage necessary care. We accept the need for an appropriate co-payment as a useful restraint on demand, as well as a source of revenue for the system. However, we propose the elimination of co-payments for low-income patients, so that the entire fee would be covered by insurance. For others, co-payment would be limited to a specified percentage of the fee, and subject to an annual cap. We would hope that as both patients and physicians become more knowledgeable about medically appropriate care, the need for co-payments will diminish and ultimately cease.

Payment reform is an essential element of managing utilization. Reimbursement continues to favor procedures over careful evaluation of the patient, and high cost technology over less expensive procedures. The new Medicare fee schedule was based on the concept of equitable payment, but its implementation has further eroded payment for evaluation and management services. Until the system is restructured so that it values general medical care, incentives to overutilize procedures will continue to drive up spending.

Finally, there should be restraint on patient self-referral to a specialist or subspecialist. We propose that most patients establish a clinical relationship with a primary care or generalist physician who would refer to specialty services as needed. We recognize that some patients need ongoing care from subspecialists.

Managing Administrative Costs

The nation must recapture the billions of dollars wasted in administrative expenditures, and redirect that spending for medical care. We predict substantial savings from administrative simplification under the ACP plan. Eliminating experience rating and fee discounts and forcing companies to compete on premium price and value is likely to result in the consolidation of health insurance companies. Eliminating case-by-case review would also save money. On the public side, replacing the many current programs would save the substantial costs of maintaining separate bureaucracies and developing and enforcing divergent sets of rules.

We propose a highly simplified claims process. Providers would file claims with a single processing agent at the state level (either a state agency or a firm under contract). That agent would make payments to providers and bill the patient's insurance plan. Patients would require only a plastic card encoded with the name of their plan and the source of the financing. We must adopt a uniform claims form, and move as rapidly as is feasible to electronic filing and computerized patient records.

Conclusions

Any proposal for change implies gains and losses for the participants in a system. One criterion of the seriousness of a plan is the degree to which it asks all parties to accept responsibility for achieving its goals. The College plan asks everyone to be responsible for ensuring access to care, improving quality, and controlling costs.

The recommendations in this paper have evolved from our philosophy on the role of a professional society that holds the public's interest primary; from listening to our members who care for and about their patients and the practice of medicine; and from our assessment of what should and, we believe, can be done.

The key change is the acceptance of limits, both philosophically and in the reality of operating within a national health care budget. In contrast to an open-ended system, squandering resources on unnecessary care or on bureaucratic excess in a limited system means that those resources are not available for patients in need and are taken from responsible colleagues and institutions in the community. Combined with a decentralized approach to the allocation of resources, the demands of providing care for all when there are limits on spending will be a powerful force to engender cooperation among all parties in meeting the community's needs.

Learning to live within limits will require sacrifices. For patients, limits imply that they cannot have everything they want; for providers, investments and incomes must know some bounds; for insurers and other administrators, no more micro-managing the system; and for employers not providing health insurance, an end to their free ride.

What are the gains? All patients are guaranteed coverage for all effective and appropriate services. No one is without care, and there is no second-class care. Our plan restores to physicians, hospitals, and other providers their central role in meeting the community's health care needs. They receive appropriate compensation for all care, and are relieved of the regulatory intrusion that characterizes the current system. Government and other payers gain predictability of expenditures and limits on the rate of growth. And employers get control of their costs and a boost in their ability to compete. They also see an end to cost-shifting—the hidden tax for uncompensated care which they have paid through their private insurance premiums.

Finally, the College insists that reform must be comprehensive. We cannot modify one element of the system without affecting others. For example, expanding access to care would be a false promise if we do not produce more generalist physicians. Attempting to control costs becomes doubly difficult if we do not eliminate pressures for defensive medicine through liability reform. Comprehensive reform does not imply that all changes must be implemented at one time. Careful transition and phasing, particularly with regard to the financial impact, will be necessary under an overall strategy that relates the components and presents a clear plan for achieving an integrated system and comprehensive reform.

The American College of Physicians offers its professional and organizational commitment to the task of reforming health care. The proposal we have offered is a conceptual outline. We recognize that important and practical details must be completed. Financial projections must be developed and tested. We are prepared to adjust our thinking as our own analysis proceeds and as the public debate continues. We look forward to participating with all others to achieve universal access to care and comprehensive reform.

Requests for Reprints: H. Denman Scott, MD, Health and Public Policy Division, American College of Physicians, Independence Mall West, Sixth Street at Race, Philadelphia, PA 19106-1572.

References

1. **American College of Physicians.** Access to health care. Ann Intern Med. 1990;112:641-61.

2. **Schwartz JS, Ball JR, Moser RH.** Safety, efficacy, and effectiveness of clinical practice: a new initiative. Ann Intern Med. 1982;96:246-7.
3. **American College of Physicians.** Hospital Clinical Privileges. Philadelphia: American College of Physicians; 1988.
4. **American College of Physicians.** Guidelines for the physician expert witness. Ann Intern Med. 1990:113:789.
5. **AMA/Specialty Society Medical Liability Project.** A Proposed Alternative to the Civil Justice System for Resolving Medical Liability Disputes: A Fault-based Administrative System. Chicago: American Medical Association; 1988.
6. **Association of American Medical Colleges.** 1991 Graduating Student Survey Results. Washington, DC: AAMC; 1992.
7. **Health Care Financing Administration, Office of the Actuary.** National health expenditures aggregate amounts and average annual percentage change, by type of expenditure: selected years 1965-2000. In: **Sonnefeld ST, Waldo DR, Lemieux JA, McKusick DR.** Projections of national health expenditures through the year 2000. Health Care Financing Review. 1991;13:1-27.
8. **Physician Payment Review Commission.** Chapter 12, Managing care: beyond the rhetoric. Annual Report 1992. Washington DC: PPRC; 1992:313-46.
9. **Evans RG, Lomas J, Barer ML, Labelle RJ, Fooks C, Stoddart GL, et al.** Controlling health expenditures: the Canadian reality. N Engl J Med. 1989;320:571-7.
10. **Iglehart JK.** Canada's health care system (Part 2). N Engl J Med. 1986;315:778-84.
11. **Reinhardt UE.** West Germany's health care and health insurance system: combining universal access with cost control. Report to United States Bipartisan Commission on Comprehensive Health Care, 1989.
12. **Kirkman-Liff BL.** Cost containment and physician payment methods in the Netherlands. Inquiry. 1989;26:468-81.
13. **Newhouse JP, Manning WG, Morris CN, Orr LL, Duan L, Keeler EB, et al.** Some interim results from a controlled trial of cost sharing in health insurance. N Engl J Med. 1981;305:1501-7.

AARON PLAN

Aaron HJ. *Serious and Unstable Condition: Financing America's Health Care.* Washington, D.C.: The Brookings Institution; 1991. [Pages 140-152 are reprinted here.]

The Universal-Access Single-Payer Health Plan

I propose a universal-access single-payer health plan that would provide acute and long-term health care insurance coverage for all U.S. residents and create a framework that can be used to limit the growth of spending. It rests on four propositions.

First, in common with most of the proposals for reform now under discussion, it presumes continuation of the system of employer-sponsored and -financed health insurance for working people and their families. Although a wholly public plan probably could achieve some additional administrative savings and some support persists for such an approach, the following plan is predicated on the unwillingness of Congress to shift the bulk of currently private health care outlays to public budgets and to displace current health care arrangements for most Americans.

Second, it presupposes that the current system can never provide coverage for people with little or no connection to the work force. The medicare system embodies such a presupposition for the elderly and disabled. The medicaid system reflects an understanding that employer-sponsored insurance will never serve more than a minority of the poor. The rest of the poor, as well as the unskilled and the long-term unemployed, can be assured access only through an extension of public coverage or through public payment for private insurance.

Third, in common with the proposals for fundamental restructuring, the plan described below posits that control over health care spending must be concentrated in one or a few hands. Efficient rationing of medical resources is more probable through some form of overall budget, rather than through controls on price per unit of service (such as the DRG system under medicare). Price limits provide no incentive to deny low-benefit care, but only avoid outlays for a given class of cases that consistently exceed some norm. A fixed budget permits physicians, hospital administrators, nurses, and other providers to implement rules for allocating limited resources to maximize medical benefits.

Fourth, the plan presented below is based on the presumption that federal action is necessary to set a floor under the provision of insurance coverage, but that in a country as large and diverse as the United States the allocation of health care spending and many elements of the design of health care benefits should be permitted to differ regionally. The federal government can use its regulatory powers, including tax rules, to achieve substantially universal coverage of working people and their families through private, employer-sponsored insurance for care during acute illness. And it will have to use its spending powers to assure coverage of people who cannot secure coverage through work. However, the case for encouraging regional variation is strong, particularly with respect to long-term care because of the large variations in costs and in the availability of home care, as well as the considerable current uncertainty about the best design for public support of long-term care.

Benefits and Plan Design

Because the system of paying for health care is likely to require major reform before the federal budget deficit has been eliminated, the plan sketched below is designed to help deal with both problems. Progress toward both goals can be achieved if reforms in the financing of health care are accompanied by measures to raise additional revenues at least sufficient to cover any added budgetary costs.

COVERAGE. The federal government would pursue a dual strategy. It would mandate that employers either sponsor coverage for all workers employed at least twenty-five hours a week and for their dependents and pay approximately three-fourths of the premium cost of this coverage, or pay a tax equal to roughly 9 percent of total payroll.[44] The requirement would apply to all employers, including the self-employed. The mandated coverage would include up to

44. This provision is taken from the plan of the National Leadership Commission on Health Care. The tax would apply whether or not particular employees were covered through another employer-sponsored plan of some relative.

120 days of hospitalization annually, unlimited physicians' services, specified preventive services (including maternity and prenatal care, routine examinations and unlimited care for preschool children, mammography, and Pap smears), inpatient and outpatient mental health benefits, and specified medications upon payment of a flat fee. All employers would be required to provide dependent coverage. Workers with low incomes would be entitled to a refundable personal income tax credit to prevent the net cost of coverage from exceeding roughly 5 percent of income. The federal government would also extend public coverage to people in families that have no one attached to the labor force and to employees of companies that elected to pay the tax instead of offering health insurance.

COST CONTROL. The federal government would establish general guidelines under which states, acting alone or jointly, would create a series of "financial agents" that would operate as the single payer for acute-care services in their areas. These agents, like those in the New York plan and unlike those in the Enthoven-Kronick plan, would be quasi-independent state regulatory agencies. Financial agents operating in standard metropolitan areas that span two or more states would be the responsibility of the states jointly; disputes among states would be settled by the federal government. Responsibility for administering limited budgets would rest with the financial agents. The financial agents would be empowered to establish and enforce payment schedules for physicians, such as the relative value scales used in medicare. They would negotiate hospital reimbursements and would be authorized to set fixed budgets as a means of controlling growth of hospital spending. They would be authorized to stipulate services that would be paid for only if rendered in hospitals and to specify which hospitals could receive payment for specified procedures. In this way, the financial agents could require the establishment of regional centers for the provision of particular services and prevent the proliferation of facilities outside the hospital setting. These powers are necessary to limit care to cases where benefits are judged sufficient to justify the costs. Without this power, entrepreneurial hospitals and physicians would continue to be reimbursed for investments in costly equipment for diagnosis or treatment, thereby making denial of low-benefit care difficult or impossible to enforce. In addition, the financial agents would be the conduit for federal payments to provide coverage for those not covered through employer-sponsored plans.

The federal government would set annual targets for the increase in total health care spending within financial agents' areas. These overall spending targets would set the limits on total spending, but the financial agents would determine how that total should be distributed among various medical services.

The financial agents would not supplant private insurers. Private insurers would cease to make payments to providers, but they would continue to market insurance to businesses. Initially, premiums for acute-care coverage would continue to be experience rated. But each financial agent would have responsibility for designing a gradual transition to a form of community rating that complied with broad and loosely drawn federal guidelines. Financial agents would be allowed to retain rate differences demonstrably related to workplace hazards or personal habits such as smoking or consumption of alcohol or other drugs. Rate variations based on workers' personal characteristics, such as age, race, sex, or disability status, would be prohibited. The financial agents could permit some local variation in the number and definition of groups. The transition from experience rating to community rates would have to be complete within five years of adoption of the plan. Companies that do not now sponsor health insurance and that would experience large proportionate increases in costs would be eligible for federally funded subsidies until the transition to community rating was complete.

PRIVATE "STOP-LOSS" PROTECTION. To strengthen the hand of the financial agents in cost control and to ease the transition to community rating, an annual limit on liabilities of private insurers should be set along the lines proposed in the New York state plan. In that way, the financial agents would be responsible for high-cost episodes of care. But the principal initial insurance responsibility of the financial agents would be to pay for acute health care for people not covered under employer-sponsored insurance, along the lines proposed by the National Leadership Commission on Health Care and other proposals to mandate workplace coverage.

The stop-loss limit would be the focus of debate on whether the United States is to retain a mixture of employer-sponsored and public insurance or will shift gradually to all-public financing, with the gradual elimination of private companies from the health insurance business.[45] If the stop-loss limit were raised as fast as medical costs, private insurers would retain a secure position in the system of paying for health care costs for most people. If the stop-loss limit were frozen, inflation would gradually lower the size of the market covered by private insurers until the remaining market was too small to support continued operations.

LONG-TERM CARE. The financial agents would also serve as the channel for financing long-term home care and nursing home care. Their role would depend on a national decision about the nature of the public role in supporting long-term care.

At least three broad courses of action are open. First, the nation might try to encourage the purchase of private health insurance through a variety of tax concessions and perhaps some direct subsidies. Unless the subsidies are quite large, many or most of the elderly who come to require long-term care will be uninsured. This course of action would require a large income- or means-tested public program for the support of long-term care. The financial agents would be the natural managers of this program. Because many financial agents would exist throughout the United States, they could retain much of the discretion now enjoyed by the states in regulating vendors of home care and nursing homes. Standards of eligibility should be established nationally, rather than locally, however, to reduce the existing wide national disparities in access to care.

Adoption of a national social insurance program is the second option for supporting long-term care. A social insurance program could provide home health services or nursing home care as a matter of right to those suffering from stipulated limitations on activities of daily living.[46] As noted earlier, a social insurance program can take many forms. Under some versions, a large income- or means-tested backup program would remain essential. The financial agents should administer any such backup program and should assume state regu-

45. Some major insurance companies, including Aetna and Teachers Insurance and Annuity Association, have elected to withdraw from the health insurance market in some or all states.

46. For illustrative plans, see Ball, *Because We're All in This Together*; and Alice M. Rivlin and Joshua M. Wiener with Raymond J. Hanley and Denise A. Spence, *Caring for the Disabled Elderly: Who Will Pay?* (Brookings, 1988).

latory functions concerning vendors of home care and nursing homes.

The third option neither institutes a new social insurance program nor relies on private insurance to provide access to long-term care. Rather, it entails grants from the federal government to state or local governments or nonprofit organizations operating under limited budgets to underwrite home care and nursing home services up to the limits of available funds. This approach could provide the same services for given total expenditures as the other options, but it would reduce the risk inherent in the social or private insurance approaches—that demand, supported by a financial entitlement, would result in much larger than anticipated costs. A new long-term-care entitlement could face such a cost "surprise" if unexpectedly large numbers of the disabled elected to use benefits to which they had become newly entitled. The grant mechanism would also create an instrument, absent from the social insurance approach, for controlling costs of providers.

Reorganization of Federal Health Care Activities

The new federal health program would assume most current health activities of the federal government, including medicare, which could be retained in its current form or folded into the larger system of paying for acute care. Medicaid would become part of the backup program for those not covered under employer-sponsored plans. Most Veterans Administration facilities should be put under the aegis of the financial agents except for special missions of this organization (treatment of spinal cord injuries, for example) that might not be adequately served in a unified framework. The federal employees health benefits program and CHAMPUS would be treated like other employer-sponsored plans and required to channel financing through the financial agents.[47] Outlays for these activities under current policy are projected to reach $205 billion in 1991 (table 5-1). But the universal-access single-payer health plan would have additional responsibilities. It would direct subsidies to the private companies required to offer health insurance that face particularly high

47. In general, the goal would be to vest a single agency with responsibility for all health care activities classified under budget accounts 551 and 553. Health research would remain a federal responsibility.

Table 5–1. *Proposed Health Care Trust Fund, 1991*
Billions of 1991 dollars

Expenditures		*Revenues*	
Current activities		*Current earmarked revenues and state payments*	
Medicaid	79	Payroll tax and medicare trust fund interest	87
Medicare	104	Contribution to medicare Part B	12
Veterans' health	13		
Other	9	State medicaid outlays (estimated)	34
Subtotal	205	Subtotal	133
Additional activities[a]		*Additional revenues*[a]	
Acute care	40	Employer payments in lieu of insurance	30
Long-term care	25	Tax on employer-financed health insurance above cap	9
		Value-added tax at 6 percent[b]	102
Total	270	Total	274
Addendum: Reduction in federal deficit relative to current policy			
Added revenue	141		
Added expenditure	65		
Deficit reduction	76		

Sources: *Budget of the United States Government, Fiscal Year 1992,* pp. 4-9, 7-55, 7-58; and *Overview of Entitlement Programs, 1990 Green Book, Background Material and Data on Programs Within the Jurisdiction of the Committee on Ways and Means: 1990 Edition,*Committee Print, House Committee on Ways and Means, 101 Cong. 2 sess. (Government Printing Office, 1990), pp. 162, 1290. Figures are rounded.

a. Author's estimates.

b. Based on Congressional Budget Office, *Reducing the Deficit: Spending and Revenue Options,* February 1990, pp. 144, 417–20, assuming full effectiveness by 1991. The VAT revenues assume the CBO "narrow base" plus medical expenditures. The inflationary effects of the VAT on medical prices are assumed to be offset by cost control measures.

costs. And it would finance the new long-term-care program. Total expenditures in 1991 would be an estimated $270 billion if the programs were all fully in effect.

The total budget of the federal health care agency that administers the universal-access single-payer health plan would exceed the current budget of all federal departments, other than the Department of Defense and the Social Security Administration. Under plausible projections, health care outlays under current policy will exceed defense outlays late in the 1990s and social security benefits after about 2009.[48] Because expenditures on health care are large and

48. *Budget of the United States Government, Fiscal Year 1991.* These crossovers would occur sooner if responsibilities for the health department were increased or if defense or social security outlays fell below projections.

certain to keep growing, it would be sound budgetary procedure to house these functions in an independent cabinet-level Department of Health and to finance federal expenditures on health care through a trust fund, like those now used for social security pensions and medicare hospital benefits.

Financing

The activities of the new Department of Health would be financed through three main sources (see table 5-1). The first and most important would be revenues currently collected to pay for medicare and funds allocated by states to medicaid;[49] and premiums now paid by individuals for part B medicare coverage ($133 billion). The second would be payments by employers who elected to pay taxes rather than sponsor insurance (approximately $30 billion) and revenues from a cap placed on the value of employer-financed insurance that employees can exclude from personal income tax ($9 billion). The cap on excludable premiums is assumed to be $100 a month for individuals and $250 a month for families. The third source would consist of new tax revenues earmarked for the finance of health care. An earmarked value-added tax of 6 percent would yield approximately $102 billion. As an alternative revenue source, an increase in the payroll tax from its current level of 15.3 percent of covered earnings to 19.3 percent would yield approximately $100 billion. Doubling federal tobacco taxes and imposing a tax of $0.25 per ounce of ethyl alcohol in beverages would yield about $10 billion a year.[50] Repealing the 1981 increase in the exemption used in calculating federal estate and gift taxes and adjusting the prior exemption for inflation would yield $1 billion, an increase which can be easily justified on the grounds that long-term-care benefits would protect estates against the devastation wrought by chronic disabling illnesses.

49. Federal legislation would be necessary to ensure that states did not reduce their outlays.

50. Whether alcohol or tobacco consumption creates financial burdens for people other than the consumers is not clear. Consumption of alcohol and tobacco increases the frequency of many illnesses, but it also shortens life expectancy, thereby reducing the incidence of other illnesses and lowering pension costs. On this issue, see Thomas C. Schelling, "Economics and Cigarettes," *Preventive Medicine*, vol. 15 (September 1986), pp. 549–60.

The additional taxes would cover added federal expenditures on acute and long-term care and also reduce the overall deficit. Because federal expenditures now financed out of general revenues would be shifted to the health trust fund, this plan would reduce the federal deficit by approximately $76 billion. The increase in taxes would be determined by the target for deficit reduction and the health care benefits—especially the range of acute-care benefits mandated under the acute-care plan and the extent of patient cost sharing; the terms of long-term-care benefits, including notably whether these benefits are financed through a new social insurance program or through grants to states, localities, and selected providers; and the size of transitional subsidies offered to employers forced to sponsor acute-care insurance.

The Federal Role: Short and Long Run

The role of the federal government as direct provider and manager of health insurance would be smaller under the universal-access single-payer health plan than under current law. Administration of health care plans would reside with state or regional bodies—the financial agents—rather than with federal agencies. But the federal government would have greatly expanded financial responsibility for raising revenues sufficient to support costs of acute-care health benefits for those not covered through work, high-outlay episodes of acute care for everyone, and long-term care. It would establish the budget constraints within which the financial agents would have to operate.

Criticisms

Major reforms of important institutions are always subject to criticism. The universal-access single-payer health plan is no exception. Like any other fundamental reform, the universal-access single-payer health plan will redistribute responsibility for financing health care, generating costs and savings in a somewhat capricious manner. Businesses that do not sponsor health insurance will be forced to do so and incur the associated costs. Eventually these costs may be offset by slowed growth in money wages or other fringes, but some businesses will suffer some competitive disadvantages in the meantime. On the other hand, companies that now sponsor plans may find their costs reduced, as providers' costs for uncompensated care decline. And taxes will go up to pay for services formerly paid by private payers and new services. Some citizens will gain and some will lose.

The answer to this criticism is that the only way to avoid such redistribution is to continue the current system, a course that I have argued is not open. Therefore the only issue concerns the pattern and amount of redistribution. The universal-access single-payer health plan would cause less redistribution than would other major alternatives, including large refundable tax credits (a centerpiece of the voluntary incrementalist strategy) or vouchers funded from tax revenues. In any event, the choice among reforms should not be driven solely by such transitional problems but should be made by weighing them against improvements in access and in the capacity to control costs.

Other criticisms of the universal-access single-payer health plan hold that it is not really necessary, because less disruptive reforms that do not impinge on free choice by businesses and individuals could ensure access and enable cost control. I have argued above that this view is hard to accept because private actions are unlikely to control the provision of low-benefit, high-cost care or assure access to all. Even if the strategy of voluntary incrementalism were eventually to work, it would take many years, during which millions would still be unable to afford care and expenditures on low-benefit, high-cost care would continue.

The most serious criticisms of the universal-access single-payer health plan concern the workability of its specific elements: mandated employer-sponsored insurance and the financial agents. The administrative problems associated with mandatory employer-sponsored insurance are real.[51] To prevent gaps in coverage, rules will be necessary to stipulate whether workers who are between jobs are covered by their old employer or the public backup plan. Some employers will undoubtedly supplement any mandated benefit package. Two-worker families will have to decide under which plan to

51. Some criticisms relate to mandates that retain experience rating and are not applicable to the universal-access single-payer health plan. Katherine Swartz, "Why Requiring Employers to Provide Health Insurance Is a Bad Idea," *Journal of Health Politics, Policy, and Law*, vol. 15 (Winter 1990), pp. 779–92.

include their children. Workers who change jobs will experience changes in their coverage. These complexities are costly and inconvenient, but they are the price of building on, rather than replacing, the current system. If the United States were designing its health care financing system from scratch, I do not think that it would choose to base it on employer-sponsored insurance. But the investment in the current system is huge. The task of reformers should be to find politically acceptable ways to improve the current system, not to argue what might be the best system if current arrangements did not exist.

Economists point out that mandating employer sponsorship and financing of health insurance is equivalent to an increase in the minimum wage and therefore threatens the jobs of some workers, especially those earning roughly the minimum wage.[52] The jobs of teenagers have been shown to be more vulnerable to increases in the minimum wage than those of mature workers. Teenagers are more likely to be working part time and hence not to be subject to an employer mandate. But the cost of some lost jobs is real. That is one of the reasons I have urged that employers should be offered the option of paying a modest tax in place of covering the costs of health insurance or that transitional subsidies should be offered to employers who would experience large increases in costs.

Another potential difficulty with the universal-access single-payer health plan is the uncertain capacity of the financial agents to make rational allocational decisions. The existence of federally imposed spending limits will require such choices if Congress uses its authority to keep the growth of spending low enough to require the denial of some beneficial care to some people. The success of the financial agents in making rational allocational decisions will depend on the progress of effectiveness research. Even more important will be the development of procedures and criteria for deciding which services provide benefits too small to justify their costs. These techniques do not yet exist. The attempt by Oregon to develop such procedures illustrates the importance and the difficulty of finding analytically and politically defensible policies.

52. Standard theory suggests that mandated health insurance will tend to cause money wages or other fringe benefits to fall. Such adjustments cannot take place for workers receiving the minimum wage or a bit more. Swartz, "Why Requiring Employers to Provide Health Insurance Is a Bad Idea," p. 788.

A Time to Begin

In brief, the universal-access single-payer health plan would provide essentially universal financial access to acute care. It would greatly expand access to long-term care. And by creating budget-constrained entities that are empowered to negotiate fees and hospital budgets, it would establish the basis for control over the growth of medical care costs. Whether this power would be used to hold down costs would hinge on national support for budget limits. That such support would be forthcoming is not assured, but other countries in which a larger part of health care spending is under governmental control have been more successful than the United States in restraining growth of health care spending.

The universal-access single-payer health plan would not automatically assure high-quality care or lead to improved information about the efficacy of various medical interventions. The achievement of this goal under any system of paying for health care hinges on continuation and expansion of publicly sponsored effectiveness research.

This plan would leave open how the U.S. health care system should evolve. If the dollar limit used to cap the liability of employer-sponsored health plans for acute care were raised annually by the rate at which health care spending rose, private insurance companies would retain a major role in the provision of employment-based insurance. Insurance companies could continue to compete for sales on the basis of service, quality monitoring, and benefits in addition to those required under law, but not on the basis of premiums, which would be set by community rating. While such competition would be attenuated by the standardization of price, it would retain some of the incentive for innovation that distinguishes the current system. The price of such competition would be a continuation of the extra selling costs and other administrative expenses associated with multiple insurers.

Alternatively, if the limit on liability of employer-sponsored plans were not adjusted for inflation, the role of private health insurance in financing acute health care would gradually shrink and eventually vanish. Although revenues of insurance companies from this source would decline, any adjustments would take place over many years and would be easily managed both for companies and employees.

The financial agents would come to finance health care entirely with revenues from public sources.

In short, the United States can achieve universal health insurance coverage now and can immediately strengthen the capacity of the system to combat rising costs, while leaving for later debate the divisive question of what role private insurance should ultimately play. Access to health care for the uninsured and control of health care costs for everyone should not be held hostage to divisions over the ultimate goals for an ideal system.

CATHOLIC HEALTH ASSOCIATION PLAN

Catholic Health Association. Setting Relationships Right: A Working Proposal for Systemic Healthcare Reform. Washington, D.C.: CHA; February 20, 1992. [Pages ix-xv, which constitute the Executive Summary, are reprinted here.]

SETTING RELATIONSHIPS RIGHT:

A WORKING PROPOSAL FOR SYSTEMIC HEALTHCARE REFORM

Adopted by the Board of Trustees
of the Catholic Health Association of the United States
February 20, 1992

EXECUTIVE SUMMARY

Today, millions of working Americans, their families, and others cannot afford or otherwise obtain health insurance, and are often excluded from the benefits of our nation's healthcare system. Hundreds of thousands go without needed care or become impoverished when they have to pay their medical bills. And large numbers die prematurely for lack of care. Paradoxically, all of this is happening at a time when national healthcare expenditures are escalating rapidly, seemingly without control, and are consuming increasing portions of the nation's wealth. These problems have been exacerbated by the abandonment of community rating in private health insurance and employers' growing resistance to cost-shifting. Together these developments are undermining our nation's voluntary social safety net in healthcare and are making it much more difficult for many of our not-for-profit healthcare institutions to meet their historic missions of community service.

Meanwhile, the healthcare delivery system is fragmented and lacks economic discipline. It is increasingly burdened by a broad range of private and public rules on prices, volume, and methods of treatment that make American healthcare providers among the most regulated in the world (Exhibit 1, p. 10).

The Catholic Health Association of the United States is responding to this crisis by proposing[1] a value-driven reform proposal that provides comprehensive, high quality care--including long-term care--for all. The CHA working proposal (Exhibit 4, p.18) combines unitary financing with multiple payors and a pluralistic delivery system. To assure equity there is universal coverage for a comprehensive package of services. To assure efficiency and innovation there is competition. To assure quality, there is informed consumer choice and state chartering of private provider networks. To assure overall expenditure control there is a national budgeting process and extensive use of managed competition.

This is not a proposal to adopt the Canadian system, nor the British, German, or Japanese. This is a proposal designed to enhance the demonstrable strengths of American healthcare while addressing its weaknesses at the opening of the 21st century. It represents a unique public/private partnership to assure high quality, innovative, and affordable healthcare to all.

I. Values in the Reform Proposal

Healthcare reform is essentially a debate about values. Defense of the status quo in healthcare and every proposal for reform are based on a set of implied or explicit values. Catholic healthcare providers have a distinctive value tradition, and much of that tradition makes

1. Adopted by the CHA Board of Trustees, February 20, 1992, as one model for systemic reform that reshapes the U.S. healthcare system in a manner consistent with the values articulated in this document.

an important appeal to a broad cross-section of contemporary Americans. Six such values are embodied in this reform proposal.

- **Healthcare Is a Service**

Care of the ill and dying is an important measure of the moral character of any society. This conviction has an important implication relevant across American healthcare: Healthcare must always be more than a business. It is an essential social good, a service to persons in need and should never be reduced to a mere commodity exchanged for profit.

- **Healthcare and Human Dignity**

Every person is the subject of human dignity. The most important secular consequence of this view is commitment to individual human rights. Many Americans have a right to healthcare through various public programs, but the importance of healthcare to human dignity insists on universality, that is, all persons have a right to basic and comprehensive healthcare.

- **Healthcare and the Common Good**

Dignity is realized only in association with others. The human person is inherently social and this entails an obligation to serve the common good. Few messages are more important in light of the excessive individualism of contemporary culture. That is, we cannot look only at the self-interest of a few. We must also look at what is in the best interest of our communities and nation. Service to the common good is not foreign to America; it is an important part of our Biblical and other national traditions that must be recovered. Rediscovery of the common good is critical to the future of healthcare if not all other American social systems.

- **Healthcare and the Poor**

The wealthy and the well should care for the poor and the sick. This conviction, the original moral premise of community-rated health insurance, is strongly reflected in many American movements that have been driven by concern for those who are less well-off. Since programs for the poor too often become poor programs, a reformed healthcare system should tie the fate of the poor to that of the average American.

- **Healthcare and Stewardship**

Each of us is required to exercise responsible stewardship over creation. This belief has a secular parallel in the widespread recognition that natural and other resources are not unlimited and must be managed wisely. Responsible healthcare reform requires the introduction of economic discipline into the healthcare delivery system and the creation of credible expenditure controls to hold overall spending within realistic financial and political limits.

- **Healthcare and Government**

Respect for the dignity of persons should be balanced with support for institutions that serve the common good. This wisdom is reflected in American political traditions and suggests that a politically prudent reform must use federal authority to create a national healthcare community, respond to local diversity through state involvement, preserve pluralism in delivery, and protect a range of choice by clients and patients.

II. The CHA Working Proposal for Reforming the Healthcare System

The CHA working proposal begins with **delivery reform**, in contrast to other proposals that focus primarily on financing issues. The current delivery system is deficient primarily because it is fragmented and too costly. Financial incentives too often encourage providers to function in isolation from one another with little integration among primary care, acute care, and long-term care settings. Some important services are excluded while others are duplicated. Health promotion and preventive care are often uncovered. The current system also lacks internal economic discipline, forcing purchasers to use costly and demoralizing external controls on physicians and healthcare facilities. Finally, access to the current delivery system is often restricted. This is especially true for the millions of individuals who have no insurance but also for many persons with insurance.

Most existing reform proposals would impose new financing and external cost controls on this inefficient delivery system. This approach is certain to fail. The CHA working proposal recognizes that effective cost and quality control can occur only in concert with a reformed delivery system.

Elements of a Reformed System

Funding for the proposed system derives from multiple sources--some presently in place, some newly gathered into a healthcare trust fund managed by a new national agency, the National Health Board (NHB) (Exhibit 2, p. 13). The NHB administers the trust, establishes annual expenditure levels, and determines a comprehensive benefits package for all. A new entity at the state level, the State Health Organization (SHO), receives NHB dollars, charters local networks of providers, assures competition among them, and allocates funding to them on a risk-adjusted, capitated basis. New private entities, Integrated Delivery Networks (IDNs) (Exhibit 3, p. 14), compete to provide a continuum of care to their enrollees and bear the financial risk of capitated payment. Clients choose their doctors and hospitals by selecting one of several locally competing IDNs during periodic open enrollment periods.

- **Clients**

All individuals select among IDNs during an open season process. No one can be refused enrollment regardless of health status. Risk-adjusted capitation helps assure that sick and high-risk individuals are not avoided by providers. Premiums are eliminated. Client cost sharing is income-based. Persons below poverty have no cost sharing, while those between 100 and 200 percent of poverty pay on a sliding fee scale. Annual cost sharing amounts are limited to $2,000 for individuals and $3,000 [2] for families. No balance billing is allowed. Supplemental benefits and care can be purchased outside the IDN system but without tax benefits.

Clients are represented at every level of the system: on the IDNs, the SHOs, and the NHB.

- **Comprehensive Benefits**

The specifics of coverage are determined by the NHB, tailored by the SHOs, and delivered by the IDNs. Categories of benefits include: preventive care, acute care, and long-term care (Exhibits 5 & 6, pp. 21 & 22).

- **Integrated Delivery Networks (IDNs)**

An IDN is a set of providers--institutions and professionals--privately organized by contract (or ownership) and publicly chartered by the SHO. IDNs assume financial risk for providing a continuum of healthcare services: preventive, primary, acute, and long-term care. Most providers will be in or contract with one or more IDNs to participate in the healthcare system. Each IDN receives a risk-adjusted capitated payment to provide care to an enrolled population. Communities will be served by several IDNs, competing for enrollees on the basis of quality and service.

Clients select from among IDNs in their community during a periodic open season and participate in network decision making.

The IDN concept is designed to create new relationships among providers in order to improve coordination, efficiency, and quality of care. IDNs ensure that patients receive appropriate levels of care in optimal settings by offering a care coordination function to all enrollees. IDNs are accountable for healthcare quality and effectiveness. Open seasons that allow individuals to change IDNs, risk adjusted capitated payments, and periodic charter review by the SHO guarantee that IDNs provide high-quality, innovative, client-centered care. In other words, they will produce good value for the healthcare dollar.

---

2. See note p. xv.

State Health Organizations (SHOs)

SHOs determine community needs, authorize or "charter" IDNs within the state, assure competition among them (wherever competition is feasible), provide IDNs with their capitated payments, and empower consumers by providing comparative information on IDN service and quality. SHOs grant charters to IDNs only when they demonstrate their responsiveness to community needs. Clients are represented on the SHO.

Each state has at least one SHO while some large states are likely to have a number of regional SHOs. The SHO administers open season for IDN enrollment and pays each IDN a risk-adjusted, capitated payment for each of its enrollees from funds allocated by the NHB. The SHO applies for targeted funding from the NHB for special state needs, determines ground rules for IDN development and competition, and ensures that IDNs remain responsive to community needs.

National Health Board (NHB)

The NHB is an **independent**, public agency modeled on the Federal Reserve Board. It is charged with overseeing the system, managing the national trust fund, recommending healthcare expenditure levels to Congress, allocating funds to the SHOs, and determining a uniform, comprehensive benefits package for all individuals.

The NHB has an autonomous board insulated from undue influence by the President or Congress. The board is comprised of 10 to 15 members appointed by the President and confirmed by the Senate.

The NHB has three critical features: First, the *independent* character of the NHB allows it to challenge purely budget-driven decisions regarding healthcare. Second, the NHB has "Boren Amendment" judicial recourse if underfunding occurs. Third, through the NHB citizens have a direct voice in the system, for the first time gauging the appropriateness of healthcare appropriations and thereby holding politicians accountable for their action or inaction on healthcare budgets and benefits. The link between healthcare and its cost is public and explicit.

Financing

Major public financing sources are maintained. Employers and employees pay their health insurance premiums through a new 6.9 percent payroll tax on all employers and a 1.7 [3] percent payroll tax on all employees. New excise taxes on alcohol and tobacco are added and federal income tax is increased. These various financing sources are combined into a *dedicated* national **trust fund** for healthcare (Exhibit 9, p. 34).

---

3. See note, p. xv.

In the short run, many employers save money under the reformed system, and the average household spends less out-of-pocket. In the long run, everyone saves money as costs are controlled even as quality and universal coverage are assured.

III. Strategic Goals Met

The proposed system assures comprehensive care for all. It also meets three additional strategic goals: 1) the system produces **value** for each additional dollar spent on healthcare; 2) the system provides an **adequate flow of dollars** to sustain the healthcare infrastructure; and 3) the system makes **providers** and **clients** primarily responsible for **cost** and **quality** control.

1. **Good value** requires striking a balance between economic discipline and society's desire for effective and comprehensive healthcare services. Annual healthcare budgeting allows the nation to deal explicitly with healthcare spending. Capitated IDNs competing on service assure efficiency, quality, and innovation. Additional administrative savings result from consolidation of multiple public programs, elimination of indemnity insurance, and uniform procedures and billing forms.

2. **Adequate flow of dollars** is assured in three ways. First, the NHB is an *independent* agency. Second, there is judicial recourse if the system is underfunded. Finally, providers and clients are joined as healthcare system advocates and are able to react to any financial gap between NHB recommendations and federal funding.

3. **Cost control and quality** are primarily assured by providers and clients. Providers help set the rules for reimbursement, internal cost containment, and quality control by managing the IDN or serving on its board. Clients participate in decision making and help contain costs through wellness efforts and by exercising informed choice in their selection of an IDN. Funding is set by the NHB and apportioned by the SHO as it oversees quality. The reformed system eliminates today's private and public regulatory controls on prices, volume, and methods of treatment by making providers and clients primarily responsible for cost and quality control.

The proposal retains the best of our pluralistic healthcare system while introducing essential incentives for economic efficiency. Maximum flexibility is retained at the local level to allow for creative arrangements among providers, efficient methods of payment and delivery, and choice for individuals. Yet unitary funding assures universal coverage and a level of financial stability that is simply not achievable in our present system.

IV. Estimated Costs and Financial Impact [4]

Estimated First Year Spending

During the first year of operation the proposed system results in an increase in spending estimated at $31 billion, or about 4.2 percent of current healthcare spending (Exhibit 7, p. 30).

Distribution of First Year Costs

Households, on average, spend less on healthcare. Private employers pay more as a group, but many employers who currently offer comprehensive insurance to their employees pay less. State and local governments pay less for healthcare. The federal government "breaks even" because the proposal is budget neutral at the national level (Exhibit 8, p. 32).

Potential Savings

The CHA working proposal will save the economy large amounts of money annually, how much cannot be predicted accurately. If the reformed system reduces the rate of spending by only two percent each year, $580 billion will be saved over the next decade.

---

4. These estimated costs and savings are preliminary, and presented for illustrative purposes only. They will change as CHA continues to examine and refine them based on such factors as CHA's reform objectives, the range and types of benefits included, the relationship between copayments/deductibles to the overall cost of the reform proposal, and levels and types of taxation.

HAGAN PLAN

Ohio House of Representatives, Hagan Outlines New Health Care Reform Package. Columbus:House of Representatives; February 10, 1993. [news release]

Hagan RF. The UHIO Health Security Act of 1993: Key Features. Columbus: House of Representatives; 1993: 1-4.

Hagan, Mallory, Sheerer, *et al.* HB 175: Universal Health Insurance for Ohio (UHIO). Columbus: House of Representatives; February 1991.

Ohio House of Representatives

Columbus
43215

FOR IMMEDIATE RELEASE
FEBRUARY 10, 1993

CONTACT: JIM WOODS
(614)466-9373

HAGAN OUTLINES NEW HEALTH CARE REFORM PACKAGE

(Columbus)-State Representative Robert F. Hagan (D-64, Youngstown) announced that he will be reintroducing an updated version of his universal health care reform initiative very soon.

"This state must get serious about health care reform. We have to break the impasse and do what the citizens of Ohio want us to do. As legislators, we need to quit bickering over ideology and get the job done," said Representative Hagan.

"The plan I am announcing today is a blended approach. It combines the best aspects of a single payer system with managed competition elements. However, it's competition is based on quality and consumer choice, not cost and provider preference."

Representative Hagan's plan would divide Ohio into three regions, roughly equal in population. In each region a Health Insurance Purchasing Cooperative (HPIC) would be established. Each HPIC would have the responsibility of bargaining contracts on behalf of large pools of subscribers with providers of "qualified plans". Such providers could be Health Maintenance Organizations (HMOs) or Preferred Provider Organizations (PPOs). The plans would offer a comprehensive standard benefits package to all Ohioans within the region. The HPIC would also be responsible for insuring at least one freedom-of-choice-of-provider plan is available in all areas of the region, urban or rural.

Once a year, the HPIC would offer an open enrollment period where each person in the region would be free to choose the plan that will serve their needs best. During this period, each individual would also be free to change plans. No person would be refused enrollment or services on the basis of a pre-existing condition, race, color, income, national origin, religion, sex, sexual orientation, disabling condition, or health status.

"Providing quality health care service is only half of the battle. We must also control costs. Our current system is bankrupting the government, business, and individuals."

In Representative Hagan's plan, costs would be contained because the Statewide UHIO Health Security Board would be responsible for setting an annual global health care budget for provision of benefits included in the comprehensive standard benefits package. This board would have the power to set the premiums, establish standards of quality assurance, and regulate the introduction of new technologies. Also, only three to five health plans, including at least one freedom-of-choice-of-provider plan, would be offered per HPIC. This is to keep duplication of efforts and administrative costs to a minimum. The UHIO Health Security Board would also oversee and fund the regional HPICs.

"When we are thinking about financing, we need to keep in mind the Clinton Administration's commitment to free Medicaid dollars from Federal regulations through the waiver process. New Jersey and Oregon are already moving on that commitment. Ohio needs to be in position to take advantage of that commitment as well." The package will also be financed through Health Security premiums which will replace current private spending for health care plans by employees, employers, and the self employed.

This proposal essentially takes employers out of the health care equation because eligibility is based on residence not employment.

Representative Hagan also called for malpractice reform. This balances the consumer's right to relief if they are mistreated, with the need to curb large settlements and cut back on "defensive medicine" practices.

The only out of pocket costs to consumers would be a $25 copay for a visit to a specialist, if the patient is not referred by a primary care physician, and a $25 copay for unnecessary emergency room services.

The UHIO Health Security Act of 1993

A single, universal, comprehensive, pro-consumer system of health care for all Ohioans at a cost our state can afford.

Key features:

(1) universal coverage for all Ohioans, old and young, healthy and sick, working and unemployed, students and retirees;

(2) a comprehensive standard benefits package including: inpatient and outpatient hospital services; physician and other provider services; preventive services; population-based disease prevention and health promotion services; prescription drugs; mental health and substance abuse treatment; health rehabilitative care; hospice care; acute and primary dental services; vision services to age 18;

(3) no pre-existing conditions or genetic screening limitations;

(4) freedom for every Ohioan to choose among between three to five health plans, including at least one freedom-of-choice-of-provider plan, with each plan providing the comprehensive standard benefits package;

(5) an annual open enrollment allowing unlimited freedom to change plans;

(6) no person to be refused enrollment or services on the basis of race, color, income level, national origin, religion, sex, sexual orientation, disabling condition, health status;

(7 establishment of a state-level UHIO Health Security Board to set standards for "qualified" health plans (only "qualified" plans may offer benefits); control costs; insure quality and appropriateness in treatment; maintain a special fund to cover the costs of catastrophic care incurred by qualified plans; operate in the interest of consumers (see 13 and 14 below for information on the UHIO Health Security Board);

(8) provision that "qualified plans" may offer UHIO Health Security Board-approved supplemental benefits at Board-approved rates;

(9) no paperwork or individual billing for individual health care consumers;

(10) no payments at time of service other than $25 co-pay for visit to specialist if not referred by a primary care provider and $25 fee for emergency room use not resulting in admission

except in medically underserved areas or times (e.g., when primary care doctors offices are closed) as designated by the UHIO Health Security Board;

(11) public regulation and accountability through the UHIO Health Security Board and through regional Health Insurance Purchasing Cooperatives, all operating on behalf of and with accountability to Ohio's health care consumers and taxpayers (see 15 and 16 below for information on the Health Insurance Purchasing Cooperatives);

(12) public information on costs, outcomes, quality, and service through the UHIO Health Security Board and the Health Insurance Purchasing Cooperatives; comprehensive data, reporting, and electronic exchange systems;

(13) establishment of the state-level UHIO Health Security Board, whose duties include:

* to act in the interests of health care consumers;
* to insure competition based on quality;
* to establish rules and regulations concerning the comprehensive standard benefits package;
* to set the premium for the comprehensive standard benefits package;
* to establish standards for quality assurance, volume control, utilization review, appropriateness review;
* to define standards for "qualified plans" (provider capacity, financial stability, minimum enrollment, data capacity, customer service, consumer information, non-discrimination, etc.); (note: only "qualified plans" will be allowed to provide health benefits);
* to establish data, reporting, and disclosure requirements (all "qualified plans" and their participating providers and facilities will be required to operate in accordance with these);
* to operate the UHIO Health Security Trust;
* to fund the Health Insurance Purchasing Cooperatives and their costs for provision of the comprehensive standard benefits package;
* to establish Ohio's annual global budget for provision of benefits included in the comprehensive standard benefits package;
* to regulate Centers of Excellence, specialty hospitals, and medical "high" technology;
* to insure adequate primary care capacity;
* to monitor and oversee Health Insurance Purchasing Cooperatives;

* to take corrective action where necessary.

(14) membership of UHIO Health Security Board to be: 4 consumer representatives; 3 business representatives; 3 labor representatives; 2 physician representatives; 2 hospital representatives; 1 representative of licensed non-physician health care professionals; plus 4 ex-officio members (State Director of Health; Director of Human Services; Superintendant of Insurance; and the Tax Commissioner); the 15 public members shall be chosen by the governor with the advice and consent of the Senate from lists submitted by organizations representing their constituencies

(15) division of Ohio into three Health Insurance Purchasing Regions and establishment of three corresponding Health Insurance Purchasing Cooperatives (HIPCs) whose duties with respect to their individual regions include:

* to provide customer education, and complaint resolution services;
* to insure adequate, appropriate, quality services;
* to establish and consult with local advisory boards;
* to insure competition based on quality;
* to contract with "qualified plans" to provide comprehensive standard benefits package to all Ohioans in the HIPC region;
* to insure at least one freedom-of-provider-choice plan option in all parts of the HIPC region;
* if in any part of a HIPC region, insufficient qualified plans bid to provide benefits, to directly provide the standard benefits package;
* to conduct annual open enrollment for all in the HIPC region;
* to collect, evaluate, and publish data on health plan costs, quality, service;
* to conduct financial, performance audits of plans in the HIPC area;
* to receive funds from the UHIO Health Security Trust and to pay capitated premiums for that package to plans on behalf of enrolled individuals;
* to guard against adverse selection, to risk-adjust the capitated premium payments as necessary;
* to review and renew plan contracts on annual basis;

(16) membership of each Health Insurance Purchasing Cooperative Board to be: 4 consumer representatives; 3 business representatives; 3 labor representatives; 2 physician representatives; 2 hospital representatives; 1 representative of

licensed non-physician health care professionals; plus 4 ex-officio members (representatives of the State Director of Health; Director of Human Services; Superintendant of Insurance; and the Tax Commissioner); the 15 public members shall be chosen by the Governor with the advice and consent of the Senate from lists submitted by organizations representing their constituencies

(17) effective cost containment through global budgeting of the comprehensive standard benefits package; through UHIO Health Security Board regulation of hospital budgets and medical technology; through a "Centers of Excellence" network for highly specialized services (such as organ transplants); and through control of capatitated health plan premium payments for comprehensive standard benefits package;

(18) major financing of the comprehensive standard benefits package through Health Security premiums, which will replace current private spending for these benefits by employees, employers, the self-employed, and others (analysis is underway to determine need for supplemental sources of revenue);

(19) fraud prevention through prohibition of self-referrals, requirements for financial and performance audits of health plans, disclosure of ownership requirements;

(20) requirement that Ohio Health Security Board and regional HIPCs acquire significant staff expertise (e.g., medical, computer, actuarial, customer service, administrative);

(21) provision that disputes concerning alleged medical malpractice be submitted to an alternate dispute resolution forum before proceeding to court; provision that adhering to Ohio Health Security Board-approved practice protocols is an affirmative defense against malpractice in court;

(22) provisions to increase primary care capacity by (1) giving the Ohio Health Security Board authority to revise practice acts governing nursing and other primary health care providers if, following public hearings, the Board certifies that the changes are needed to provide appropriate primary care capacity; and (2) providing that the Board of Regents and the state funded medical schools will, within a year and subject to the approval of the Ohio Health Security Board, develop a plan to increase the number of primary care physicians without increasing the overall number of physicians;

(23) a study committee on long term care with a requirement to develop a plan, including financing, within five years of the effective date of this plan.

rev. 2/8/93

H.B. 175
(As Introduced)

Reps. Hagan, Mallory, Sheerer, Hartley, Mottl, Czarcinski, Lucas, Seese, Gerberry, Boggs, Koziura, Cain, McLin, Rankin, Colonna, Sykes, Abel, Roberts, Malone, James, Bara, Campbell, Pringle, Skeen, Krupinski, Prentiss, Vukovich, Whalen, C. Jones, Wise

Effective January 1, 1992, creates the Ohio Universal Health Insurance Plan to provide a publicly financed insurance program covering health care services for all Ohio residents.

Authorizes Ohio residents to select any participating health care provider.

Prohibits providers from refusing to furnish services on the basis of race, color, income level, national origin, religion, sex, sexual orientation, disabling condition, or any other nonmedical criteria.

Levies a 9% payroll tax, a 1 and 1/4% wage tax, a 10% tax on self-employment income, a payroll tax based on number of employees and a specified tax rate schedule, and additional tobacco and liquor taxes to finance the Plan.

Requires that the Plan be administered by a 19-member Board of Governors composed of representatives of consumers, labor, business, hospitals, physicians, and nonphysician health care professionals, and four directors of state departments.

Prohibits insurers, health maintenance organizations, and other third-party payers from offering benefits that duplicate coverage under the Plan.

CONTENT AND OPERATION

<u>The Ohio Universal Health Insurance Plan; board of governors (secs. 3961.02, 3961.03, and 3961.05(A)(5) and Sections 2 and 8)</u>

On January 1, 1992, the bill creates the Ohio Universal Health Insurance Plan, which consists of a single, publicly financed statewide insurance program to make available to all Ohio residents comprehensive health care services.

The Ohio Universal Health Insurance Plan is to be administered by a 19-member Board of Governors. Four of the members are the Director of Health, the Director of Human Services, the Superintendent of Insurance, and the Tax Commissioner. The other 15 members must, by reason of previous training and experience, be knowledgeable in matters pertaining to health care and health care administration. Those 15 members must be appointed by the Governor, with the advice and consent of the Senate, as follows:

(1) Four members representing consumers and appointed from a list of eight nominees submitted by the Advisory Council of Consumer Organizations (see "Advisory councils" below);

(2) Three members representing labor and appointed from a list of six nominees submitted jointly by organizations representing labor;

(3) Three members representing business and appointed from a list of six nominees submitted jointly by organizations representing employers;

(4) Two members representing hospitals and appointed from a list of four nominees submitted jointly by organizations representing hospitals;

(5) Two members representing physicians and selected from a list of four nominees submitted jointly by organizations representing physicians;

(6) One member representing licensed nonphysician health care professionals and appointed from a list of two nominees submitted by the Advisory Council of Licensed Nonphysician Health Care Professionals (see "Advisory councils" below).

If the Governor elects not to make an appointment for a position on the Board of Governors from a list of nominees submitted to him, or if the Senate does not give its advice and consent for an appointment, another list of nominees for that position must be resubmitted in the same manner as the original list. This appointment must also be made with the advice and consent of the Senate.

The bill requires the Governor to make the initial appointments to the Board of Governors by February 29, 1992. Of the initial appointments, three are for a term ending December 31, 1992, three are for a term ending December 31, 1993, three are for a term ending December 31, 1994, three are for a term ending December 31, 1995, and three are for a term ending December 31, 1996. Subsequent terms of office are for five years with each term ending on December 31.

The bill requires each member to hold office from the date of appointment until the end of his appointed term. Any member appointed to fill a vacancy occurring prior to the expiration of the term for which his predecessor was appointed must hold office for the remainder of that term. Each member is required to continue in office after the expiration date of his term until a successor takes office or until a period of 60 days has elapsed, whichever occurs first. The bill authorizes the Governor, at any time after notice and opportunity for a hearing, to remove for cause any member appointed by him.

The bill requires the Board members to annually select a chair and secretary of the Board from among its membership. Meetings are to be held upon the call of the chair and as may be provided for by the Board.

A quorum consists of 10 Board members and the affirmative vote of 10 members is necessary for the Board to take any action. Members serve without compensation, but are reimbursed for mileage and their necessary and actual expenses associated with Board business.

<u>Eligibility for, and services covered under, the Plan; role of insurers and other third-party payers</u> (secs. 3961.01, 3961.10, and 3961.11)

Every Ohio resident is eligible to receive benefits for covered services under the Plan, and is considered a "plan member" for purposes of the bill. Every plan member is entitled to receive benefits for any covered service furnished within this state by a participating provider, if the service is necessary or appropriate for maintaining the person's health, or for the diagnosis or treatment of or rehabilitation following an injury, disability, or disease. "Participating provider" is defined by the bill to mean any person that is authorized to furnish covered services pursuant to the Ohio Universal Health Plan Law and rules adopted by the Plan's Board of Governors.

The bill identifies certain health care services that the Plan must cover, but permits coverage of other services. The required services include the following:

(1) Inpatient and outpatient services;

(2) Provider services;

(3) Preventive services;

(4) Laboratory tests and imaging procedures;

(5) Short-term home health services;

(6) Prescription drugs, at no cost, that are approved by the Federal Drug Administration and are included in a formulary established by the Board of Governors of the Plan. Plan members may purchase a brand-name prescription drug that is not included in the formulary for an amount representing the difference between the cost of the brand-name drug and the average cost of

comparable drugs in that class that are included in the formulary.

(7) Ambulatory mental health care services and substance abuse treatment services, subject to quality assurance and appropriateness reviews;

(8) Medically necessary primary and acute dental services;

(9) Vision appliances, including lenses, frames, and medically necessary contact lenses, for plan members who are 18 years of age or younger;

(10) Medical supplies, durable medical equipment, and selected assistive devices.

The Plan does not cover any of the following services:

(1) Cosmetic surgery other than reconstructive surgery;

(2) Medical examinations and medical reports prepared for the purposes of purchasing or renewing life insurance or participating in a civil action for the recovery or settlement of damages;

(3) Basic care in a nursing home;

(4) Cosmetic dental services;

(5) Vision appliances, including lenses, frames, and contact lenses, for plan members who are older than 18.

Insurers, health maintenance organizations, employers, and other health plans and third-party payers are permitted to offer benefits that do not duplicate coverage offered by the Plan, but are prohibited from offering benefits that duplicate the Plan's coverage.

<u>Obligations of and payments to health care providers</u> (secs. 3961.12 and 3961.13)

The bill prohibits participating providers from denying services to a plan member on the basis of race, color, income level, national origin, religion, sex, sexual orientation, disabling condition, or other nonmedical criteria. A plan member is free to choose any participating provider, including any physician practicing on an independent basis, in a small group, or in a capitated (payment on a per patient basis) practice. A plan member enrolled in a capitated practice may disenroll from that practice only after a specified interval of at least 90 days after enrollment.

The Plan is required to reimburse participating providers located outside Ohio at Plan rates for care rendered to plan members while they were out of the state.

The Plan is required to pay each institutional provider of services, including providers of inpatient care and ambulatory facilities for diagnosis, treatment, and surgery, on the basis of a single, comprehensive, annual budget approved by the Board of Governors. Each institutional provider must negotiate with the Plan an annual budget to cover anticipated services based on past performance and projected changes in prices and service levels. Every physician or other provider employed by an institutional provider funded under such a budget must be paid through and in a manner determined by the institutional provider. This budgeting procedure also applies to institutions that provide plan services and that are funded by a political subdivision or an agency or instrumentality of a political subdivision. No later than June 30, 1992, no political subdivision or agency or instrumentality of a political subdivision can fund these institutions.

The bill requires independent health care providers to be reimbursed on a fee-for-service basis. The Plan must negotiate the fee schedule annually with each appropriate professional group. The fee schedule must be applied to health care services rendered by independent providers throughout the state. The fee schedules may take into account recognized differences among geographical areas regarding cost of practice and, to the greatest feasible extent, fee schedule categories must include payment for all procedures routinely performed for a given diagnosis. The bill allows the Board to specify that certain technical procedures will be reimbursed only when performed in certain institutions or by designated providers.

Providers are prohibited from charging rates higher than the negotiated reimbursement level, and from charging separately for covered services. The bill allows health maintenance organizations and other multispecialty organizations of providers to elect to be reimbursed on a capitation (per person) basis rather than according to the fee schedule. If the organization meets the Board's enrollment requirements, the organization may elect to have included in its capitation payments inpatient services provided by institutions funded under a single, comprehensive, annual budget (described above). Upon that election, the institutional budgets of these institutions must be adjusted accordingly.

The bill requires participating providers to furnish any information the Board of Governors reasonably required for utilization review, cost containment, quality assurance, payment of providers, and statistical or other studies of the Plan. The providers also must permit the Board to examine their records as necessary to verify payment.

<u>Plan coverage for nonresidents and members while in another state</u> (secs. 3961.05(A)(19), 3961.14, and 3961.15)

The bill allows any private or state college, university, or other institution of higher education situated in Ohio to purchase coverage under the Plan for students who are not residents of this state. In addition, any employer located in Ohio may purchase Plan coverage for employees in Ohio who are residents of another state. The Board of Governors of the Plan is required to bill employers located in another state for covered services rendered in Ohio to their employees who are Ohio residents.

The bill requires the Board to establish and operate an indemnity plan to provide payments for services, at rates negotiated by the Board for benefits for comparable services provided by the Plan in Ohio, under the following circumstances:

(1) If a Plan member receiving a pension, benefit, or allowance from a private or public retirement system in Ohio establishes residence in another state, the Board of Governors must pay for services comparable to the benefits for covered services provided by the Plan to plan members residing in Ohio and receiving a pension, benefit, or allowance from a private or public retirement system in this state. The Board may establish a schedule of partial payments for services based on accumulation of service credit under a retirement system. The bill applies to the following public retirement systems: the Police and Firemen's Disability and Pension Fund, the Public Employees Retirement System, the School Employees Retirement System, the State Highway Patrol Retirement System, the State Teachers Retirement System, and any municipal retirement system.

(2) If a plan member is temporarily in another state and receives services, the Board must pay for such services.

(3) If a plan member receives services in another state, the Board may pay for such services for compelling reasons relating to the suitability of medical care, the nature of the condition, and personal circumstances.

<u>Financing the Plan</u> (sec. 3961.16 and Section 6)

Effective January 1, 1993, the bill imposes the following taxes to provide revenue for the Ohio Universal Health Insurance Plan:

(1) On each employer, a 9% payroll tax. Any employer whose employee health benefit costs on January 1, 1993 exceed 9% of its payroll is permitted to continue its existing coverage until they expire, and then must convert to coverage under the Plan. Employers whose health benefit costs on January 1, 1993 are less than 9% of its payroll must pay to the Ohio Health Care Trust Fund the amount by which its then current payments are less than 9%. Employers who on January 1, 1993 are not making any payments for employee health care are allowed to pay a 3% payroll tax in 1993, a 6% payroll tax in 1994, and pay the 9% tax thereafter.

"Employer" is defined to mean the state of Ohio, its instrumentalities, and its political subdivisions and their instrumentalities, any individual, partnership, association, corporation, business trust, or any person or group of persons, acting in the interest of an employer in relation to an employee.

(2) On each employee who is a resident, a 1 and 1/4% tax on gross salary or wage. "Employee" is defined to mean any individual who works for an employer. "Resident" has the same meaning as in the Ohio Income Tax Law.

(3) On each self-employed individual, a 10% tax on the individual's self-employment income, subject to the limit on taxable self-employment income for Medicare Hospital Insurance under the Federal Insurance Contributions Act.

(4) On each employer, a payroll tax based on the number of employees, in accordance with the following tax rate schedule:

Number of Employees			Tax Rate
Column One		Column Two	Column Three
1	-	9	0.00%
10	-	49	0.50
50	-	99	1.00
100	-	249	1.75
250	-	499	2.50
500	-	999	3.20
1000 and greater			4.00

If the number of employees is equal to or greater than the number in Column One and less than or equal to the corresponding number in Column Two, the tax rate is the corresponding percentage of the employer's payroll as set forth in Column Three.

(5) An additional 10% tax on the retail price of cigarettes, cigars, snuff, and other tobacco products. "Price" is defined to mean the total cost of the property purchased at retail sale including any other taxes included in that cost.

(6) An additional 10% tax on the retail price of wine, sparkling and carbonated wine and champagne, vermouth, beer, malt liquor, mixed beverages, and spirituous liquor.

The bill requires the Board of Governors to adopt rules pursuant to the Administrative Procedure Act regarding the levy and collection of these taxes and allows the Board to enter into contracts with the Departments of Taxation and Liquor Control and the Industrial Commission for the collection of these taxes.

The Ohio Health Care Trust Fund; the Health Professional Education and Training Fund (secs. 3961.05(A)(6) and 3961.07 to 3961.09 and Sections 3 and 4)

All tax revenues are to be deposited in the Ohio Health Care Trust Fund, which the bill creates. The Fund is to be administered by the Board of Governors, which is required by the bill to conduct a quarterly review of the expenditures from and revenues received by the Fund. The Board can invest the Fund only in investments that are authorized by Ohio law for the investment of the capital, surplus, and accumulations of domestic life insurance companies. The bill specifies that the limitations set forth in those laws apply to the investment of the Fund.

The Department of Human Services is required to do the following by March 31, 1992:

(1) Apply to the Secretary of Health and Human Services for all waivers of Medicare and Medicaid requirements that are necessary to allow Ohio to deposit all federal payments under those programs in the Ohio Health Care Trust Fund.

(2) Identify other federal programs that make payments for health care services to individuals in Ohio, and comply with the requirements under those programs and apply for any waivers of those requirements that are necessary to allow Ohio to deposit the federal payments in the Ohio Health Care Trust Fund.

The Board of Governors and the Department of Human Services, no later than December 31, 1992, are required to pursue any reasonable course of action with the Secretary of Health and Human Services to establish procedures and conditions under which:

(1) The Department can pay to the Fund amounts that are equivalent to those amounts that are paid on behalf of Ohio residents for health benefits under Medicare and Medicaid.

(2) The Plan can impose and collect for payment into the Fund a surcharge on Ohio residents in amounts necessary to replace payments made by Ohio residents under the cost-sharing provisions of Medicare.

In addition to these tax revenues, federal payments, surcharges, and other amounts, the Ohio Health Care Trust Fund consists of all of the following:

(1) Federal and state funds in an annual amount equal to those federal funds appropriated for expenditure in federal

fiscal year 1991 and those state funds appropriated for expenditure in state fiscal year 1991, for purposes of the federal block grant program for social services, which the Departments of Human Services, Mental Health, and Mental Retardation and Developmental Disabilities used to provide services that would otherwise be covered under the Plan. The funds paid into the Trust Fund must increase in proportion to any increase in the federal or state funds appropriated for purposes of the block grant program for social services.

(2) State moneys in an annual amount equivalent to the money appropriated for expenditure in fiscal year 1991 for purposes of the Medicaid program. The moneys must increase in proportion to any increase in the federal payments received by the Plan.

(3) State moneys in an annual amount equal to the money appropriated for expenditure in fiscal year 1991 to the Departments of Human Services, Mental Health, and Mental Retardation and Developmental Disabilities, and to all other state departments or agencies, that was used to provide funding for services that would otherwise be covered under the Plan. The moneys must increase in proportion to any increase in the money appropriated to the Department of Human Services, Mental Health, or Mental Retardation and Developmental Disabilities, or to any other state department or agency, if the department or agency would otherwise provide funding for services covered under the Plan. The remaining portions of the budgets of these departments and agencies are to remain separate from the Fund.

Money in the Ohio Health Care Trust Fund is not subject to appropriation or allotment by the state or any political subdivision. Beginning on January 1, 1997, the amount of reserves in the Fund at any time must equal at least the total amount of expenditures from the Fund in the three preceding months.

The bill requires that the money in the Fund be placed in the following accounts and used for the following purposes, in accordance with rules established by the Board of Governors:

(1) The Prevention Account, which is used solely to establish and maintain primary community prevention programs, including selective preventive screening tests not performed as part of routine care. Every two years, the Board of Governors must determine the amount to be allocated to this account. From January 1, 1992, to December 31, 1996, the bill requires that moneys in the account equal at least one-half of 1% of the moneys in the Trust Fund. Thereafter, moneys in the account must equal at least 1% of the moneys in the Trust Fund. The Board also is required to administer the account.

(2) The Health Services Account, which is used solely to pay providers participating in the Plan.

(3) The Capital Account, which is used solely to pay for: (a) construction, renovation, and equipping of health care institutions, including institutional providers of inpatient care and ambulatory facilities for diagnosis, treatment, and surgery; and (b) establishment and maintenance of a loan program for facilities and equipment for use by health care professionals who establish practices in areas of Ohio in which, according to criteria established by the Board, the delivery of health care services is inadequate.

(4) The Communication and Transportation Account, which is used solely to cover the transportation of plan members from one institution funded under a single, comprehensive, annual budget, described in "Obligations of and payments to health care providers" above, to another for the provision of covered services and to effect cooperation and communication between such institutions.

The bill also creates the Health Professional Education and Training Fund, which consists of all moneys received from federal health professions training funds. This Fund is used solely to pay for educating and training health professionals. During the five-year period beginning January 1, 1992, and ending December 31, 1996, the annual state expenditures for such education and training cannot be reduced below the level of the expenditures in calendar year 1991.

[SUBSEQUENT MATERIAL OMITTED]

MCDERMOTT/WELLSTONE PLAN

Wellstone P. The American Health Security Act of 1993: Bill Summary (S-491). Washington, D.C. 1993.

Himmelstein DU, Woolhandler S, Writing Committee of the Working Group on Program Design. (1989). A National Health Program for the United States: A Physicians' Proposal. *N Eng J Med.* 320:102-108.

THE AMERICAN HEALTH SECURITY ACT OF 1993, S. 491

Senator Paul Wellstone (D-MN)

Introduced March 3, 1993

BILL SUMMARY

This bill would establish a national American Health Security Program to provide affordable, comprehensive, high quality health care to all Americans. The state-based national Program would simplify and streamline the administration and financing of health care, and administrative costs would drop dramatically. Consumers could choose their own providers from the same broad array of health providers available in the current system, including private and public providers, and accountable managed care plans.

There would be no gaps in coverage and no barriers to care. The government would become the sole health insurer. Consumers would simply show their national health card to receive health care from the health provider of their choice. Everyone would be entitled to the same benefits, and these would not change when a person changed jobs or moved to a different state. No one would lose coverage because he or she got sick.

The bill would control costs while improving the quality and efficiency of our health care system. It encourages training in primary and preventive care for doctors and midlevel practitioners, teamwork through multidisciplinary practices, the use of outcomes research and practice guidelines, and the integration of existing public health services with community-based primary care. States can decide how to distribute high-tech care and specialty centers on a local and regional basis, and to extend care into underserved rural and inner-city areas. Providers would compete based on quality of care.

Annual health care budgets could not increase faster than the growth of the Gross Domestic Product. Global institutional budgets, rate-setting for practitioners, and control of prescription drug prices, would further contain costs.

Major Provisions

- Universal access to health care through a single program, administered by the states.
- Comprehensive benefits, including primary and preventive care, hospital and practitioner care, treatment for mental illness and substance abuse, long-term care, and prescription drugs.
- Freedom of choice so that everyone can choose his or her own physician or other source of care, including managed care plans.
- Effective cost control through annual budgets, national fee schedules, and streamlined administration.
- Progressive financing, so that health care is affordable for all.
- Control over medical fraud and abuse.
- Re-shaping the health care delivery system to emphasize primary care, and to expand services to medically underserved rural and inner city areas.

Benefits and Eligibility

Health insurance would be provided for all citizens and legal residents of the United States. Everyone would receive a health insurance card entitling him or her to benefits covered under the American Health Security Program. The National Board can also cover undocumented workers, or states can do so at their own expense.

The covered benefits include:

- Primary and preventive services, including screening exams, well-child care, immunizations, and reproductive health care.
- Pre-natal, post-natal and well-baby care.
- Services of health care professionals who are authorized to provide such services under state law.
- Inpatient and outpatient hospital care.
- Diagnostic tests.
- Prescription drugs and biologicals.
- Nursing facility services.
- Home care and community-based services for individuals unable to perform at least two activities of daily living (ADL's).
- Hospice care.
- Mental health and substance abuse services, subject to care coordination, and to regulated utilization review after 15 days of inpatient care and 20 outpatient visits a year.
- Expanded services by community clinics and migrant health centers.
- Other medical or health care items or services as the National Health Board determines to be appropriate.

Consumers would be free to choose their own health providers.

What Is Not Covered

Over-the-counter drugs (aspirin, cold medicine), surgery performed only for cosmetic purposes, physicals for purposes of litigation or obtaining life insurance would not be covered under the Plan.

Cost Containment

The Program would contain costs in a variety of ways. It would reduce administrative waste, cap provider payments by global budgets and negotiated fees, continue consumer-oriented managed care plans, re-shape the service delivery system to emphasize primary care, control prescription drug prices, set separate budgets for costly new equipment, and control fraud and abuse.

No Cost Sharing

There would be no coinsurance, deductibles or copayments for benefits covered under the American Health Security Plan.

High Quality Care

The bill would improve the quality and efficiency of the service delivery system.

It would promote and expand the use of outcomes research and practice guidelines, including research on primary and preventive care, and encourage the integration of public health principles and services to improve the community's health.

Within five years, 50% of doctors in training would have to be in primary care programs, compared to the current 20%, and an advisory council would set goals for training more midlevel practitioners and non-professionals such as outreach workers.

It would encourage training programs and practices that include multidisciplinary teams, an important feature of high quality group practices such as the Mayo Clinic. Accountable managed care systems, called Community Health Service Organizations (CHSO's), could compete based on the quality of their integrated services.

States could concentrate specialty care in centers of excellence to promote better outcomes while containing costs.

States would control health care fraud and abuse, assisted by a national data base.

Underserved Rural and Inner City Areas

The bill would double funding for community clinics and migrant health centers, and greatly increase funding through public health block grants for services such as maternal and child health care, and care for people with AIDS under the Ryan White Act.

It would also expand funding for the National Health Service Corps, which sends doctors and midlevel practitioners into underserved area for two years, in exchange for help with educational expenses.

States could plan how to distribute services on a local or regional basis, to address current inequities.

Payments to Providers

Hospitals and nursing homes would be paid based on global budgets established annually through negotiations with the designated state agency and reviewed by state advisory boards.

Community Health Service Organizations (CHSO's) could offer comprehensive, integrated services for an annual, capitated rate.

Other facility-based services, including hospice care, outpatient services, and home, school-based and community-based services would be paid through one of the following options:

- Annual operating budgets.
- Fee schedules.
- A capitation payment.
- An alternative prospective payment method.

A professional board would classify prescription drugs into categories, as a basis for the Board to negotiate prices for similarly-classified drugs. The Board would establish price limits.

Health care professionals would be reimbursed according to fee schedules negotiated at the state level.

Payments for capital items, such as new buildings and equipment, would be budgeted and allocated separately.

The payments from the states to providers would constitute the payment in full for covered benefits. No additional payments or charges would be permitted.

Administration and Budgets

The American Health Security Standards Board would implement guidelines for national benefits, and national and state budgets. The budget could not increase more than the annual percentage increase in the Gross Domestic Product.

Each state would administer the program at the state level.

The budget would act as an expenditure target, so that if the budget for a service were exceeded, the state and the Board could lower payments for that service the following year.

Each state and national budget would include an amount for total expenditures for capital-related items, operating expenses, health professional education, and administration.

The state health budgets would be determined based solely on the following factors:

- The population of the state.
- Reasonable differences in the prices for goods and services.
- Any special social, environmental, or other condition affecting health status or the need for health care services.

- The geographic distribution of the state's population, particularly the proportion of the population residing in rural or medically underserved areas.

The state could enter into a contract with a fiscal intermediary to process claims. Only one contract would be allowed for each state.

Advisory boards representing both consumers and health care providers would advise on the implementation of the Program at the local, state and federal levels.

Financing

All revenues collected for health care would be placed into an American Health Security Trust Fund and could only be used for health care expenses.

The Program would be financed by collecting at the federal level all funds currently spent on health care.

The national insurance program would be financed through a 7.9% payroll tax on employers, increasing the existing 1.45% Medicare payroll tax by 6.45%; an increase in corporate income tax from 34% to 38% for businesses with more than $75,000 in profits; increases in the personal income tax from 15%-28%-31% to 15%-30%-34%, with a top rate of 38% for families with incomes over $200,000, and a health premium equal to about .5% of income (or 7.5% of income taxes paid); reforms to close loopholes in the tax code; a long term care premium equal to the Medicare Part B premium plus $25 a month for the elderly above 120% of poverty; an increase in the amount of Social Security benefits included as taxable income from 50% to 85%; state and federal spending will remain the same as current health care payments, with increases limited to growth in the Gross Domestic Product.

A NATIONAL HEALTH PROGRAM FOR THE UNITED STATES

A Physicians' Proposal

David U. Himmelstein, M.D., Steffie Woolhandler, M.D., M.P.H.,
and the Writing Committee of the Working Group on Program Design*

Abstract Our health care system is failing. Tens of millions of people are uninsured, costs are skyrocketing, and the bureaucracy is expanding. Patchwork reforms succeed only in exchanging old problems for new ones. It is time for basic change in American medicine. We propose a national health program that would (1) fully cover everyone under a single, comprehensive public insurance program; (2) pay hospitals and nursing homes a total (global) annual amount to cover all operating expenses; (3) fund capital costs through separate appropriations; (4) pay for physicians' services and ambulatory services in any of three ways: through fee-for-service payments with a simplified fee schedule and mandatory acceptance of the national health program payment as the total payment for a service or procedure (assignment), through global budgets for hospitals and clinics employing salaried physicians, or on a per capita basis (capitation); (5) be funded, at least initially, from the same sources as at present, but with all payments disbursed from a single pool; and (6) contain costs through savings on billing and bureaucracy, improved health planning, and the ability of the national health program, as the single payer for services, to establish overall spending limits. Through this proposal, we hope to provide a pragmatic framework for public debate of fundamental health-policy reform. (N Engl J Med 1989; 320:102-8.)

OUR health care system is failing. It denies access to many in need and is expensive, inefficient, and increasingly bureaucratic. The pressures of cost control, competition, and profit threaten the traditional tenets of medical practice. For patients, the misfortune of illness is often amplified by the fear of financial ruin. For physicians, the gratifications of healing often give way to anger and alienation. Patchwork reforms succeed only in exchanging old problems for new ones. It is time to change fundamentally the trajectory of American medicine — to develop a comprehensive national health program for the United States.

We are physicians active in the full range of medical endeavors. We are primary care doctors and surgeons, psychiatrists and public health specialists, pathologists and administrators. We work in hospitals, clinics, private practices, health maintenance organizations (HMOs), universities, corporations, and public agencies. Some of us are young, still in training; others are greatly experienced, and some have held senior positions in American medicine.

As physicians, we constantly confront the irrationality of the present health care system. In private practice, we waste countless hours on billing and bureaucracy. For uninsured patients, we avoid procedures, consultations, and costly medications. Diagnosis-related groups (DRGs) have placed us between administrators demanding early discharge and elderly patients with no one to help at home — all the while glancing over our shoulders at the peer-review organization. In HMOs we walk a tightrope between thrift and penuriousness, too often under the pressure of surveillance by bureaucrats more concerned with the bottom line than with other measures of achievement. In public health work we are frustrated in the face of plenty; the world's richest health care system is unable to ensure such basic services as prenatal care and immunizations.

Despite our disparate perspectives, we are united by dismay at the current state of medicine and by the conviction that an alternative must be developed. We hope to spark debate, to transform disaffection with what exists into a vision of what might be. To this end, we submit for public review, comment, and revision a working plan for a rational and humane health care system — a national health program.

We envisage a program that would be federally mandated and ultimately funded by the federal government but administered largely at the state and local level. The proposed system would eliminate financial barriers to care; minimize economic incentives for both excessive and insufficient care, discourage administrative interference and expense, improve the distribution of health facilities, and control costs by curtailing bureaucracy and fostering health planning. Our plan borrows many features from the Canadian national health program and adapts them to the unique circumstances of the United States. We suggest that, as in Canada's provinces, the national

From the Working Group on Program Design, Physicians for a National Health Program, Center for National Health Program Studies, Cambridge Hospital–Harvard Medical School, 1493 Cambridge St., Cambridge, MA 02139, where reprint requests should be addressed to Dr. Himmelstein.

*This proposal was drafted by a 30-member Writing Committee, then reviewed and endorsed by 412 other physicians representing virtually every state and medical specialty. A full list of the endorsers is available on request. The members of the Writing Committee were as follows: David U. Himmelstein, M.D., Cambridge, Mass. (cochair); Steffie Woolhandler, M.D., M.P.H., Cambridge, Mass. (cochair); Thomas S. Bodenheimer, M.D., San Francisco; David H. Bor, M.D., Cambridge, Mass.; Christine K. Cassel, M.D., Chicago; Mardge Cohen, M.D., Chicago; David A. Danielson, M.P.H., Newton, Mass.; Alan Drabkin, M.D., Cambridge, Mass.; Paul Epstein, M.D., Brookline, Mass.; Kenneth Frisof, M.D., Cleveland; Howard Frumkin, M.D., M.P.H., Philadelphia; Martha S. Gerrity, M.D., Chapel Hill, N.C.; Jerome D. Gorman, M.D., Richmond, Va.; Michelle D. Holmes, M.D., Cambridge, Mass.; Henry S. Kahn, M.D., Atlanta; Robert S. Lawrence, M.D., Cambridge, Mass.; Joanne Lukomnik, M.D., Bronx, N.Y.; Arthur Mazer, M.P.H., Cambridge, Mass.; Alan Meyers, M.D., Boston; Patrick Murray, M.D., Cleveland; Vicente Navarro, M.D., Dr.P.H., Baltimore; Peter Orris, M.D., Chicago; David C. Parish, M.D., M.P.H., Macon, Ga.; Richard J. Pels, M.D., Boston; Leonard S. Rodberg, Ph.D., New York City; Jeffrey Scavron, M.D., Springfield, Mass.; Gordon Schiff, M.D., Chicago; Isaac M. Taylor, M.D., Boston; Howard Waitzkin, M.D., Ph.D., Anaheim, Calif.; Paul H. Wise, M.D., M.P.H., Boston; and William Zinn, M.D., Cambridge, Mass.

Reprinted from the *New England Journal of Medicine*
320:102-108 (January 12), 1989

health program be tested initially in statewide demonstration projects. Thus, our proposal addresses both the structure of the national health program and the transition process necessary to implement the program in a single state. In each section below, we present a key feature of the proposal, followed by the rationale for our approach. Areas such as long-term care; public, occupational, environmental, and mental health; and medical education need much more development and will be addressed in detail in future proposals.

Coverage

Everyone would be included in a single public plan covering all medically necessary services, including acute, rehabilitative, long-term, and home care; mental health services; dental services; occupational health care; prescription drugs and medical supplies; and preventive and public health measures. Boards of experts and community representatives would determine which services were unnecessary or ineffective, and these would be excluded from coverage. As in Canada, alternative insurance coverage for services included under the national health program would be eliminated, as would patient copayments and deductibles.

Universal coverage would solve the gravest problem in health care by eliminating financial barriers to care. A single comprehensive program is necessary both to ensure equal access to care and to minimize the complexity and expense of billing and administration. The public administration of insurance funds would save tens of billions of dollars each year. The more than 1500 private health insurers in the United States now consume about 8 percent of revenues for overhead, whereas both the Medicare program and the Canadian national health program have overhead costs of only 2 to 3 percent. The complexity of our current insurance system, with its multiplicity of payers, forces U.S. hospitals to spend more than twice as much as Canadian hospitals on billing and administration and requires U.S. physicians to spend about 10 percent of their gross incomes on excess billing costs.[1] Eliminating insurance programs that duplicated the national health program coverage, though politically thorny, would clearly be within the prerogative of the Congress.[2] Failure to do so would require the continuation of the costly bureaucracy necessary to administer and deal with such programs.

Copayments and deductibles endanger the health of poor people who are sick,[3] decrease the use of vital inpatient medical services as much as they discourage the use of unnecessary ones,[4] discourage preventive care,[5] and are unwieldy and expensive to administer. Canada has few such charges, yet health costs are lower than in the United States and have risen slowly.[6,7] In the United States, in contrast, increasing copayments and deductibles have failed to slow the escalation of costs.

Instead of the confused and often unjust dictates of insurance companies, a greatly expanded program of technology assessment and cost-effectiveness evaluation would guide decisions about covered services, as well as about the allocation of funds for capital spending, drug formularies, and other issues.

Payment for Hospital Services

Each hospital would receive an annual lump-sum payment to cover all operating expenses — a "global" budget. The amount of this payment would be negotiated with the state national health program payment board and would be based on past expenditures, previous financial and clinical performance, projected changes in levels of services, wages and other costs, and proposed new and innovative programs. Hospitals would not bill for services covered by the national health program. No part of the operating budget could be used for hospital expansion, profit, marketing, or major capital purchases or leases. These expenditures would also come from the national health program fund, but monies for them would be appropriated separately.

Global prospective budgeting would simplify hospital administration and virtually eliminate billing, thus freeing up substantial resources for increased clinical care. Before the nationwide implementation of the national health program, hospitals in the states with demonstration programs could bill out-of-state patients on a simple per diem basis. Prohibiting the use of operating funds for capital purchases or profit would eliminate the main financial incentive for both excessive intervention (under fee-for-service payment) and skimping on care (under DRG-type prospective-payment systems), since neither inflating revenues nor limiting care could result in gain for the institution. The separate appropriation of funds explicitly designated for capital expenditures would facilitate rational health planning. In Canada, this method of hospital payment has been successful in containing costs, minimizing bureaucracy, improving the distribution of health resources, and maintaining the quality of care.[6-9] It shifts the focus of hospital administration away from the bottom line and toward the provision of optimal clinical services.

Payment for Physicians' Services, Ambulatory Care, and Medical Home Care

To minimize the disruption of existing patterns of care, the national health program would include three payment options for physicians and other practitioners: fee-for-service payment, salaried positions in institutions receiving global budgets, and salaried positions within group practices or HMOs receiving per capita (capitation) payments.

Fee-for-Service Payment

The state national health program payment board and a representative of the fee-for-service practitioners (perhaps the state medical society) would negotiate a simplified, binding fee schedule. Physicians would submit bills to the national health program on a simple form or by computer and would receive extra payment for any bill not paid within 30 days. Payments to physicians would cover only the services provided by physicians and their support staff and would exclude reimbursement for costly capital purchases of equipment for the office, such as CT scanners. Physicians who accepted payment from the national health program could bill patients directly only for uncovered services (as is done for cosmetic surgery in Canada).

Global Budgets

Institutions such as hospitals, health centers, group practices, clinics serving migrant workers, and medical home care agencies could elect to receive a global budget for the delivery of outpatient, home care, and physicians' services, as well as for preventive health care and patient-education programs. The negotiation process and the regulations covering capital expenditures and profits would be similar to those for inpatient hospital services. Physicians employed in such institutions would be salaried.

Capitation

HMOs, group practices, and other institutions could elect to be paid fees on a per capita basis to cover all outpatient care, physicians' services, and medical home care. The regulations covering the use of such payments for capital expenditures and for profits would be similar to those that would apply to hospitals. The capitation fee would not cover inpatient services (except care provided by a physician), which would be included in hospitals' global budgets. Selective enrollment policies would be prohibited, and patients would be permitted to leave an HMO or other health plan with appropriate notice. Physicians working in HMOs would be salaried, and financial incentives to physicians based on the HMO's financial performance would be prohibited.

The diversity of existing practice arrangements, each with strong proponents, necessitates a pluralistic approach. Under all three proposed options, capital purchases and profits would be uncoupled from payments to physicians and other operating costs — a feature that is essential for minimizing entrepreneurial incentives, containing costs, and facilitating health planning.

Under the fee-for-service option, physicians' office overhead would be reduced by the simplification of billing.[1] The improved coverage would encourage preventive care.[10] In Canada, fee-for-service practice with negotiated fee schedules and mandatory assignment (acceptance of the assigned fee as total payment) has proved to be compatible with cost containment, adequate incomes for physicians, and a high level of access to and satisfaction with care on the part of patients.[6,7] The Canadian provinces have responded to the inflationary potential of fee-for-service payment in various ways: by limiting the number of physicians, by monitoring physicians for outlandish practice patterns, by setting overall limits on a province's spending for physicians' services (thus relying on the profession to police itself), and even by capping the total reimbursement of individual physicians. These regulatory options have been made possible (and have not required an extensive bureaucracy) because all payment comes from a single source. Similar measures might be needed in the United States, although our penchant for bureaucratic hypertrophy might require a concomitant cap on spending for the regulatory apparatus. For example, spending for program administration and reimbursement bureaucracy might be restricted to 3 percent of total costs.

Global budgets for institutional providers would eliminate billing, while providing a predictable and stable source of income. Such funding could also encourage the development of preventive health programs in the community, such as education programs on the acquired immunodeficiency syndrome (AIDS), whose costs are difficult to attribute and bill to individual patients.

Continuity of care would no longer be disrupted when patients' insurance coverage changed as a result of retirement or a job change. Incentives for providers receiving capitation payments to skimp on care would be minimized, since unused operating funds could not be devoted to expansion or profit.

Payment for Long-Term Care

A separate proposal for long-term care is under development, guided by three principles. First, access to care should be based on need rather than on age or ability to pay. Second, social and community-based services should be expanded and integrated with institutional care. Third, bureaucracy and entrepreneurial incentives should be minimized through global budgeting with separate funding for capital expenses.

Allocation of Capital Funds, Health Planning, and Return on Equity

Funds for the construction or renovation of health facilities and for purchases of major equipment would be appropriated from the national health program budget. The funds would be distributed by state and regional health-planning boards composed of both experts and community representatives. Capital projects funded by private donations would require approval by the health-planning board if they entailed an increase in future operating expenses.

The national health program would pay owners of for-profit hospitals, nursing homes, and clinics a reasonable fixed rate of return on existing equity. Since virtually all new capital investment would be funded by the national health program, it would not be included in calculating the return on equity.

Current capital spending greatly affects future operating costs, as well as the distribution of resources. Effective health planning requires that funds go to high-quality, efficient programs in the areas of greatest need. Under the existing reimbursement system, which combines operating and capital payments, prosperous hospitals can expand and modernize, whereas impoverished ones cannot, regardless of the health needs of the population they serve or the quality of services they provide. The national health program would replace this implicit mechanism for distributing capital with an explicit one, which would facilitate (though not guarantee) allocation on the basis of need and quality. Insulating these crucial decisions from distortion by narrow interests would require the rigorous evaluation of the technology and assessment of needs, as well as the active involvement of providers and patients.

For-profit providers would be compensated for existing investments. Since new for-profit investment would be barred, the proprietary sector would gradually shrink.

Public, Environmental, and Occupational Health Services

Existing arrangements for public, occupational, and environmental health services would be retained in the short term. Funding for preventive health care would be expanded. Additional proposals dealing with these issues are planned.

Prescription Drugs and Supplies

An expert panel would establish and regularly update a list of all necessary and useful drugs and outpatient equipment. Suppliers would bill the national health program directly for the wholesale cost, plus a reasonable dispensing fee, of any item in the list that was prescribed by a licensed practitioner. The substitution of generic for proprietary drugs would be encouraged.

Funding

The national health program would disburse virtually all payments for health services. The total expenditure would be set at the same proportion of the gross national product as health costs represented in the year preceding the establishment of the national health program. Funds for the national health program could be raised through a variety of mechanisms. In the long run, funding based on an income tax or other progressive tax might be the fairest and most efficient solution, since tax-based funding is the least cumbersome and least expensive mechanism for collecting money. During the transition period in states with demonstration programs, the following structure would mimic existing funding patterns and minimize economic disruption.

Medicare and Medicaid

All current federal funds allocated to Medicare and Medicaid would be paid to the national health program. The contribution of each program would be based on the previous year's expenditures, adjusted for inflation. Using Medicare and Medicaid funds in this manner would require a federal waiver.

State and Local Funds

All current state and local funds for health care expenditures, adjusted for inflation, would be paid to the national health program.

Employer Contributions

A tax earmarked for the national health program would be levied on all employers. The tax rate would be set so that total collections equaled the previous year's statewide total of employers' expenditures for health benefits, adjusted for inflation. Employers obligated by preexisting contracts to provide health benefits could credit the cost of those benefits toward their national health program tax liability.

Private Insurance Revenues

Private health insurance plans duplicating the coverage of the national health program would be phased out over three years. During this transition period, all revenues from such plans would be turned over to the national health program, after the deduction of a reasonable fee to cover the costs of collecting premiums.

General Tax Revenues

Additional taxes, equivalent to the amount now spent by individual citizens for insurance premiums and out-of-pocket health costs, would be levied.

It would be critical for all funds for health care to flow through the national health program. Such single-source payment (monopsony) has been the cornerstone of cost containment and health planning in Canada. The mechanism of raising funds for the national health program would be a matter of tax policy, largely separate from the organization of the health care system itself. As in Canada, federal funding could attenuate inequalities among the states in financial and medical resources.

The transitional proposal for demonstration programs in selected states illustrates how monopsony payment could be established with limited disruption of existing patterns of health care funding. The employers' contribution would represent a decrease in costs for most firms that now provide health insurance and an increase for those that do not currently pay for benefits. Some provision might be needed to cushion the impact of the change on financially strapped small businesses. Decreased individual spending for health care would offset the additional tax burden on individual citizens. Private health insurance, with its attendant inefficiency and waste, would be largely eliminated. A program of job placement and retraining for insurance and hospital-billing employees would be an important component of the program during the transition period.

Discussion

The Patient's View

The national health program would establish a right to comprehensive health care. As in Canada, each person would receive a national health program card entitling him or her to all necessary medical care without copayments or deductibles. The card could be used with any fee-for-service practitioner and at any institution receiving a global budget. HMO members could receive nonemergency care only through their HMO, although they could readily transfer to the non-HMO option.

Thus, patients would have a free choice of providers, and the financial threat of illness would be eliminated. Taxes would increase by an amount equivalent to the current total of medical expenditures by individuals. Conversely, individuals' aggregate payments for medical care would decrease by the same amount.

The Practitioner's View

Physicians would have a free choice of practice settings. Treatment would no longer be constrained by the patient's insurance status or by bureaucratic dicta. On the basis of the Canadian experience, we anticipate that the average physician's income would change little, although differences among specialties might be attenuated.

Fee-for-service practitioners would be paid for the care of anyone not enrolled in an HMO. The entrepreneurial aspects of medicine — with the attendant problems as well as the possibilities — would be limited. Physicians could concentrate on medicine; every patient would be fully insured, but physicians could increase their incomes only by providing more care. Billing would involve imprinting the patient's national health program card on a charge slip, checking a box to indicate the complexity of the procedure or service, and sending the slip (or a computer record) to the physician-payment board. This simplification of billing would save thousands of dollars per practitioner in annual office expenses.[1]

Bureaucratic interference in clinical decision making would sharply diminish. Costs would be contained by controlling overall spending and by limiting entrepreneurial incentives, thus obviating the need for the kind of detailed administrative oversight that is characteristic of the DRG program and similar schemes. Indeed, there is much less administrative intrusion in day-to-day clinical practice in Canada (and most other countries with national health programs) than in the United States.[11,12]

Salaried practitioners would be insulated from the financial consequences of clinical decisions. Because savings on patient care could no longer be used for institutional expansion or profits, the pressure to skimp on care would be minimized.

The Effect on Other Health Workers

Nurses and other health care personnel would enjoy a more humane and efficient clinical milieu. The burdens of paperwork associated with billing would be lightened. The jobs of many administrative and insurance employees would be eliminated, necessitating a major effort at job placement and retraining. We advocate that many of these displaced workers be deployed in expanded programs of public health, health promotion and education, and home care and as support personnel to free nurses for clinical tasks.

The Effect on Hospitals

Hospitals' revenues would become stable and predictable. More than half the current hospital bureaucracy would be eliminated,[1] and the remaining administrators could focus on facilitating clinical care and planning for future health needs.

The capital budget requests of hospitals would be weighed against other priorities for health care investment. Hospitals would neither grow because they were profitable nor fail because of unpaid bills — although regional health planning would undoubtedly mandate that some expand and others close or be put to other uses. Responsiveness to community needs, the quality of care, efficiency, and innovation would replace financial performance as the bottom line. The elimination of new for-profit investment would lead to a gradual conversion of proprietary hospitals to not-for-profit status.

The Effect on the Insurance Industry

The insurance industry would feel the greatest impact of this proposal. Private insurance firms would have no role in health care financing, since the public administration of insurance is more efficient[1,13] and single-source payment is the key to both equal access and cost control. Indeed, most of the extra funds needed to finance the expansion of care would come from eliminating the overhead and profits of insurance companies and abolishing the billing apparatus necessary to apportion costs among the various plans.

The Effect on Corporate America

Firms that now provide generous employee health benefits would realize savings, because their contribution to the national health program would be less than their current health insurance costs. For example, health care expenditures by Chrysler, currently $5,300 annually per employee,[14] would fall to about

$1,600, a figure calculated by dividing the total current U.S. spending on health by private employers by the total number of full-time-equivalent, nongovernment employees. Since most firms that compete in international markets would save money, the competitiveness of U.S. products would be enhanced. However, costs would increase for companies that do not now provide health benefits. The average health care costs for employers would be unchanged in the short run. In the long run, overall health costs would rise less steeply because of improved health planning and greater efficiency. The funding mechanism ultimately adopted would determine the corporate share of those costs.

Health Benefits and Financial Costs

There is ample evidence that removing financial barriers to health care encourages timely care and improves health. After Canada instituted a national health program, visits to physicians increased among patients with serious symptoms.[15] Mortality rates, which were higher than U.S. rates through the 1950s and early 1960s, fell below those in the United States.[16] In the Rand Health Insurance Experiment, free care reduced the annual risk of dying by 10 percent among the 25 percent of U.S. adults at highest risk.[3] Conversely, cuts in California's Medicaid program led to worsening health.[17] Strong circumstantial evidence links the poor U.S. record on infant mortality with inadequate access to prenatal care.[18]

We expect that the national health program would cause little change in the total costs of ambulatory and hospital care; savings on administration and billing (about 10 percent of current health spending[1]) would approximately offset the costs of expanded services.[19,20] Indeed, current low hospital-occupancy rates suggest that the additional care could be provided at low cost. Similarly, many physicians with empty appointment slots could take on more patients without added office, secretarial, or other overhead costs. However, the expansion of long-term care (under any system) would increase costs. The experience in Canada suggests that the increased demand for acute care would be modest after an initial surge[21,22] and that improvements in health planning[8] and cost containment made possible by single-source payment[9] would slow the escalation of health care costs. Vigilance would be needed to stem the regrowth of costly and intrusive bureaucracy.

Unsolved Problems

Our brief proposal leaves many vexing problems unsolved. Much detailed planning would be needed to ease dislocations during the implementation of the program. Neither the encouragement of preventive health care and healthful life styles nor improvements in occupational and environmental health would automatically follow from the institution of a national health program. Similarly, racial, linguistic, geographic, and other nonfinancial barriers to access would persist. The need for quality assurance and continuing medical education would be no less pressing. High medical school tuitions that skew specialty choices and discourage low-income applicants, the underrepresentation of minorities, the role of foreign medical graduates, and other issues in medical education would remain. Some patients would still seek inappropriate emergency care, and some physicians might still succumb to the temptation to increase their incomes by encouraging unneeded services. The malpractice crisis would be only partially ameliorated. The 25 percent of judgments now awarded for future medical costs would be eliminated, but our society would remain litigious, and legal and insurance fees would still consume about two thirds of all malpractice premiums.[23] Establishing research priorities and directing funds to high-quality investigations would be no easier. Much further work in the area of long-term care would be required. Regional health planning and capital allocation would make possible, but not ensure, the fair and efficient allocation of resources. Finally, although insurance coverage for patients with AIDS would be ensured, the need for expanded prevention and research and for new models of care would continue. Although all these problems would not be solved, a national health program would establish a framework for addressing them.

Political Prospects

Our proposal will undoubtedly encounter powerful opponents in the health insurance industry, firms that do not now provide health benefits to employees, and medical entrepreneurs. However, we also have allies. Most physicians (56 percent) support some form of national health program, although 74 percent are convinced that most other doctors oppose it.[24] Many of the largest corporations would enjoy substantial savings if our proposal were adopted. Most significant, the great majority of Americans support a universal, comprehensive, publicly administered national health program, as shown by virtually every opinion poll in the past 30 years.[25,26] Indeed, a 1986 referendum question in Massachusetts calling for a national health program was approved two to one, carrying all 39 cities and 307 of the 312 towns in the commonwealth.[27] If mobilized, such public conviction could override even the most strenuous private opposition.

References

1. Himmelstein DU, Woolhandler S. Cost without benefit: administrative waste in U.S. health care. N Engl J Med 1986; 314:441-5.
2. Advisory opinion regarding House of Representatives Bill 85-H-7748 (No. 86-269-MP, R.I. Sup. Ct. Jan 5, 1987).
3. Brook RH, Ware JE Jr, Rogers WH, et al. Does free care improve adults' health? Results from a randomized controlled trial. N Engl J Med 1983; 309:1426-34.

4. Siu AL, Sonnenberg FA, Manning WG, et al. Inappropriate use of hospitals in a randomized trial of health insurance plans. N Engl J Med 1986; 315:1259-66.
5. Brian EW, Gibbens SF. California's Medi-Cal copayment experiment. Med Care 1974; 12:Suppl 12:1-303.
6. Iglehart JK. Canada's health care system. N Engl J Med 1986; 315:202-8, 778-84.
7. *Idem.* Canada's health care system: addressing the problem of physician supply. N Engl J Med 1986; 315:1623-8.
8. Detsky AS, Stacey SR, Bombardier C. The effectiveness of a regulatory strategy in containing hospital costs: the Ontario experience, 1967-1981. N Engl J Med 1983; 309:151-9.
9. Evans RG. Health care in Canada: patterns of funding and regulation. In: McLachlan G, Maynard A, eds. The public/private mix for health: the relevance and effects of change. London: Nuffield Provincial Hospitals Trust, 1982:369-424.
10. Woolhandler S, Himmelstein DU. Reverse targeting of preventive care due to lack of health insurance. JAMA 1988; 259:2872-4.
11. Reinhardt UE. Resource allocation in health care: the allocation of lifestyles to providers. Milbank Q 1987; 65:153-76.
12. Hoffenberg R. Clinical freedom. London: Nuffield Provincial Hospitals Trust, 1987.
13. Horne JM, Beck RG. Further evidence on public versus private administration of health insurance. J Public Health Policy 1981; 2:274-90.
14. Cronin C. Next Congress to grapple with U.S. health policy, competitiveness abroad. Bus Health 1986; 4(2):55.
15. Enterline PE, Salter V, McDonald AD, McDonald JC. The distribution of medical services before and after "free" medical care — the Quebec experience. N Engl J Med 1973; 289:1174-8.
16. Roemer R, Roemer MI. Health manpower policy under national health insurance: the Canadian experience. Hyattsville, Md.: Health Resources Administration, 1977. (DHEW publication no. (HRA) 77-37.)
17. Lurie N, Ward NB, Shapiro MF, et al. Termination of Medi-Cal benefits: a follow-up study one year later. N Engl J Med 1986; 314:1266-8.
18. Institute of Medicine. Preventing low birthweight. Washington, D.C.: National Academy Press, 1985.
19. Newhouse JP, Manning WG, Morris CN, et al. Some interim results from a controlled trial of cost sharing in health insurance. N Engl J Med 1981; 305:1501-7.
20. Himmelstein DU, Woolhandler S. Free care: a quantitative analysis of the health and cost effects of a national health program. Int J Health Serv 1988; 18:393-9.
21. LeClair M. The Canadian health care system. In: Andreopoulos S, ed. National health insurance: can we learn from Canada? New York: John Wiley, 1975:11-92.
22. Evans RG. Beyond the medical marketplace: expenditure, utilization and pricing of insured health care in Canada. In: Andreopoulos S, ed. National health insurance: can we learn from Canada? New York: John Wiley, 1975:129-78.
23. Danzon PM. Medical malpractice: theory, evidence, and public policy. Cambridge, Mass.: Harvard University Press, 1985.
24. Colombotas J, Kirchner C. Physicians and social change. New York: Oxford University Press, 1986.
25. Navarro V. Where is the popular mandate? N Engl J Med 1982; 307:1516-8.
26. Pokorny G. Report card on health care. Health Manage Q 1988; 10(1):3-7.
27. Danielson DA, Mazer A. Results of the Massachusetts Referendum on a national health program. J Public Health Policy 1987; 8:28-35.

SECTION 7

BIBLIOGRAPHY

BIBLIOGRAPHY

This Bibliography presents additional sources of information on U.S. health care reform. The sources are grouped under the topic headings listed below. Some of the articles and documents touch on several aspects of health care reform and are cited under more than one heading.

Access 657

Cost Containment 658

Effect on Small Businesses . . . 660

Ethics and Values 660

Health Care Reform: Overview . . . 661

Health Care Reform: Focused Discussion . 664

History 668

Insurance 669

International Health Care Systems . . 669

Managed Competition 670

Political Action Committees (PACs) . . 672

Public Opinion 672

Statewide Reforms 673

Statistics 674

ABBREVIATED PERIODICAL NAMES

Periodical	Abbreviation
Annals of Internal Medicine	Ann Intern Med
Archives of Internal Medicine	Arch Intern Med
Consumer Reports	Consumer Rep
Health Care Financing Review	Health Care Financing Rev
Health Maintenance Quarterly	Health Maintenance Q
Health Services Management	Health Services Manage
Health Systems Review	Health Systems Rev
Iowa Law Review	Iowa Law Rev
Journal of the American Medical Assoc.	JAMA
Journal of American Health Policy	J Am Health Policy
Journal of the National Medical Assoc.	J Natl Med Assoc
Medical Care Review	Med Care Rev
Medical Group Management	Med Group Manage
New England Journal of Medicine	New Engl J Med

ACCESS

American Hospital Association. (July 1992). *Selected Resources: Health Care Reform.* Washington D.C.: AHA.

Aukerman GF. (1991). Access to Health Care for the Uninsured: The Perspective of the American Academy of Family Physicians. *JAMA.* 265:2856-2858.

Brooks DD, Smith DR, Anderson RJ. (1991). Medical Apartheid: An American Perspective. *JAMA.* 266:2746-2749.

Burke M. (1992). Hawaii's Health Care Plan Stirs Capitol Hill Debate Over Access. *Hospitals.* 66:32-36.

Cornelius LJ. (1991). Access to Medical Care for Black Americans with an Episode of Illness. *J Natl Med Assoc.* 83:617-626.

Davidson RJ. (1992). Community Care Networks: Cornerstone of Health Care Reform. *J Am Health Policy.* 2(3):12-15.

Fraser I. Health Policy and Access to Care. In: Litman TJ, Robins LS. *Health Politics and Policy.* 2nd ed. Albany, NY: Delmar Publishers, 1991:302-319.

Friedman E. (1991). The Uninsured: From Dilemma to Crisis. *JAMA.* 265:2491-2495.

Ginzberg E., Ostow M. (1991). Beyond Universal Health Insurance to Effective Health Care. *JAMA.* 265:2559-2562.

Health Care Advisory Board. *America's Uninsured: Special Report for Civic and Business Leaders.* Washington D.C.: HCAB, 1992.

Johnson C. (1991). Access to Health Care in America. *J Natl Med Assoc.* 83:197-200.

Morrisey MA, Kletke PR, Marder WD. (Spring 1991). The Role of Local Hospitals in Physician Rural Location Decisions. *Inquiry.* 28:7-18.

Olsen CM. (1991). Hospital Admission Through the Emergency Department: The Obstructed Pathway. *JAMA.* 266:2274.

Stern RS, Weissman JS, Epstein AM. (1991). The Emergency Department as a Pathway to Admission for Poor and High-Cost Patients. *JAMA.* 266:2238-2243.

Todd JS, Seekins SV, Krichbaum JA, Harvey LK. (1991). Health Access America - Strengthening the US Health Care System. *JAMA.* 265:2503-2506.

Weissman JS, Stern R, Fielding SL, *et al.* (1991). Delayed Access to Health Care: Risk Factors, Reasons, and Consequences. *Ann Intern Med.* 114:325-331.

COST CONTAINMENT

Coles R. How to Improve America's Medical Care. *Fortune* May 4, 1992 (Special Advertising Section).

Custer WS. (Spring 1991). Employer Health Care Plan Design and Its Effect on Plan Costs. *Inquiry.* 28:81-86.

Dentzer S. How to Fight Killer Health Costs. *U.S. News and World Rep.* September 23, 1991:50-58.

Eddy DM. (1990). Connecting Value and Costs: Whom Do We Ask and What Do We Ask Them? *JAMA.* 1264:1737-1739.

Eddy DM. (1990). What Do We Do About Costs? *JAMA.* 264:1161-1170.

Enthoven AC. (1991). Market Forces and Health Care Costs. *JAMA.* 266:2751-2754.

Fleming ST. (Spring 1991). The Relationship Between Quality and Cost: Pure and Simple? *Inquiry.* 28:29-38.

Frank RG. Salkever DS, Sharfstein SS. (Summer 1991). A New Look at Rising Mental Health Insurance Costs. *Health Affairs.* 10:116-123.

Greene J. (March 9, 1992). Systems Geared Up For Coming Reforms. *Modern Healthcare.* 22(10):24-28.

Holahan J, Dor A, Zuckerman S. (1990). Understanding the Recent Growth in Medicare Physician Expenditures. *JAMA.* 263:1658-1661.

Levit KR, Lazenby HC, Cowan CA, Letsch SW. (1991). National Health Expenditures, 1990. *Health Care Financing Rev.* 13(1):29-54.

Rice T. (1992). Containing Health Care Costs in the United States. *Med Care Rev.* 49(1):19-65.

Schwartz WB, Mendelson DN. (1991). Hospital Cost Containment in the 1980s -- Hard Lessons Learned and Prospects for the 1990s. *New Engl J Med.* 324:1037-1042.

Sonnefeld ST, Waldo DR, Lemieux JA, McKusick DR. (1991). Projections of Health Expenditures Through the Year 2000. *Health Care Financing Rev.* 13:1-27.

Witkin G, Friedman D, Gutman M. Health Care Fraud. *U.S. News & World Rep.* February 24, 1992: 34-43.

Woolhandler S, Himmelstein DU. (1991). The Deteriorating Administrative Efficiency of the U.S. Health Care System. *New Engl J Med.* 324:1253-1258.

EFFECT ON SMALL BUSINESSES

Cantor JC, Barrand NL, Desonia RA, *et al.* (Spring 1991). DataWatch: Business Leaders' Views on Health Care. *Health Affairs.* 10:98-105.

Edwards JN, Blendon RJ, Leitman R, Morrison E, Morrison I, Taylor H. (Spring 1992). Small Businesses and the National Health Care Reform Debate. *Health Affairs.* 164-173.

Nemes J. (1992). Making Their Voices Clearly Heard: Investor-Owned Facilities Are Working Hard to Share Their Opinions on Healthcare Reform. *Modern Healthcare.* 23(13):37-44.

Thompson R. (1992). States Take Lead in Health Reform. *Nation's Business.* 18-26.

Zedlewski SR, Acs GP, Winterbottom CW. (Spring 1992). Play-or-Pay Employer Mandates: Potential Effects. *Health Affairs.* 62-83.

ETHICS AND VALUES

Binstock RH, Post SG. *Too Old For Health Care?* Baltimore, MD: The Johns Hopkins University Press, 1991.

Botelho RJ. (1991). Overcoming the Prejudice Against Establishing a National Health Care System. *Arch Intern Med.* 151:863-869.

Callahan D. (1991). The Oregon Initiative: Ethics and Priority Setting. *Health Matrix.* 1(2):157-170.

Center for Biomedical Ethics. *The Community Dialogue on Values and Health Care: The Medically Underserved.* Cleveland, OH: 1990.

Daniels N. (1991). Is the Oregon Rationing Plan Fair? *JAMA.* 265(17):2232-2235.

Darr K. *Ethics in Health Services Management.* New York, NY: Praeger Publishers, 1987.

Dougherty CJ. (1992). The Excesses of Individualism. *Health Progress.* 73:22-28.

Eddy DM. (1991). The Individual vs Society: Is There A Conflict? *JAMA.* 265(11):1446, 1449-1450.

Eddy DM. (1991). The Individual vs Society: Resolving the Conflict. *JAMA.* 265(18):2399-2406.

Ellwood DT. *Poor Support: Poverty in the American Family.* New York, NY: Basic Books, Inc. 1988.

Looking for the Ethical Basis in Health Care Reform Plans. (1992). *Hospital Ethics.* 8(2):1-4.

Lundberg GD. (1992). National Health Care Reform: The Aura of Inevitability Intensifies. *JAMA.* 267(18):2521-2524.

Priester R. (Spring 1992). A Values Framework for Health System Reform. *Health Affairs.* 11:84-107.

Ross JW. *Handbook for Hospital Ethics Committees.* Chicago: American Hospital Publishing, Inc. 1986.

Witkin G, Friedman D & Gutman M. Health Care Fraud. *U.S. News & World Rep.* February 24, 1992:34-43.

HEALTH CARE REFORM: OVERVIEW

Association of American Medical Colleges. *Avenues to Access: A Resource Guide to Health Care Reform.* Washington D.C.: 1992.

Blendon RJ, Donelan K. (1990). The Public and the Emerging Debate Over National Health Insurance. *New Engl J Med.* 323:208-212.

Blendon RJ, Edwards JN, Hyams AL. (1992). Making the Critical Choices. *JAMA.* (267)18:2509-2520.

Blumenthal D. (1991). The Timing and Course of Health Care Reform. *New Engl J Med.* 325:198-200.

Bromberg MD. (1991). Health Care Reform: The Issue is Trust. *Health Systems Rev.* 24:3.

Buckley J. Clinton's Big Test: The Fate of the Budget, The Economy and His First Term Rests on Containing Medical Costs. *U.S. News &World Rep.* November 23, 1992:26-39.

Burke M. (1992). Business and Labor Move Forward Via Joint Health Care Reform Plan. *Hospitals.* 66:52-55.

Burke M. (1992). Comprehensive vs. Incremental Reform: The Debate Intensifies. *Hospitals.* 66:38-42.

Castro J. Condition Critical. *Time.* November 25, 1991:34-42.

Coddington DC, Keen DJ, Moore KD, Clarke RL. *The Crisis in Health Care: Costs, Choices, and Strategies.* San Francisco: Jossey-Bass Publishers, 1990.

Committee on Ways and Means, U.S. House of Representatives. *U.S. Health Care Spending: Trends, Contributing Factors, and Proposals for Reform.* Washington D.C.: U.S. GAO, June 1991; GAO publication no. (HRD)91-102.

Committee on Ways and Means, U.S. House of Representatives. *Health Care Coverage and Costs: Major Legislative Proposals.* Washington D.C.: October 4, 1991.

Congress of the United States. *Universal Health Insurance Coverage Using Medicare's Payment Rates.* Washington D.C.: Congressional Budget Office, December 1991.

Congress of the United States. *Rising Health Care Costs: Causes, Implications, and Strategies.* Washington D.C.: Congressional Budget Office, April 1991.

Health Care Information Center. *Insuring the Uninsured: A Guide to the Proposals and Players.* Faulkner & Gray, Inc., Washington D.C.: 1992.

Health Care Information Center. *Medicine & Health.* [newsletter] Faulkner & Gray, Inc., Washington D.C.

Frieden J. (1991). Many Roads Lead to Health System Reform. *Business and Health.* 9(11):38-44,46-55,58.

Fuchs VR. (1991). National Health Insurance Revisited. *Health Affairs.* 10(4):7-17.

Garland SB. The Health Care Crisis: A Prescription for Reform. *Business Week.* October 7, 1991:59-66.

Greene J. (1992). Systems geared up for coming reforms. *Modern Healthcare.* 22(10):24-28.

Health Care System Meltdown by 1996? *Health Business.* May 22, 1992; 7(21):4.

Hopkins K. (1992). Business and the Future of American Health Care. *Business Week* (Special Advertising Section) 1-15.

Kinzer DM. (1990). Universal Entitlement to Health Care: Can We Get There From Here? *N Engl J Med.* 322:467-470.

Long RE. *The Crisis in Health Care.* New York: The H.W. Wilson Company, 1991.

Lundburg GD. (1991). National Health Care Reform: An Aura of Inevitability is Upon Us. *JAMA.* 265:2566-2567.

Lundberg GD. (1992). National Health Care Reform: The Aura of Inevitability Intensifies. *JAMA.* 267:2521-2524.

Monroe JA. The Politics of Health Care Reform. In: Litman TJ, Robins LS. *Health Politics and Policy.* 2nd ed. Albany: Delmar Publishers, 1991:273-286.

Prospective Payment Assessment Commission. *Medicare and the American Health Care System: Report to the Congress.* Washington D.C.: June 1992.

Randall A. (1992). The Health Debate USA. *Health Services Manage.* 88(3):10-14.

Wasted Health Care Dollars. *Consumer Rep.* July 1992:435-448.

HEALTH CARE REFORM: FOCUSED DISCUSSION

Aaron HJ. (1991). Choosing From the Health Care Reform Menu. *J Am Health Policy.* 1:23-27.

Benham L, Dennis WJ, Ferrara PJ, *et al. An Agenda for Solving America's Health Care Crisis.* Report No. 151. Dallas: National Center for Policy Analysis, May 1990.

Bigelow V, Trees CB. (1991). A Model for Primary Care Delivery to a Widely Dispersed Medically Indigent Population. *JAMA.* 266:563-564.

Blendon RJ, Edwards JN. *System in Crisis: The Case for Health Care Reform.* Washington D.C.: Faulkner & Gray; Health Care Information Center, 1991.

Brumbach K, Bodenheimer T, Himmelstein DU, Woolhandler S. (1991). Liberal Benefits, Conservative Spending: The Physicians for a National Health Program Proposal. *JAMA.* 265:2549-2554.

Butler SM. (1991). A Tax Reform Strategy to Deal With the Uninsured. *JAMA.* 265-2541-2544.

Claiborne W. Out of the Frying Pan, Into Canada: When it Comes to Health Care, The U.S. Should Look Before it Leaps. *Washington Post* August 12-18, 1991:6-7.

Committee on Ways and Means, U.S. House of Representatives. *Health Care Coverage and Costs: Major Legislative Proposals.* Washington D.C.: October 4, 1991.

Committee on Ways and Means, U.S. House of Representatives. *U.S. Health Care Spending: Trends, Contributing Factors, and Proposals for Reform.* Washington D.C.: U.S. GAO, June 1991; GAO publication no. (HRD)91-102.

Congress of the United States. *Rising Health Care Costs: Causes, Implications, and Strategies.* Washington D.C.: Congressional Budget Office, April 1991.

Congress of the United States. *Universal Health Insurance Coverage Using Medicare's Payment Rates.* Washington D.C.: Congressional Budget Office, December 1991.

Daniels N. (1991). Is the Oregon Rationing Plan Fair? *JAMA.* 265:2232-2235.

Davidson RJ. (1992). Community Care Networks: Cornerstone of Health Care Reform. *J Am Health Policy* 2(3):12-15.

Davis K. (1991). Expanding Medicare and Employer Plans to Achieve Universal Health Insurance. *JAMA.* 265:252-2528.

Dukakis MS, Roseman C. (1992). Learning from the Aloha State. *J Am Health Policy.* 2(2):11-14.

Enthoven A, Kronick R. (1989). A Consumer-Choice Health Plan for the 1990s: Universal Health Insurance in a System Designed to Promote Quality and Economy, I. *N Engl J Med.* 320(1):29-37.

Enthoven A, Kronick R. (1989). A Consumer-Choice Health Plan for the 1990s: Universal Health Insurance in a System Designed to Promote Quality and Economy, II. *N Engl J Med.* 320(1):94-101.

Enthoven AC, Kronick R. (1991). Universal Health Insurance Through Incentives Reform. *JAMA.* 265:2532-2536.

Faltermayer E. Let's Really Cure the Health System. *Fortune.* March 23, 1992:46-58.

Feder J. Testimony Before the Committee on Labor and Human Resources. Center for Health Policy Studies, Washington D.C.: March 4, 1992.

Feder J. Testimony before the Subcommittee on Education and Health. Center for Health Policy Studies, Washington D.C.: October 2, 1991.

Fein R. (1991). The Health Security Partnership: A Federal-State Universal Insurance and Cost-Containment Program. *JAMA.* 265:2555-2558.

Ferrara J. *Averting the Medicare Crisis: Health IRAs.* Policy Analysis No. 62 Washington, D.C.: Cato Institute, October 1985.

Friedman E. (1991). What's Ahead for Managed Care? *Business and Health.* 9(13):42-49.

Goodman JC, Ferrara PA, Musgrave GL, Rahn R. *Solving the Problem of Medicare.* Report No. 109. Dallas: National Center for Policy Analysis, January 1984.

Goodman JC, Musgrave GL. *Patient Power: Solving America's Health Care Crisis.* Washington D.C.: Cato Institute, 1992.

Hagland MM. (1992). The Sagging Safety Net: Emergency Departments on the Brink of Crisis. *Hospitals.* 66(4):26-32.

Hard R. (1991). Pharmaceutical Prices Continue to Drive up Supply Costs. *Hospitals.* 65(24):26-29.

Health Care Information Center. *Insuring the Uninsured: A Guide to the Proposals and Players.* Faulkner & Gray, Inc., Washington D.C.: 1992.

Himmelstein DU. (1991). The Case for a National Health Program. *J Natl Med Assoc.* 83:1049-1053.

Holahan J, Moon M, Welch WP, Zuckerman S. (1991). An American Approach to Health System Reform. *JAMA.* 265:2537-2540.

The Kansas Employer Coalition on Health, Task Force on Long-term Solutions. (1991). A Framework for Reform of the US Health Care Financing and Provision System. *JAMA.* 265:2529-2531.

Lamm RD. (1992). Rationing: The Unspoken Issue. *Foundation News.* January/February:27-29.

Nutter DO, Helms CM, Whitcomb ME, Weston WD. (1991). Restructuring Health Care in the United States: A Proposal for the 1990s. *JAMA.* 265:2516-2520.

Priester R. (Spring 1992). A Values Framework for Health System Reform. *Health Affairs.* 11:84-107.

Reinhardt U. (Summer 1991). Breaking American Health Policy Gridlock. *Health Affairs.* 10:96-103.

Rockefeller JD. (1991). A Call for Action: The Pepper Commission's Blueprint for Health Care Reform. *JAMA.* 265:2507-2510.

Thier SO. (1991). Health Care Reform: Who Will Lead? *Ann Intern Med.* 115(1):54-58.

Weissenstein E. (1992). Long-term Care Begins to Emerge as an Issue in Health Reform Debate. *Modern Healthcare.* 22(16):26-30.

Wilensky GR. (1991). Treat the Causes, Not the Symptoms of the Health Care Cost Problems. *J Am Health Policy.* 1(2):15-17.

Zedlewski SR, Acs GP, Winterbottom CW. (Spring 1992). Play-or-Pay Employer Mandates: Potential Effects. *Health Affairs.* 11:62-83.

HISTORY

Anderson OW. Health Services in the United States: A Growth Enterprise for a Hundred Years. In: Litman TJ, Robins LS. *Health Politics and Policy.* 2nd ed. Albany, NY: Delmar Publishers, 1991:38-52.

Anderson OW. *Health Services in the United States: A Growth Enterprise Since 1875.* Ann Arbor, MI: Health Administration Press, 1985.

Fawley IL. (1992). A Historical Perspective on Health Reform. *Med Group Manage J.* 39:44-49.

Rosenberg CE. *The Care of Strangers: The Rise of America's Hospital System.* New York, NY: Basic Books, Inc., 1987.

Starr P. *The Social Transformation of American Medicine.* New York, NY: Basic Books, Inc., 1983.

Weller CD. (1984). Free Choice as a Restraint of Trade in American Health Care Delivery and Insurance. *Iowa Law Rev.* 69(5):1351-1392.

INSURANCE

Cotton P. (1991). Preexisting Conditions 'Hold Americans Hostage' to Employers and Insurance. *JAMA.* 265:2451-2453.

Health Insurance Association of America. *Source Book of Health Insurance Data.* Washington D.C.: 1991.

Kolata G. An Old Health Insurance Idea Returns: Sharing the Risk. *New York Times.* June 28, 1992:6E.

Wagner L. Report Links Poor Care to Level of Insurance. *Modern Healthcare.* September 28, 1992:35.

Weller CD. (1984). Free Choice as a Restraint of Trade in American Health Care Delivery and Insurance. *Iowa Law Rev.* 69(5):1351-1392.

INTERNATIONAL HEALTH CARE SYSTEMS

Altman S, Jackson T. (Fall 1991). Health Care in Australia: Lessons From Down Under. *Health Affairs.* 10:129-146.

American Hospital Association. *Briefing: Canadian Health Care.* Washington D.C.: January 1990.

Blendon RJ, Taylor H. (1989). Views on Health Care: Public Opinion in Three Nations. *Health Affairs.* 8(1):150-157.

Day P, Rudolf K. (Fall 1991). Britain's Health Care Experiment. *Health Affairs.* 10:39-59.

Doherty K. (1989). Is the Canadian System as Good as it Looks for Employers? *Business and Health.* 7(7):31-34.

Fuchs VR, Hahn JS. (1990). How Does Canada Do It? A Comparison of Expenditures for Physicians' Services in the United States and Canada. *New Engl J Med.* 323:884-890.

Goodman JC, Musgrave GL. *Patient Power: Solving America's Health Care Crisis.* Washington D.C.: Cato Institute, 1992.

Hurst JK. (Spring 1991). Reform of Health Care in Germany. *Health Care Financing Rev.* 12:73-86.

Ikegami, N. (1992). The Economics of Health Care in Japan. *Science.* 258:614-618.

Kirkman-Liff BL. (1991). Health Insurance Values and Implementation in the Netherlands and the Federal Republic of Germany. *JAMA* 265:2496-2502.

Schieber GJ, PoullierJ-P. (Spring 1991). International Health Spending: Issues and Trends. *Health Affairs.* 10:106-116.

Schneider M. (1991). Health Care Cost Containment in the Federal Republic of Germany. *Health Care Financing Rev.* 12:87-101.

Starfield B. (1991). Primary Care and Health: A Cross-National Comparison. *JAMA.* 266:2268-2271.

White JH. (1991). U.S. Healthcare Reform: Lessons From Other Countries. *Health Progress.* 72(8):14-16.

MANAGED COMPETITION

Aaron HJ, Schwartz WB. (1993). Managed Competition: Little Cost Containment Without Budget Limits. *Health Affairs.* 12(Supp.):204-215.

Bergthold LA. (1993). Benefit Design Choices Under Managed Competition. *Health Affairs.* 12(Supp.):99-109.

Enthoven AC. (1993). The History and Principles of Managed Competition. *Health Affairs.* 12(Supp.):24-48.

Faltermayer E. Yes, The Market Can Curb Health Costs. *Fortune.* December 28, 1992:84-88.

Fielding JE, Rice T. (1993). Can Managed Competition solve the Problems of Market Failure? *Health Affairs.* 12(Supp.):216-228.

Hillman AL, Greer WR, Goldfarb N. (1993). Safeguarding Quality in Managed Competition. *Health Affairs.* 12(Supp.):110-122.

Hudson T. (1992). Health Care Reform Advocates Urge Changes to Antitrust Laws. *Hospitals.* 66(7):40-42.

Johnsson J. (1992). Managed Care in the 1990s: Providers' New Role For Innovative Health Delivery. *Hospitals* 66:26-30.

Kongstvedt PR. *The Managed Health Care Handbook.* Gaithersburg, MD: Aspen Publishers, Inc., 1989:11-18, 329-334.

Robinson JC. (1993). A Payment Method for Health Insurance Purchasing Cooperatives. *Health Affairs.* 12(Supp.):65-75.

Schlesinger M, Mechanic D. (1993). Challenges for Managed Competition from Chronic Illness. *Health Affairs.* 12(Supp.):123-137.

Sofaer S. (1993). Informing and Protecting Consumers Under Managed Competition. *Health Affairs.* 12(Supp.):76-86.

Starr P. (1993). Design of Health Insurance Purchasing Cooperatives. *Health Affairs.* 12(Supp.):58-64.

Starr P, Zelman WA. (1993). A Bridge to Compromise: Competition Under a Budget. *Health Affairs.* 12(Supp.): 7-23.

Winslow R. 'Managed-Care Networks' Show Promise. *Wall Street J.* March 24, 1992:B1.

Zelman WA. (1993). Who Should Govern the Purchasing Cooperative? *Health Affairs.* 12(Supp.):49-57.

POLITICAL ACTION COMMITTEES (PACS)

HIAA's Gamble to Block National Health Insurance. (May 1992). *Health Business.* 7(21):4.

Kemper V, Novak V. (October 1991). A Plague on Both Their Houses. *Common Cause Magazine.* 1-8.

Kemper V, Novak V. (Jan-Mar 1992). What's Blocking Health Care Reform? *Common Cause Magazine.* 8-25.

PUBLIC OPINION

Burke M. (1992). Health Care Surveys: Pollsters Present Debatable Results. *Hospitals.* 66(13):38-42.

Hagland M. (1992). Voices of the People. *Hospitals.* 66(13):32-36.

Health Care For America Policy Institute. *Guide to Health Care Reform.* Washington D.C.: 1992.

Health Care Information Center. *The Healthcare 500.* Faulkner & Gray, Inc., Washington D.C.: 1992.

Hudson T. (1992). Educating the Public. *Hospitals.* 66(13):38-42.

Melville K. *The Health Care Crisis: Containing Costs, Expanding Coverage.* New York: McGraw-Hill, 1992.

Project Vote Smart. *The Voter's Self-Defense Manual.* Corvallis, Oregon: 1992.

Project Vote Smart. *Reporter's Source Book.* Corvallis, Oregon: 1992.

Public Agenda Foundation. *Condition Critical: The American Health Care Forum.* New York, NY: 1992.

Public Agenda Foundation. *Faulty Diagnosis: Public Misconception About Health Care Reform.* New York, NY: 1992.

Reiser SJ. (1992). Consumer Competence and the Reform of American Health Care. *JAMA.* 267(11):1511-1515.

Rochefort DA, Pezza PE. Public Opinion and Health Policy. In: Litman TJ, Robins LS. *Health Politics and Policy.* 2nd ed. Albany NY: Delmar Publishers, 1991:247-269.

Yankelovich D. *Coming to Public Judgment: Making Democracy Work in a Complex World.* Syracuse, New York: Syracuse University Press, 1991.

Yankelovich D, Immerwahr J. (1991). A Perception Gap. *Health Maintenance Q.* 10(3)11-14.

STATEWIDE REFORMS

Beauchamp DE, Rouse RL. (1990). Universal New York Health Care -- A Single-Payer Strategy Linking Cost Control and Universal Access. *New Eng J Med.* 323:640.

Brown LD. (Summer 1991). The National Politics of Oregon's Rationing Plan. *Health Affairs.* 10:28-51.

Dixon J, Welch H. (1991). Priority Setting: Lessons From Oregon. *The Lancet.* 337:891-894.

Fox DM, Leicher HM. (Summer 1991). Rationing Care in Oregon: The New Accountability. *Health Affairs.* 10:7-27.

Kronick R. (Spring 1991). Can Massachusetts Pay For Health Care For All? *Health Affairs.* 10:26-44.

Lipson DJ. An Overview of State Roles in Health Care Policy. In: Litman TJ, Robins LS. *Health Politics and Policy.* 2nd ed. Albany: Delmar Publishers, 1991:170-189.

National Governors' Association. *A Healthy America: The Challenge for the States.* Washington, D.C.: NGA, 1991.

Pallarito K. (1992). States in the Eye of Reform. *Modern Healthcare.* 22(21):26-28.

Weissenstein E. (1992). Proposal to Streamline States' Waiver Process. *Modern Healthcare.* 22(25):4.

STATISTICS

Committee on Ways and Means, U.S. House of Representatives. *1991 Green Book: Background Material and Data on Programs Within the Jurisdiction of the Committee on Ways and Means.* U.S. Government Printing Office: Washington D.C.: 1991.

Committee on Ways and Means, U.S. House of Representatives. *Health Care Coverage and Costs: Major Legislative Proposals.* Washington D.C.: October 4, 1991.

Committee on Ways and Means, U.S. House of Representatives. *U.S. Health Care Spending: Trends, Contributing Factors, and Proposals for Reform.* Washington D.C.: U.S. GAO, June 1991; GAO publication no. (HRD)91-102.

Congress of the United States. *Economic Implications of Rising Health Care Costs.* Washington D.C.: Congressional Budget Office, October 1992.

Congress of the United States. *Projections of National Health Expenditures.* Washington D.C.: Congressional Budget Office, October 1992.

Congress of the United States. *Rising Health Care Costs: Causes, Implications, and Strategies.* Washington D.C.: Congressional Budget Office, April 1991.

Congress of the United States. *Universal Health Insurance Coverage Using Medicare's Payment Rates.* Washington D.C.: Congressional Budget Office, December 1991.

Health Insurance Association of America. *Source Book of Health Insurance Data.* Washington D.C.: 1991.

Nelson C, Short K. (1990). Health Insurance Coverage 1986-1988 (SIPP). Series P-70, No. 17.

Prospective Payment Assessment Commission. *Medicare and the American Health Care System: Report to the Congress.* Washington D.C.: June 1992.

Sonnefeld ST, Waldo DR, Lemieux JA, McKusick DR. (1991). Projections of National Health Expenditures Through the Year 2000. *Health Care Financing Rev.* 13(1):1-27.

SECTION 8

INDEX

INDEX

A

Aaron, Henry J., 265, 593-607

Aaron Plan
- Summaries and Key Concepts, 263-268; Refining Key Concepts, 86, 100, 103, 107, 144, 150-151; Original Text, 593-607

Accountable Health Plan
- definition of, 9; Jackson Hole Group, 214; Conservative Democratic Forum, 221

acute care
- definition of, 10

adverse selection
- definition of, 10-11

American Association of Retired Persons Plan
- Summaries and Key Concepts, 229-236; Refining Key Concepts, 94, 97, 102, 129, 130-131, 135, 142, 149; Original Text, 505-514

American College of Physicians Plan
- Summaries and Key Concepts, 255-261; Refining Key Concepts, 85, 89, 100, 103, 110, 117, 1 29, 144; Original Text, 581-591

American Hospital Association, 491, 501-504
American Hospital Association Plan
Summaries and Key Concepts, 205-212; Refining Key Concepts, 89, 91, 94, 96, 98, 105, 128, 134, 138, 142; Original Text, 451-459
American Nurses Association Plan
Summaries and Key Concepts, 193-197; Refining Key Concepts, 87, 91, 96, 98, 102, 116; Original Text, 421-436
antitrust
definition of, 11-12; Chart of the Debate, 71, 75; Refining Key Concepts, 119; Bush Plan, 173

B

balance billing
definition of, 12
Bibliography, 653-675
bundling
definition of, 12
Bush Plan
Summaries and Key Concepts, 169-174; Refining Key Concepts, 83, 99, 103, 109, 111, 113, 119, 120, 136, 153; Original Text, 339-371
Bush, President George
See "Bush Plan"
Butler, Stuart M., 176-177, 373-388
buy into
definition of, 13

C

capitation
definition of, 13-14; Catholic Health Association Plan, 270
catastrophic care
definition of, 14
Catholic Health Association Plan
Summaries and Key Concepts, 269-276; Refining Key Concepts, 87-88, 90, 95, 100-101, 131, 135, 144, 148, 151; Original Text, 609-618
cautionary principles
Chart of the Debate, 69, 75; Refining Key Concepts, 83-90
certificate of need
definition of, 14-15
CHAMPUS
definition of, 15

Chart of the Debate, 63-75
description, 65-67; fold-out, 75
chronic care
definition of, 15
Citizen Action, 286
claim
definition of, 16
Clinton Plan
Summaries and Key Concepts, 237-241; Refining Key Concepts, 100, 112, 114, 117, 127, 137, 143; Original Text, 515-537
Clinton, President Bill
See "Clinton Plan"
closed panel
definition of, 16
coinsurance
definition of, 16
community care networks, 205-206
community rating
definition of, 17
Conservative Democratic Forum Plan
Summaries and Key Concepts, 221-228; Refining Key Concepts, 92, 108, 109, 112, 114, 116, 29, 135, 137, 140, 141; Original Text, 491-504
Continuous Quality Improvement (CQI)
definition of, 17-18
Cooper, Congressman Jim, 224
coordinated care
definition of, 18
copayments
definition of, 19
cost containment
definition of, 19
cost sharing
definition of, 20
cost shifting
definition of, 20

D
deductible
definition of, 21
Diagnosis-Related Grouping System (DRG)
definition of, 21-22
disability
definition of, 22

E
Ellwood, Paul M., 215-216, 461-482
employer-sponsored insurance
Chart of the Debate, 70, 75; Refining Key Concepts, 102-105; Oregon Plan,

165; Health Insurance Association of America Plan, 199; American Hospital Association Plan, 206; American College of Physicians Plan, 255
Enthoven, Alain C., 215, 217, 461-482, 483-485
ERISA
definition of, 23
Hawaii Plan, 159
Etheredge, Lynn, 215, 217, 461-482
excise tax, 271, 277
exclusion
definition of, 23
Exclusive Provider Organization (EPO)
definition of, 24
expenditure targets
Chart of the Debate, 73, 75; Refining Key Concepts, 142-148; American Association of Retired Persons Plan, 229
experience rating
definition of, 24-25

F

federal poverty level
definition of, 25
fee-for-service
definition of, 26

G

Garland, Michael J., 305-324
gatekeeper
definition of, 26-27
global budget
definition of, 27; Chart of the Debate, 73, 75; Refining Key Concepts, 142-148; Clinton Plan, 237; Stark Plan, 243; Shortell Plan, 249; American College of Physicians Plan, 255; Aaron Plan, 263; Catholic Health Association Plan, 269; Hagan Plan, 277; McDermott/Wellstone Plan, 283
Glossary, 9-62
Gross Domestic Product (GDP)
definition of, 27
Gross National Product (GNP)
definition of, 28

H

Hagan Plan
Summaries and Key Concepts, 277-282; Refining Key Concepts, 138, 145, 152; Original Text, 619-636
Hagan, Representative Robert F., 279-280, 619-636

Hawaii Plan
Summaries and Key Concepts, 159-164; Refining Key Concepts, 87, 104, 111, 115, 138, 139, 145; Original Text, 295-303
Hawaii's Prepaid Health Care Act, 159, 161
Health Care Financing Administration (HCFA)
definition of, 28
health care provider
definition of, 28
health insurance
definition of, 28
Health Insurance Association of America Plan
Summaries and Key Concepts, 199-204; Refining Key Concepts, 104, 112, 113, 116, 118126, 128, 133, 139; Original Text, 437-450
health insurance network, 169
Health Insurance Purchasing Cooperative (HIPC)
definition of, 30; Clinton Plan, 237
Health Maintenance Organization (HMO)
definition of, 29-30
health outcomes, 221,
Health Plan Purchasing Cooperative (HPPC)
definition of, 30; Jackson Hole Group, 214; Conservative Democratic Forum, 221-222; Stark Plan, 244
Health Promotion and Accountability Region (HPAR), 249-250; Chart of the Debate, 73, 75; Shortell Plan, 249; Catholic Health Association Plan, 269
Heritage Plan
Summaries and Key Concepts, 175-180; Refining Key Concepts, 83, 86, 93, 115, 120, 124, 146; Original Text, 373-388
high-risk insurance pools, 165
Himmelstein, David U., 645-651
hospice
definition of, 31

I

Independent Practice Association (IPA)
definition of, 31-32
individual perspective
Chart of the Debate, 69, 75; Refining Key Concepts, 91-101

insurable risk
definition of, 32
insurance
Chart of the Debate, 71, 75; Refining Key Concepts, 113-118; preexisting conditions, 71, 75; experience rating, 71, 75; cost-shifting, 71, 75
integrated health care plans, 249, 269
International Classification of Disease, Ninth Revision, Clinical Modification (ICD-9-CM)
definition of, 33

J

Jackson Hole Group Plan
Summaries and Key Concepts, 213-220; Refining Key Concepts, 94, 113, 126, 128, 132, 134, 137, 138, 140, 146; Original Text, 461-489
job lock
definition of, 33
Joint Commission on Accreditation of Healthcare Organizations (JCAHO)
definition of, 34

K

Key Concepts
Chart of the Debate, 63-75; Refining Key Concepts, 77-154; Summaries and Key Concepts, 155-290; unrefined Concepts, 65-67, 79-80
Kitzhaber, John, 166

L

Lewin, John C., 161-162, 295-303
lock-in
definition of, 33
long-term care
definition of, 34-35; Chart of the Debate, 72, 75

M

Magaziner, Ira, 239, 515-531
malpractice
Chart of the Debate, 70, 75; Refining Key Concepts, 111-112
managed care
definition of, 35-36
managed competition
definition of, 37; Chart of the Debate, 72, 75; Refining Key Concepts, 126-141; Jackson Hole Group Plan, 213-214; Conservative Democratic

Forum Plan, 221; Clinton Plan, 237; Stark Plan, 243
Mason, Tom, 305, 325-328
McDermott, Congressman Jim, 285-287, 637-643
McDermott/Wellstone Plan
Summaries and Key Concepts, 283-290; Refining Key Concepts, 95, 101, 110, 131, 145, 152-153; Original Text, 637-651
Medicaid
definition of, 38-39; Chart of the Debate, 70, 75; Refining Key Concepts, 106-108; Hawaii Plan, 160-161; American Hospital Association Plan, 206; Stark Plan, 245
Medical IRA, 170
Medicare
definition of, 39; Chart of the Debate, 73, 75; Refining Key Concepts, 149; American Hospital Association Plan, 206; American Association of Retired Persons Plan, 229-230; Stark Plan, 245
Medigap
definition of, 40
multiple payer system
definition of, 40

O

Office of Technology Assessment, 305, 329-338
open panel
definition of, 41; Catholic Health Association Plan, 270
Oregon Plan
Summaries and Key Concepts, 165-168; Refining Key Concepts, 87, 106, 115, 132, 136; Original Text, 305-338
outcomes management
definition of, 42

P

Pauly, Mark V., 182, 389-409
Pauly Plan
Summaries and Key Concepts, 181-186; Refining Key Concepts, 83, 91, 99, 121, 122-123, 124, 153; Original Text, 389-409
payer
definition of, 42
Peer Review Organization (PRO)
definition of, 43

Physician-Hospital Organization (PHO)
play-or-pay
 definition of, 44; American Nurses Association Plan, 193-194; American Association of Retired Persons Plan, 229; Shortell Plan, 249; American College of Physicians Plan, 256; Aaron Plan, 263
point-of-service plan
 definition of, 45
Political Action Committee (PAC)
 definition of, 46
portability
 definition of, 46
preexisting condition
 definition of, 47
Preferred Provider Organization (PPO)
 definition of, 48-49
primary care physician
 definition of, 49-50
primary caregiver
 definition of, 49-50
Prospective Payment System (PPS)
 definition of, 50

Q

quality assurance
 definition of, 51

R

rationing
 definition of, 51-52; Chart of the Debate, 70, 75; Oregon Plan, 165-166
Reinhardt Plan
 Summaries and Key Concepts, 187-192; Refining Key Concepts, 93-94, 99, 105, 123, 125, 133, 136; Original Text, 411-420
Reinhardt, Uwe E., 189, 411-420
reinsurance
 definition of, 52
Resource-Based Relative Value System (RBRVS)
 definition of, 52-53
risk pool
 definition of, 53

S

Scott, H. Denman, 581-591
self-insurance
 definition of, 53
Shapiro, Howard B., 581-591
single payer system
 definition of, 54; Chart of the Debate, 73, 75;

Refining Key Concepts, 150-154; American Association of Retired Persons Plan, 229-230; Aaron Plan, 263; Catholic Health Association Plan, 269; Hagan Plan, 277; McDermott/Wellstone Plan, 283

Shortell Plan

Summaries and Key Concepts, 249-253; Refining Key Concepts, 100, 135, 143, 147-148; Original Text, 559-580

Shortell, Stephen M., 250-251, 559-580

skilled nursing facility

definition of, 54

Stark, Congressman Pete, 245-246

Stark Plan

Summaries and Key Concepts, 243-248; Refining Key Concepts, 108, 114, 117, 137, 143; Original Text, 539-558

State Health Insurance Plan (SHIP), 159-161

State Health Organization (SHO), 269

stop loss

definition of, 55

supplemental insurance

definition of, 55

T

tax credit

definition of, 56; Chart of the Debate, 71, 75; Refining Key Concepts, 120-125; Bush Plan, 169-170; Heritage Plan, 175-176; Pauly Plan, 181-182

tax deduction

definition of, 56; Bush Plan, 169-170

tax exclusion

definition of, 57

tax exemption

definition of, 57

third party payer

definition of, 58

Toner, Robin, 487-489

Total Quality Management (TQM)

definition of, 58

U

UCR (usual, customary and reasonable)

definition of, 59

uncompensated care

definition of, 59-60

underserved areas
Chart of the Debate, 70, 73, 75; Refining Key Concepts, 109-110, 150-154
underwriting
definition of, 60
uninsurable risk
definition of, 60
universal access
definition of, 60
unrefined Concepts
description, 65-67, 79-80; Summaries and Key Concepts, 155-290
utilization review (UR)
definition of, 61

V

value-added tax
definition of, 62

W

Wellstone, Senator Paul, 285, 287, 637-643
Woolhandler, Steffie, 645-651

About the Author

Frederick I. (Rick) Taft is a lawyer and public policy enthusiast. A graduate of Yale College and Yale Law School, he practices business law in Cleveland, Ohio with Spieth, Bell, McCurdy & Newell. His public policy interest has been nurtured in recent years through involvement in the Cleveland Heights schools, which his two children attend, and work on the City Club Forum, a nationally broadcast radio show featuring speakers on matters of public import. He and his wife, a nursing school professor, share a long-standing interest in the health care field.